D1758266

MWITPSY

08006316

Responses to Victimizations
and Belief in a Just World

CRITICAL ISSUES IN SOCIAL JUSTICE

Published in association with the International Center for Social Justice Research, Department of Psychology, Washington University, St. Louis, Missouri.

Series Editors: **MELVIN J. LERNER** and **RIËL VERMUNT**
University of Waterloo   University of Leiden
Waterloo, Ontario, Canada   Leiden, The Netherlands

A Continuation Order Plan is available for this series. A continuation order will bring delivery of each new volume immediately upon publication. Volumes are billed only upon actual shipment. For further information please contact the publisher.

3017958

Responses to Victimizations and Belief in a Just World

Edited by

LEO MONTADA

University of Trier
Trier, Germany

and

MELVIN J. LERNER

University of Waterloo
Waterloo, Ontario, Canada

SHORT LOAN

UNIVERSITIES AT MEDWAY LIBRARY

303.
372
RES

Plenum Press • New York and London

Library of Congress Cataloging-in-Publication Data

Responses to victimizations and belief in a just world / edited by Leo
Montada and Melvin J. Lerner.
    p.   cm. -- (Critical issues in social justice)
  Includes bibliographical references and index.
  ISBN 0-306-46030-0
  1. Social justice--Psychological aspects. 2. Belief and doubt.
3. Victims of crimes--Psychology.   I. Montada, Leo. II. Lerner,
Melvin J., 1929-   . III. Series.
HM216.R47 1998
303.3'72--dc21   98-34332
                                                         CIP

ISBN 0-306-46030-0

© 1998 Plenum Press, New York
A Division of Plenum Publishing Corporation
233 Spring Street, New York, N.Y. 10013

http://www.plenum.com

10 9 8 7 6 5 4 3 2 1

All rights reserved

No part of this book may be reproduced, stored in a data retrieval system, or transmitted in any
form or by any means, electronic, mechanical, photocopying, microfilming, recording, or
otherwise, without written permission from the Publisher

Printed in the United States of America

Contributors

VICTOR BISSONNETTE, Southeastern Louisiana University, Box 401, Hammond, Louisiana, 70402

THOMAS BURROUGHS, Department of Psychology, Washington University, 1 Brookings Drive, Box 1125, St. Louis, Missouri 63130-4899

ALISON L. CHASTEEN, Department of Psychology, Washington University, 1 Brookings Drive, Box 1125, St. Louis, Missouri 63130-4899

CLAUDIA DALBERT, Department of Psychology, University of Kaiserslautern, D-67653 Kaiserslautern, Germany

ADRIAN FURNHAM, Department of Psychology, University College London, 26 Bedford Way, London, WC1, Great Britain

CAROLYN L. HAFER, Department of Psychology, Brock University, St. Catharines, Ontario, Canada L2S 3A1

ALAN J. LAMBERT, Department of Psychology, Washington University, 1 Brookings Drive, Box 1125, St. Louis, Missouri 63130-4899

MELVIN J. LERNER, Department of Psychology, University of Waterloo, Waterloo, Ontario N2L 3G1, Canada

ISAAC M. LIPKUS, Duke University Medical Center, Box 2949, Durham, North Carolina 27710

JÜRGEN MAES, Department of Psychology, University of Trier, D-54286 Trier, Germany

CHANGIZ MOHIYEDDINI, Psychologisches Institut, Universität Mainz (FB 12), Staudingerweg 9, D-55099 Mainz, Germany

LEO MONTADA, Department of Psychology, Universität Trier, D-54286 Trier, Germany

JAMES M. OLSON, Department of Psychology, University of Western Ontario, London, Ontario, Canada N6A 5L2

BARBARA REICHLE, Department of Psychology, Universität Trier, D-54286 Trier, Germany

MANFRED J. SCHMITT, Department of Psychology, Universität Trier, D-54286 Trier, Germany

ANGELA SCHNEIDER, Department of Psychology, Universität Trier, D-54286 Trier, Germany

Preface

The preparation of this volume began with a conference held at Trier University, approximately thirty years after the publication of the first Belief in a Just World (BJW) manuscript. The location of the conference was especially appropriate given the continued interest that the Trier faculty and students had for BJW research and theory. As several chapters in this volume document, their research together with the other contributors to this volume have added to the current sophistication and status of the BJW construct. In the 1960s and 1970s Melvin Lerner, together with his students and colleagues, developed his justice motive theory. The theory of Belief in a Just World (BJW) was part of that effort. BJW theory, meanwhile in its thirties, has become very influential in social and behavioral sciences. As with every widely applied concept and theory there is a natural developmental history that involves transformations, differentiation of facets, and efforts to identify further theoretical relationships. And, of course, that growth process will not end unless the theory ceases to develop. In this volume this growth is reconstructed along Furnham's stage model for the development of scientific concepts.

The main part of the book is devoted to current trends in theory and research. One such trend is the effort to differentiate various facets of BJW, for instance, the distinction between belief in a just world and belief in an unjust world, the distinction between belief in immanent justice and belief in ultimate justice, the hope for justice, and the belief in one's ability, described as self-efficacy, to eliminate or reduce injustices. As revealed in several chapters, the operationalizations of these various facets have led to very fruitful research, and provided the bases for innovative theoretical contributions.

From its inception the BJW theory was intended to explain observers' coping with injustices suffered by other people. In a few chapters, new evidence is provided revealing that BJW motivates people to cope with unjust victimizations. When restoration of injustice is costly, people tend to deny injustice by blaming the victims or by minimizing their hardships and disadvantages. In this manner, BJW-based motivation merges with people's self-interest. It has been demonstrated, for the first time, that using strategies to deny injustices enables observers to maintain their BJW. In a sense BJW functions as a resource helping observers to maintain confidence in their world and life in general.

A rather new line of research describes the functions of BJW in victims' coping with their own hardships and problems. Several contributors report evidence that BJW helps to protect people against a stressful negative view of their situation, especially their fears of being unjustly victimized. In this manner, BJW seems to function as a resource for victims, too.

The majority of investigations during the 1980s and the 1990s are questionnaire or vignette studies where BJW and its various facets are considered to vary individually in strength. The interaction of this dispositional motivational variable with situational information about injustices is an important empirical as well as theoretical issue. Methodological issues with the interaction of personality and situational variables and the corresponding problems of validation of personality measures are extensively discussed in this volume.

The use of assessment scales also raises the question at which level of psychological functioning BJW exerts its impact—a rational cognitivistic or an intuitive emotional one. There are good reasons to believe that BJW as a fundamental belief gains its strongest impact at the intuitive emotional level of functioning. The more rational reflection is induced, the less the impact of BJW on the person's reaction. As a consequence, it is important to be aware of the level of functioning which is induced by the design and instrumentation of research: The more the instrumentation and method used induce people to engage in rational reflection, the greater the probability that they will reveal normatively appropriate "rational" reactions to injustices. However, irrational reactions such as blaming victims are most likely to appear when their responses are less censored and more directly shaped by their emotion-based intuitions.

Leo Montada and Melvin J. Lerner

Contents

Chapter 1

An Overview

ADVANCES IN BELIEF IN A JUST WORLD
THEORY AND METHODS

MELVIN J. LERNER and LEO MONTADA

It is over 30 years since the publication of Lerner & Simmons (1966). The research reported in that manuscript arose, initially, out of the efforts to explain why scientifically trained university students insisted on condemning poverty stricken victims as "lazy and no good" while denying the evidence of their victimization by overwhelming economic changes. The explanation offered for that seemingly motivated resistance was that people, for the sake of their security and ability to plan for the future, need to believe they live in an essentially "just" world where they can get what they deserve, at least in the long run. It was further reasoned that being confronted with innocent victims of undeserved suffering poses a threat to that fundamental belief, and as a consequence, people naturally develop and employ ways of defending it. This may involve acting to eliminate injustices. But failing that, by blaming, rejecting, or avoiding the victim, or having faith that the victim will eventually be appropriately compensated, people are able to maintain their confidence in the justness of the world in which they must live and work for their future security.

MELVIN J. LERNER • Department of Psychology, University of Waterloo, Waterloo, Ontario N2L 3G1, Canada. LEO MONTADA • Department of Psychology, Universität Trier, D-54286 Trier, Germany.

Responses to Victimizations and Belief in a Just World, edited by Montada and Lerner. Plenum Press, New York, 1998.

To test these theoretical conjectures university students were led to believe that as part their participation in a study of "cues of emotional arousal" they were witnessing the actual suffering of another student who had been essentially trapped in to receiving electric shocks as part of a separate experiment in human learning. The procedure succeeded in creating "innocent observers" who were emotionally moved by witnessing the suffering of an "innocent victim." The vast majority of observers in this experimental situation subsequently report being extremely upset, initially, by the victim's unjust suffering. As expected, however, those feelings often change as the suffering continues and the observers are unable to intervene. Comparing their reactions across various experimental conditions, revealed that the observers' evaluations of the victim were reliably affected by the extent of her undeserved suffering: The greater the injustice the greater the tendency to denigrate her. And as expected, this devaluation of the victim's character was precluded if the observers believed she would be appropriately compensated for her suffering in the future.

Within the next decade, additional research with the same or very similar experimental situation revealed that giving observers instructions to empathize with the victim (imagine it is happening to you) seemed to prevent their victim derogation (Aderman, Brehm & Katz, 1974), as did reminding the observers that they were not supposed to condemn innocent victims (Simons & Piliavin, 1972), and that highly religious observers were less likely than less religious observers to derogate the innocent victim (Sorrentino & Hardy, 1974). Using a rather different experimental paradigm, it was possible to test the hypothesis that people would be constrained not to derogate victims highly similar to themselves. Instead, however, they would attempt to cope with the heightened threat to their own security by extra efforts to avoid the highly similar victim of drug addiction (Lerner & Agar, 1972) or mental illness (Novak & Lerner, 1968) in comparison with one who was less similar to them. Also, the various ingenious experiments of Zuckerman and his colleagues illustrated people's use of the belief in a just world as a way of coping with threatening events (Zuckerman, 1975) as well as the distinctive aspects of people's just world beliefs and their control beliefs (Zuckerman & Gerbasi, 1977).

But even with the auspicious finding of these early experiments, it was clear that much more needed to be done, both to find the limits of these coping responses, as well as to generate and answer a host of related important questions. For example, the experiments offered a limited range of victims and instances of injustice, leaving open the question of the generalizability, i.e., external validity, of the research findings. Also, the subjects' reactions to the victims in these experiments varied within each of the experimental conditions. Not all observers condemned or avoided the innocent victim they were not able to help. Some, instead, appeared to blame the experimenters and expressed compassion for the victim. So, there clearly were individual differences in the way observers in the various experimental conditions reacted. How could one explain and predict those differences? Were they attributable to differences in the extent or ways in which people believed in the justness of their world? Would people react differently to different kinds of victims?

Although the early findings on the influence of religiosity as a personal dimension and the perception of similarity or identification with a victim were beginning attempts to recognize the role of individual differences, it was only after Rubin & Peplau (1973, 1975) introduced their face valid questionnaire to measure the extent to which people professed to believe in just world that researchers began to address these and other related issues in a systematic manner. All of the research described in this volume, the first compendium of just world research since Lerner, 1980, employs one or another form of questionnaire to measure some aspect of the belief in a just world or a set of related beliefs. Taken together, they offer compelling evidence of the investigative power of individual difference measures of meaningful dimensions. At the least, it is possible to gain considerable information from relatively large numbers of people regarding large numbers of issues.

And as the various chapters clearly demonstrate, in this manner, with the use of various means of assessing covariation, and apportioning of common and differing amounts of variance among several variables, it is possible to raise and answer important theoretical questions. To begin with, one has to be impressed with the vast array of converging and replicating evidence concerning the way people's beliefs about justice are consistently related to the way they react to a wide variety of victims.

Several chapters in this volume, include reports of a fairly strong association between the extent to which people ascribe to items on one or another scale that indicate degrees of just world beliefs and other items that indicate the blaming of visible victims in their midst and elsewhere. The respondents range from samples of university students to representative samples of larger communities. The victims include economically deprived people in the third world, Russians, asylum applicants, foreign guest workers, unemployed, physically handicapped, and victims of AIDS, rape, and traffic accidents, etc. Although the participant in these studies were typically German, the findings are congruent with those reported by investigators in North America, UK and various other countries (see Furnham, this volume). However, the findings reported in these chapters are somewhat different in that they are based upon more recent and refined measures of the just world beliefs. The strongest associations, for example, are between beliefs about the justness of the victims "worlds" and the blaming of those victims (Montada et al., this volume). At the same time, Schmitt and his students (Schmitt, this volume) were unable to find consistent associations between measured just world beliefs, victims' fates, and victim derogation. That remains a puzzle for Schmitt and anyone else who wishes to integrate his results with the array of findings reported by his German colleagues and the other contributors to this volume. Several explanations, some rather elaborate and others rather simple, remain as likely explanations.

Montada (this volume) describes several studies that conceptually replicate the early experimental findings. Using questionnaire generated data they found consistent relations between respondents' just world beliefs, and their tendency to find victims to blame for their own suffering and deprivation. However, that association did not appear among samples or respondents who were situationally "similar" to particular victims(see Lerner & Agar, 1972, Novak & Lerner, 1968, Sorrentino & Boutilier, 1974). For example there was no relation between homosexuals' belief in the justness of their world and the blaming of AIDS victims. And similarly there was no relation between the just world beliefs of unemployed respondents and the blaming of victims of unemployment. Also, advancing the earlier work of Zuckerman & Gerbasi (1977) they were able to show that observers just world beliefs predicted the blaming of victims, even when the respondents' beliefs in control and social desirability measures were partialled out of the associations.

Finally, the research of Juergen Maes (this volume) and Mohiyeddini & Montada (this volume) provide elaborate and highly sophisticated confirmation of the initial hypothesis that many people resort to the belief in ultimate justice as a way of coping with evidence of undeserved suffering (Lerner, 1980; Lerner & Simmons, 1966; Lerner & Miller, 1978). Maes' respondents clearly demonstrated that the belief in immanent, but not ultimate, justice was associated with victim blaming. And Mohiyeddini & Montada (this volume) demonstrated that similar to the subjects in Lerner & Simmons' experiment (1966), but in a much more general form, their German respondents who felt able to eliminate injustices did not derogate societal victims especially those who scored low on BJW. The respondents were most ready to support the victims.

Along with these validity enhancing replications, these investigators provided extremely important advances in the assessment and conceptualization of the domain of beliefs associated with justice and victims. Mohiyeddini & Montada developed highly reliable measures of the hope for justice and the belief that one is able to correct injustices and were able to show that the latter is related to helping victims rather than blaming them. Maes' measures of the beliefs in ultimate and intimate justice enabled him and hopefully many others to follow to test their expected relations to various forms of victimization, including illness. Also, the development of measures of victim specific just world beliefs yielded much stronger associations with peoples reactions to those victims than did more general just world beliefs. Furnham's construction of a scale assessing the belief in an "unjust world" enabled him to pursue highly sophisticated hypotheses concerning when and why such beliefs might coexist with beliefs in a just world.

Reichle, Schneider and Montada's panel study (Reichle et al., this volume) yielded a most exciting theoretically significant finding. They demonstrated, through the analyses of cross lag associations, that people who engaged in cognitive defenses of the BJW, i.e., blaming victims, at the time of the initial testing had higher BJW ratings at the later assessment than did those who did not engage in such defenses. This held true after the corrections for auto correlations among the variables. The clear implication of this finding is that condemning victims not only is a consequence of just world beliefs, but it also functions as an effective means of defending and even strengthenging that belief. That is the first, and rather elegant, test of a central hypothesis in just world theory. It should be much cited in subsequent research. Of similar theoretical significance, following a carefully reasoned analysis of the relation between justice motivation and self-interest, Montada (this volume) was able to document the distinctive influence of these motives, on their respondents' reactions to victims. Lerner (this volume) employs the distinction between "rational" and "experiential" processes to describe the manifestations of two forms of just world beliefs. According to this theory, self-interest appears as a dominant theme in peoples' conscious normatively shaped decisions. But when people are "seized by their emotions" and engage in direct acts, simple, and often irrational and personally costly, justice considerations influence their reactions.

Other chapters examine important issues not addressed in the early experiments. Although it was initially proposed that belief in a just world was fundamental to a person's security and sanity, only recently have investigators considered whether or not just world beliefs enabled people to cope with their own victimization.

Hafer and Olson (this volume) report the results of an experiment where students are confronted with unjust outcomes, a study of students' reactions to poor grades, and a panel study of full time working women, some of whom are dissatisfied with various aspects of their jobs. Hafer & Olson found that in general a stronger belief in a just world is associated with greater acceptance and less dissatisfaction with the negative outcomes one experiences.

Lipkus & Bissonnette (this volume) discovered that married couples with a strong belief in a just world were much likely to make accommodating responses to their spouses disappointing behaviors than those with weaker just world beliefs. Remarkably, this was true even after controlling for such variables as the level of "trust" in their relationship. Probably the result that will be most cited in the future was the finding that the well documented relationship between trust and accommodating relations in married couples is actually mediated by the person's level of just world beliefs. Although it was not true among dating partners, removing the belief in a just world eliminates the relation between trust and accommodating relations between married couples.

Lambert & Chasteen discovered that people holding right wing authoritarian beliefs who also held strong just world beliefs were considerably less likely to believe that a life threatening event might happen to them, than people with similar political orientations but with low just world beliefs. The authors reasoned that high authoritarians are rather anxiety ridden folks needing something like the belief in a just world to help them feel secure.

Claudia Dalbert, working with victims of unemployment and mothers of handicapped children discovered, after careful analytic efforts, that those victims were differentially helped in coping by their just world beliefs depending upon whether they raised and how they answered the "why me" question. Taken together these chapters raise and answer some of the most fundamental questions about the belief in a just world and how it fits in to people's lives. The reader will soon discover that the findings described above are illustrative rather than an exhaustive description of the theoretical and methodological innovations contained in this volume.

REFERENCES

Aderman, D., Brehm, S.S. & Katz, L.B. (1974). Empathic observation of an innocent victim: The just world revisited. Journal of Personality and Social Psychology, 29, 342–347.

Lerner, M.J. (1971). Observer's evaluation of a victim: Justice, guilt,and veridical perception. Journal of Personality and Social Psychology, 20, 127–135.

Lerner, M.J. (1980). The belief in a just world. A fundamental delusion. New York: Plenum Press

Lerner, M.J. & Agar, E. (1972). The consequences of perceived similarity:Attraction and rejection, approach and avoidance. Journal of Experimental Research in Personality, 6, 69–75.

Lerner, M.J. & Miller, D.T. (1978). Just world research and the attribution process: looking back and ahead. Psychological Bulletin, 85, 1030–1051.

Lerner, M.J. & Simmons, C.H. (1966). The observer's reaction to the "innocent victim": Compassion or rejection? Journal of Personality and Social Psychology, 4, 203–210.

Novak, D.W. & Lerner, M.J. (1968). Rejection as a consequence of perceived similarity. Journal of Personality and Social Psychology, 9,147–152.

Rubin, Z. & Peplau, L.A. (1973). Belief in a just world and reactions to another's lot: A study of participants in the National Draft Lottery. Journal of Social Issues, 29(4), 73–93.

Rubin, Z., & Peplau, L.A. (1975). Who believes in a just world? Journal of Social Issues, 31(3), 65–89.

Simons, C., & Piliavin, J.A. (1972). The effect of deception on reactions to a victim. Journal of Personality and Social Psychology, 21, 56–60.

Sorrentio, R.M. & Boutilier, R.G. (1974). Evaluation of a victim as a function of fate similarity/dissimilarity. Journal of Experimental Social Psychology 10, 83–92.

Sorrentino, R.M., & Hardy, J.E. (1974). Religiousness and derogation of an innocent victim. Journal of Personality, 42, 372–382.

Zuckerman, M. (1975). Belief in a just world and altruistic behavior Journal of Personality and Social Psychology, 31, 972–976.

Zuckerman, M., & Gerbasi, K.C. (1977). Belief in internal control or belief in a just world: The use and misuse of the I-E- scale in prediction of attitudes and behavior. Journal of Personality, 45, 356–378.

Chapter 2

Immanent Justice and Ultimate Justice
TWO WAYS OF BELIEVING IN JUSTICE

JÜRGEN MAES

1. THEORETICAL BACKGROUND

1.1. Belief in a Just World: Experimental and Survey Studies

In a series of sophisticated experiments beginning in 1965, Melvin Lerner was able to demonstrate impressively how beliefs regarding justice can alter human reactions toward the innocent victims of misfortune—instead of sympathizing and helping the victim, subjects can be made to belittle his plight and even scorn him (for a summary, see Lerner, 1970; Lerner, Miller & Holmes, 1976). According to Lerner's theory of just-world motivation, people assume that they live in a just world, in which each person gets what he deserves and deserves what he gets. Should a person witness clear injustice, this (potentially vital) belief in the justice of the world becomes threatened. Thus, people are motivated to maintain or reaffirm their belief in a just world, perhaps through personal or active engagement in the preservation of justice. Because the latter may often prove costly (if not impossible), people attempt to maintain their belief

JÜRGEN MAES • Department of Psychology, Universität Trier, D-54286 Trier, Germany.

Responses to Victimizations and Belief in a Just World, edited by Montada and Lerner. Plenum Press, New York, 1998.

in a just world by simply ignoring injustice or reinterpreting the results of events such that the consequences appear to be just. If, for example, the victim himself has contributed to his misfortune, or appears to be a bad person, one might argue that he doesn't deserve any better; in this manner, an incident of obvious injustice might paradoxically become evidence supporting a just world, and thus validate the observer's belief system. In his theoretical analyses of the topic, however, Melvin Lerner (1980) expressly points out that the devaluation of innocent victims is not the only strategy by which belief in a just world is preserved. Other strategies include the construction of many different worlds, of which only one—the one most relevant for the observer—must be just, or the assumption of various time perspectives.

The just world hypothesis was developed within experimental social psychology and originates in laboratory research. In order to investigate the essential assumptions of his theory, Lerner constructed experimental situations with various degrees of (in)justice. Virtually all of his experiments produced the same main result: The more unjust a situation appeared, the greater the devaluation of the innocent victim involved. Lerner traced the variance in victim-devaluation (the dependent variable in these experiments) back to his subjects' need to believe that there is justice in the world. In these experiments, Lerner did not assess the decisive motive, belief in a just world, directly; rather, he deduced the presence of this motivation indirectly through alterations in subjects' behavior across different combinations of experimental conditions.

It is not unusual for a phenomenon discovered by experimental research to be considered as personality construct later on (Furnham, 1990). Do all people react similarly, or are some people more prone to show the phenomenon? Furnham (1990) demonstrated how the development of personality constructs follows a typical sequence which can be described in eight stages. According to this sequence a phenomenon is discovered by experimental research (stage 1), replicated and tested for its robustness and generalizability (stage 2), until then an unidimensional self-report measure is developed on the third stage. A similar pattern can be observed in the development of just world research: Almost a decade after Lerner's first publication on this topic (Lerner, 1965), a questionnaire designed to measure belief in a just world as an interindividual trait was constructed by Rubin & Peplau (1973, 1975). An opportunity for validating the questionnaire occurred in 1971 during the "National Draft Lottery," which was used to select soldiers for deployment in Vietnam from among 20-year-old students in the United States. The results showed a tendency for those with high scores on the belief in a just world scale to conceive random outcomes as intended and to portray draftees as having deserved selection. Further experiments (see, e.g., Zuckerman et al., 1975; Miller, 1977) confirmed the validity of the instrument. Since then, more than a hundred studies conducted in England and America have relied upon the instrument developed by Rubin and Peplau. German translations and further development of the questionnaire (Dalbert, 1982; Dalbert, Montada & Schmitt, 1987; Schneider, 1988; Montada & Schneider, 1989, 1991) have also proved themselves to be valid instruments; these authors generally differentiate between general and domain-specific scales of just-world belief.

While the number of just world correlational studies increased impressively since the early eighties, less experiments were conducted since then. This development went along with a certain shift in research questions and with a gradual restriction of theoretical background. Authors using the Rubin-and-Peplau questionnaire often supposed a direct connection between the degree of belief in a just world and the derogation of victims and the denial of injustice. There are many studies which provide support for such a connection (i.e. MacLean & Shown, 1988; Dalbert & Katona-Sallay, 1993; Harper & Manasse, 1992; Connors & Heaven, 1990; Glennon & Joseph, 1993; Montada & Schneider, 1989; Murphy-Berman & Berman, 1990), but there are as well studies which failed to show the derogation effect or even report positive evaluations of victims going along with belief in a just world (Kerr & Kurtz, 1977; Thornton, Ryckman & Robbins, 1982; Sherman, Smith & Cooper, 1982; Weir & Wrightsman, 1990; Ambrosio & Sheehan, 1991; Bush, Krebs & Carpendale, 1993; Zucker & Weiner, 1993; O'Quin & Vogler, 1990; Schmitt et al., 1991; Bierhoff, Klein & Kramp, 1991).

The ambiguity of results must not surprise and is in accordance with Lerner's initial assumptions. Lerner had never claimed that there was a direct and inevitable path from belief in a just world to the derogation of innocent victims. Rejection of victims is only one possibility persons have to defend their belief in a just world against threats. They might as well actively restore justice or—if this is not possible or too costly—they might change the perspective of their perception of a just world: If what is apparently happening is not just, justice will be restored in another domain of life or in another space of time. The present situation is unjust but sometime in the future justice will be restored. The early experiment conducted by Lerner and Simmons (1966) demonstrates different ways to maintain one's belief in a just world. It is true that their subjects devalued an "innocent victim" that got electric shocks in a pretended learning experiment but only if they believed that injustice would continue to exist in the next experimental session. If the subjects could decide that the victim would receive reward instead of shock in the next session they did so by voting for reward. Such a voting procedure was not sufficient to stop the devaluation of the victim; but if they were told that the victim would receive reward in the next session (and justice would be restored this way), they would not devalue him any more.

It seems that these results have fallen into oblivion when the research efforts shifted to correlational studies. The availability of an unidimensional measure has made research more unidimensional. The initial just world formulations include different ways of maintaining one's belief in a just world. Lerner and Simmons introduced the expectation of justice in the future as a situational variable: In situations which imply the restoration of justice in early future the evaluation of victims is different from situations which do not imply any salient hint that justice will be restored soon. One may suggest that subjects´ behavior in situations with justice concern is not only influenced by situational determinants. Situations may be conceived differently by subjects, there may be biases and habits to filter situational features differently. Some people may fundamentally expect a just compensation in the future, other people won't share this opinion. Therefore, the expectation of justice in the future can be introduced as a dispositional variable. A multi-dimensional self-report measure is needed in order to investigate such different biases and habits to perceive justice in the world.

1.2. A Suggested Differentiation between Two Variants of Belief in a Just World

Which are important subdimensions of belief in a just world? One might differentiate the perception of present situations as just and the expectation of just compensation in the future (soon or far away), realizability and desirability of a just world, different degrees of influence on the production of a just world, and so on. The present article is limited to the differentiation between two dimensions: the tendency to perceive or see justice in the events that have occurred and the tendency to believe that forthcoming events will settle any injustice that occurs. The first tendency is related to the phenomenon observed by Piaget (1932), in which children view events as the direct and just payment for previous actions; hence, I shall call it "Belief in Immanent Justice." The second tendency is associated with certain religious doctrines, in which consolation for the present injustice on Earth is provided through the promise of higher justice—perhaps in another world or within a larger time frame; hence, I shall call this second tendency "Belief in Ultimate Justice."

Both variants can be traced far back to the cultural roots of Judeo-Christianity; consequently, the Bible provides numerous examples of each type of belief: "Tell the righteous that it shall be well with them, for they shall eat the fruit of their deeds. Woe to the wicked! It shall be ill with him, for what his hands have done shall be done to him" Isaiah (3:10–11). "But Er, Judah's first-born, was wicked in the sight of the Lord; and the Lord slew him" (Genesis 38:7). "No ill befalls the righteous, but the wicked are filled with trouble" (Proverbs 12:21). "Think now, who that was innocent ever perished? Or where were the upright cut off?" (Job 4:7). Psalm 92 praises God's creation as wonderful, unmarred, and just; perceived injustice in the world, it is argued, is due to man's imperfect understanding of God's justice: "How great are thy works, O Lord! Thy thoughts are very deep! The dull man cannot know, the stupid cannot understand this: that, though the wicked sprout like grass and all evildoers flourish, they are doomed to destruction forever. . . . The righteous flourish like the palm tree, and grow like a cedar in Lebanon."

Whereas the first quotes could be understood as examples of immanent justice, the last quote bases its conception of justice within an expanded time frame, thus referring to ultimate justice. The botanical allegory drawn by the psalmist—which would be familiar to anyone in his cultural sphere—is used to show that evil in the world is surely not evidence of God's justice. When grass seeds and palm seeds are planted in the earth at the same time, the grass will sprout much more quickly. Only those unfamiliar with horticultural processes, however, would conclude that grass is hardier than the palm. The initial head start achieved by the grass lasts only momentarily; it eventually withers and fades, while the palm tree grows slowly, but becomes large and sturdy, surviving through the generations (see Kushner, 1981).

Belief in ultimate justice allows one to endure injustice without having to give up a fundamental belief in a just world. Note that there is no arbitrary limit regarding when justice must be reestablished; the time frame employed might encompass this lifetime or even extend beyond. The differentiation of various time perspectives, which would appear to be quite sensible in studies on the psychology of religion, was not accounted for in the present investigation. However, since immanent and ultimate justice should have different effects upon the evaluation of victims, future research would do well to make the fundamental distinction between these two constructs.

2. METHODS

2.1. Construction of a Questionnaire

In order to assess these variants of belief in a just world, a questionnaire was created using 19 items and employed in a study of attitudes towards cancer and cancer patients. The questionnaire contained items for four hypothetical subscales, namely:

1. the assessment of immanent justice, as described by Piaget, according to which everything that happens is the just payment for previous (mis)deeds;

2. the assessment of ultimate justice, according to which all injustice is reconciled in the long run by future justice;
3. the assessment of a generalized belief in a just world;
4. the assessment of a generalized belief in an unjust world.

The two variants of just-world beliefs were assessed using items that were domain-specific in their formulation and examined responses toward "severe illness," whereas the two general scales were unspecific in their formulation.

The items categorized under belief in ultimate justice reflect the expectation that sometime in the future, every injustice suffered will receive reparation and due compensation. Conversely, the items categorized under belief in immanent justice explain the occurrence of misfortune on the basis of previous mistakes, sins, or other reprehensible acts committed by the victim. One might venture that ultimate justice projects justice into the future, whereas immanent justice is deduced on the basis of past events. Both versions of belief in a just world help one endure injustice; however, only belief in immanent justice forces the subject to reproach the victim. Conversely, belief in ultimate justice, allows the subject to perceive the victim as the (deserved) receiver of forthcoming compensation; the victim is no longer a victim in the typical sense of the word and thus reproach becomes inappropriate.

A more precise description of the questionnaire can be found in Maes (1992).

2.2. Sample

The questionnaire was used in a larger self report study assessing attitudes to cancer and cancer patients. The sample size is N = 326 (77.6 percent of the distributed questionnaires). The mean age is 27.5 (range from 15 to 66). 60 percent of the respondents are students, 40 percent employed. 62.5 percent are female, 37.5 percent are male.

3. RESULTS

The data presented herein have a partial overlap with papers submitted for publication in journals but many of them are exclusively used for the present article.

3.1. Dimensional Analyses

A main component analysis with varimax rotation was performed upon the 19 items of the questionnaire. According to the size of the eigenvalue, a four-factorial solution was found to explain 61.6 percent of the total item variance, and furthermore, corresponding precisely with the four dimensions hypothesized. A closer analysis of item and scale properties can be found in Maes (1992). However, Tables 1 and 2 provide information regarding the item content, the internal consistency, and item-related scores for both dimensions of interest. Internal consistency (alpha = .83 for belief in immanent justice, and alpha = .86 for belief in ultimate justice) can be considered satisfactory.

3.2. Immanent and Ultimate Justice: Validation and Differentiation of Two Scales

Although the scales were derived on the basis of a main component analysis with varimax rotation, the summed values were significantly and positively correlated with one another as manifest variables. The intercorrelations between just-world subscales are shown in Table 3. Belief in

TABLE 1. Item Analysis of the Scale *Belief in Immanent Justice* (N = 289)

Item content	M_x[a]	s_x	r_{it}	α_{del}[b]
Severe illnesses are often a punishment for one´s way of life	0.94	1.20	0.61	0.80
Illness often follows at the heels of improper living.	0.81	1.13	0.74	0.75
Hardly anyone becomes seriously ill without having deserved it.	0.75	1.11	0.64	0.79
Many ill persons can only blame themselves for their suffering.	1.28	1.26	0.61	0.80
A truly good person will seldom become very ill.	0.40	0.88	0.53	0.82
Subscale's alpha: 0.83				

[a]The scale ranges from 0–5 (0 = don´t agree at all; 5 = agree very strongly).
[b]Alpha coefficients for the internal consistency of the scale when one removes this item.

TABLE 2. Item Analysis of the Scale *Belief in Ultimate Justice* (N = 289)

Item content	M_x[a]	s_x	r_{it}	α_{del}[b]
Even persons who suffer from severe misfortune can expect that, in the end, something good will happen to balance everything out.	1.64	1.47	0.72	0.81
Even amidst the worse suffering, one should not lose faith that justice will prevail and set things right.	2.49	1.65	0.63	0.85
In the long run, the injustice imposed by illnesses receive appropriate reparation.	1.27	1.41	0.74	0.81
Even terrible illnesses are often compensated for by fortunate happenstance later in life.	1.37	1.47	0.73	0.81
Subscale's alpha: 0.86				

[a]The scale ranges from 0–5 (0 = don´t agree at all; 5 = agree very strongly).
[b]Alpha coefficients for the internal consistency of the scale when one removes this item.

ultimate justice correlated most highly with the general just-world scale
(r = .67). The slight positive correlation between belief in a just and in an
unjust world contradicts commonsense notions of these concepts, but has
been found now and then in studies on just-world beliefs. Immanent and
ultimate justice are also positively correlated with one another (r = .39).

In Table 3, the abbreviation "Notrust" denotes the item "One cannot
trust on justice in life," which had to be removed from the Belief in an
Unjust World scale due to low item–scale intercorrelation.

Despite the positive correlation between immanent and ultimate
justice, it was assumed that both variants of just-world beliefs could be
differentiated in terms of their relation to other variables. The variables
assessed in the questionnaire study on cancer offer a multitude of opportunities for establishing the construct validity of the scales derived by
factor analysis. Immanent justice and ultimate justice were assumed to be
two different variants of just-world beliefs with different, and in some
respects, contrary effects. The operationalization of the scales was based
upon the idea that one variant would be associated with motivation to
reestablish justice (and hence a tendency to evaluate the victim more
positively), while the other variant would be associated with acceptance
of existing injustice (and hence a tendency to evaluate the victim more
negatively). Thus, the hypothesis stated that immanent and ultimate justice are associated with positive and negative perception of the victims,
respectively. Accordingly, a set of experimental hypotheses were constructed and tested for a wide array of other relevant variables. The main
results from this investigation are presented below.

All of the tables presented share the same format. The bivariate
correlations between type of just-world belief (immanent or ultimate) and
the validation variables of interest are presented in the first row. First-order
partial correlations—calculated by partialling out the contribution of one
of the just-world belief variables toward the correlation with a third
variable—are presented in the second row. In the relationship between
belief in immanent justice and a third variable, belief in ultimate justice
has been partialled out. Similarly, in the relationship between belief in
ultimate justice and a third variable, belief in immanent justice has been
partialled out. A statistical comparison of the bivariate correlations is

TABLE 3. Intercorrelations between Just-World Subscales

	BJW	Immanent	Ultimate	BUJW
Immanent	.5094**			
Ultimate	.6663**	.3920**		
BUJW	.1463*	.2185**	.1623**	
Notrust	−.2195**	−.0374	−.1656**	.2410**

*p < .05; **p < .01.

presented in the column to the right in order to demonstrate whether the differences observed between correlations are significant; error probability was set at five percent. A formula from Olkin (1967) was applied in the calculations (Bortz, 1977, p. 265).

3.2.1. Immanent Justice, Ultimate Justice, and Victim Evaluation

Belief in ultimate justice and belief in immanent justice were expected to correlate positively and negatively with evaluations of the victims, respectively. In order to test this hypothesis, one section of the questionnaire—in which cancer victims were compared with healthy persons using 24 adjectives—was examined. The 24 adjectives included some rather neutral words (such as lonely, happy, stressed), but also many clearly positive ones (attractive, respectable, reasonable) and negative ones (selfish, boring, disturbed).

Analyses were conducted at three different levels: (1) at the level of scale variables, (2) at the level of count variables, and (3) at the individual item level.

1. No clear interpretation could be made based upon the results of the factor analysis. In the search for a more stable factorial structure, eight clearly positive adjectives (intelligent, meticulous, reasonable, helpful, well-balanced, respectable, friendly, and attractive) and seven clearly negative adjectives (impatient, restless, aggressive, hectic, disturbed, selfish, boring) were incorporated into positive and negative scales, respectively. All of the other questionnaire items could only be categorized as positive or negative with the greatest difficulty. Through this aggregation, very reliable scales (alpha = .81) could be constructed for positive and negative evaluation tendencies.

2. The evaluation measures *Sumopop, Sumonep, Sumonew* and *Sumopow* are count variables. There are four principal ways in which the evaluation of cancer patients can differ from the evaluation of healthy persons. Unfavorable perception of the patients can be expressed by the use of less positive and/or more negative characterization (compared to the healthy subject group). Conversely, favorable perception of the patients can be expressed by more positive and/or less negative characterization (again, compared to the healthy subject group). The four measures applied here are compound variables: The frequency with which cancer patients were perceived as more (*Sumopop*) and less (*Sumopow*) positive, as well as more (*Sumonep*) and less (*Sumonew*) negative, was examined.

3. In addition, the tables show the bivariate and partial correlations for several individual items with clear positive/negative valence.

The pattern of results confirmed expectations at all three levels of analysis (Table 4). The positive evaluation of victims correlates positively with beliefs in ultimate justice and negatively with beliefs in immanent justice (five percent level of significance). These correlational relationships all become stronger when the effects of the opposing just-world belief variable have been partialled out. Similarly, significant differences were observed with regards to the negative evaluation scale. The same pattern occurs again in the correlations among the four aggregated variables: As belief in ultimate justice rises, positive characterization of cancer patients increases (*Sumopop*) and negative characterization decreases (*Sumonew*). Conversely, as belief in immanent justice rises, negative characterization increases (*Sumonep*) and positive characterization decreases (*Sumopow*).

With regards to the positive characteristics, the correlational differences are also significant. In a similar vein, differences were found in the adjectives with clear positive/negative valency. While belief in ultimate justice was accompanied by a tendency to view cancer victims as more reasonable and less boring, belief in immanent justice was associated with a tendency to view cancer victims as more boring and less attractive. In sum, the statistical relationships observed support the notion that immanent and ultimate justice clearly influenced the evaluation of victims in the expected manner.

3.2.2. Immanent Justice, Ultimate Justice, and the Ascription of Responsibility

The evaluation of victims by means of adjective lists and ascriptions of responsibility are often considered parallel means of assessing the influence of justice beliefs or control motives on the evaluation of random misfortune. It is thus plausible to assume that, similar to the evaluation of victims, belief in immanent justice will be accompanied by higher ascription of responsibility to the victim than belief in ultimate justice.

Table 5 shows the bivariate and partial correlations for 11 categories of responsibility. The questionnaire item reads: "To what extent are the agents in question responsible for the spread of cancerous disease?" Note that the hypothesis concerning the differentiation between ultimate and immanent just-world beliefs was made only with regards to the first category listed (persons afflicted with cancer); the other analyses were purely exploratory. The hypothesis could be confirmed: Persons with belief in ultimate justice ascribed significantly less responsibility for cancer to the cancer victims than persons with belief in immanent justice. The correlation between belief in ultimate justice and ascription of responsibility disappears completely when the variance shared by belief in immanent justice is partialled out. The high positive correlation between belief in immanent justice and ascription of responsibility, however, remains virtually unchanged when belief in ultimate justice is partialled out.

TABLE 4. Partial Correlational Analysis: Immanent and Ultimate Justice with Victim Evaluation (271 < N < 306)

Variable	Order	Variables		Comparison of correlations	
		Immanent	Ultimate	z_{emp}	z_{theo}
Scales:					
Positive	0	−.0400	.1618**	3.21 > 1.96*	
	1a		.1930**		
	1b	−.1139			
Negative	0	.1506*	.0244	2.01 > 1.96*	
	1a		−.0381		
	1b	.1534**			
Count variables:					
Sumonop	0	.0709	.2061**	2.15 > 1.96*	
	1a		.1943**		
	1b	−.0110			
Sumonep	0	.1914**	.1108	1.31	
	1a		.0396		
	1b	.1618**			
Sumonow	0	.1779**	.0205	2.49 > 1.96*	
	1a		−.0544		
	1b	.1847**			
Sumonew	0	.0312	.1204*	1.42	
	1a		.1176		
	1b	−.0176			
Single items:					
Reasonable	0	.0148	.1684**	2.43 > 1.96*	
	1a		.1768**		
	1b	−.0565			
Attractive	0	−.1188*	.0694	2.98 > 1.96*	
	1a		.1270		
	1b	−.1591**			
Selfish	0	.0315	−.0990	2.06 > 1.96*	
	1a		−.1211		
	1b	.0768			
Boring	0	.1449*	−.0734	3.47 > 1.96*	
	1a		−.1431**		
	1b	.1893**			
Aimless	0	.0528	−.1050	2.58 > 1.96*	
	1a		−.1368		

a) Belief in Immanent Justice held constant
b) Belief in Ultimate Justice held constant
*p ≤ .05; **p ≤ .01

In addition to attributing responsibility to the victim, belief in immanent justice was also highly associated with attributing responsibility to
other people; however, other significant relationships could not be found.
Apparently, it is not necessary to hold many other sources accountable

TABLE 5. Partial Correlational Analysis: Immanent and Ultimate
Justice with Ascription of Responsibility (289 < N < 303)

Variable	Order	Variables		Comparison of correlations	
		Immanent	Ultimate	z_{emp}	z_{theo}
Responsible agent:					
Person afflicted	0	.3508**	.1687**	3.01 > 1.96*	
with cancer	1a		.0362		
	1b	.3139**			
Society	0	.0877	.1166*	0.44	
	1a		.0897		
	1b	.0460			
Fellows	0	.2569**	.1616**	1.54	
	1a		.0685		
	1b	.2132**			
Industry	0	−.0100	−.0220	0.19	
	1a		−.0197		
	1b	−.0015			
Science	0	.1247*	.1245*	0.00	
	1a		.0828		
	1b	.0831			
The church	0	.1321*	.2150**	1.33	
	1a		.1789**		
	1b	.0533			
Media	0	.1443*	.1796**	0.57	
	1a		.1352		
	1b	.0816			
Destiny	0	.0226	.1641**	2.23 > 1.96*	
	1a		.1688**		
	1b	−.0460			
God´s will	0 .	.0725	.2666**	3.13 > 1.96*	
	1a		.2596**		
	1b	−.0361			
Nature	0	.0091	.0256	0.27	
	1a		.0239		
	1b	−.0010			
Chance	0	.0540	.0324	0.34	
	1a		.0123		
	1b	.0449			

a) Belief in Immanent Justice held constant.
b) Belief in Ultimate Justice held constant.
*p ≤ .05; **p ≤ .01

when one knows quite precisely which personal agents carry the lion's share of responsibility.

Furthermore, the exploratory analyses showed that belief in ultimate justice is associated with a strong tendency to attribute responsibility for cancer to predetermined fate or God's will. When one considers the integration of ultimate justice in various religious systems of belief, this finding is not surprising; the specific mental associations that might be drawn between belief in ultimate justice and God's responsibility or fate, however, can only be speculated upon. Possibly, cancer is viewed as a kind of trial or test which one must pass in order to receive a just reward. Ultimate justice and the spread of cancer might also be understood in terms of punishment—in the long run, justice may be served by allowing the "right" to suffer while the "false" remain unharmed. Whatever the explanation, only a finer microanalysis of the relationship is liable to produce results; the present study was not designed to do so.

Just as a hypothesis was made with regards to the ascription of responsibility, one might predict significant differences between immanent/ultimate just-world beliefs and other, related variables. Such variables include the extent to which the victim is the object of reproach, the extent of sanctions against the victim, the general tendency to blame the victim, and the disposition toward self-discipline and/or stoicism regarding health norms. The functional importance of understanding the cause of cancer was also assessed in the questionnaire. Subjects indicated how important an understanding of the causes of cancer was for the prevention, cure, maintenance of health, and punishment of guilty parties. Persons with strong belief in immanent justice were expected to reproach cancer victims more, to advocate stronger sanctions, to blame the victim more, and to demonstrate more self-discipline regarding health norms. Persons with strong belief in immanent justice were also assumed to view the punishment of guilty parties as the most important function of understanding the cause of cancer.

Table 6 shows the results: reproach of victims and advocacy of stronger sanctions were significantly and positively correlated with immanent justice, whereas the slight, positive correlation shown by ultimate justice became negative when the variance shared by immanent justice was partialled out. A similar pattern of results was found with regards to the functional importance of understanding the cause of cancer: The significant positive correlation increased even further when the influence of ultimate justice was partialled out, while the negative correlation with ultimate justice became significant when immanent justice was partialled out. Belief in immanent as well as ultimate justice showed significant positive correlations with the general tendency to blame the victim, although the correlations differed significantly in their relative strength.

TABLE 6. Partial Correlational Analysis: Immanent and Ultimate Justice
with Reproach, Sanctioning, and Attribution of Blame (291 < N < 303)

Variable	Order	Variables		Comparison of correlations	
		Immanent	Ultimate	z_{emp}	z_{theo}
Reproaching victims	0	.3266**	.0870	3.93 > 1.96*	
	1a		−.0472		
	1b	.3192**			
Measures against victims	0	.2479**	.0687	2.88 > 1.96*	
	1a		−.0319		
	1b	.2407**			
Reasons for punishment	0	.1295*	−.0892	3.49 > 1.96*	
	1a		−.1534**		
	1b	.1795**			
Tendency to attribute blame	0	.3642**	.1666**	3.29 > 1.96*	
	1a		.0279		
	1b	.3295**			
Norm: health-related self-discipline	0	.2211**	.0320	3.02 > 1.96*	
	1a		−.0609		
	1b	.2268**			

a) Belief in Immanent Justice held constant.
b) Belief in Ultimate Justice held constant.
*p ≤ .05; **p ≤ .01

In partial correlations, the positive relationship between ultimate justice
and attribution of blame disappeared completely. The significant positive
correlation between immanent justice and health-related self-discipline
remained constant in the partial correlation, while the insignificant positive correlation between ultimate justice and health-related self-discipline
became negative when immanent justice was partialled out.

It is a relatively simple matter to blame or reproach a victim in the
abstract manner described above as long as no consequences are attached
to doing so. A rather weightier question concerns whether subjects are also
inclined to carry through with the consequences of those judgements at
the expense of the victims (instead of whether they simply levy their
judgements in order to preserve a sense of justice). Once again, the variables assessed in the present study offer opportunities for verification. In
one section of the questionnaire, subjects were surveyed regarding which
measures should be employed in fighting cancer as well as how these
measures should be properly financed.

Socially initiated measures (such as better funding for cancer research, expanded social health services, informational campaigns on the
prevention of cancer, or the promotion of alternative medical treatments)
are appropriate methods of curing or preventing illness and thus reestab-

lishing justice. One would thus expect the acceptance of such methods to correlate with belief in ultimate justice. Conversely, when cancer is traced back to the victim's lifestyle, the tasks of prevention and cure become delegated to the victim. Thus, immanent justice was not expected to correlate with the advocacy of such measures.

The suggested financial alternatives for such measures ranged from donations and charitable activities to taxation (mandatory support from the public at large) to the placement of financial burden upon the patient himself or upon risk groups (e.g., smokers). It was expected that the amount of financial burden placed upon the victim would increase with belief in immanent justice. On the other hand, donations and charitable activities were expected to increase with belief in ultimate justice.

Table 7 shows the correlations observed regarding these hypotheses. With respect to the promotion of various research measures, no significant differences were found between the two variants of just-world beliefs. With regards to the expansion of social health care, belief in immanent justice demonstrated a significantly negative relationship, whereas belief in ultimate justice did not. (The difference between both correlations was also significant.) The promotion of alternative medical treatments was significantly correlated with ultimate justice (but not with immanent justice), and once again, the difference between correlations was significant. Regarding the financing of measures against cancer, correlations tended in the expected direction, although none of the differences were significant. Correlations with taxation hardly deviated from zero and only differed with respect to sign. The correlation with financing through risk groups was higher for immanent justice than for ultimate justice; the correlation for immanent justice remained significant when ultimate justice was partialled out, but not vice versa. The same pattern was found regarding financing through the patients themselves. The correlation regarding financing through charitable activities was higher for ultimate justice than for immanent justice, but the difference between correlations failed to reach limits of significance. Clearly significant differences, however, were found for correlations with respect to donations. Here, significant positive correlations were found for ultimate justice, which clearly exceeded the negligible correlation between financing through donations and immanent justice.

3.2.3. Immanent Justice, Ultimate Justice, and Draconian Beliefs

The relationships discussed so far have pertained to domain-specific measures of responsibility, sanctions, and blame; however, it is plausible to assume that immanent and ultimate justice also temper the severity of the judgment levied upon other people in general. The disposition to do

TABLE 7. Partial Correlational Analysis: Immanent and Ultimate Justice
with Measures and the Financing of Measures (284 < N < 306)

Variable	Order	Immanent	Ultimate	z_{emp}	z_{theo}
		Variables		Comparison of correlations	
Measures:					
Promotion of research	0	-.0369	.0423	1.24	
	1a		.0618		
	1b	-.0582			
Expansion of health	0	-.1394*	-.0158	1.96 > 1.96*	
services	1a		.0426		
	1b	-.1448**			
Promotion of alternate	0	-.0399	.1306*	2.71 > 1.96*	
medical treatment	1a		.1591**		
	1b	-.0999			
Financing the measures:					
General taxation	0	-.0111	.0325	0.69	
	1a		.0401		
	1b	-.0260			
Financing through risk	0	.1896**	.1217*	1.08	
groups	1a		.0524		
	1b	.1554**			
Patients pay their own way	0	.1662**	.0740	1.46	
	1a		.0097		
	1b	.1496**			
Charity	0	.1169*	.2057**	1.44	
	1a		.1750**		
	1b	.0403			
Voluntary donations	0	.0436	.1758**	2.09 > 1.96*	
	1a		.1727**		
	1b	-.0280			

a) Belief in Immanent Justice held constant.
b) Belief in Ultimate Justice held constant.
*$p \leq .05$; **$p \leq .01$

so can be conceived of as a more general, trait-like measure. The questionnaire contained a scale with items designed to assess fundamental attitudes toward dealing with the mistakes made by fellow human beings.
Attitudes were assumed to range from those emphasizing strictness and
firmness (draconian beliefs) to mildness and reconciliation (Maes, 1994).
Table 8 shows the bivariate and partial correlations between four such
scales and immanent/ultimate justice. *Draconity 1* measured the need for
moral accountability; items reflect the belief that people must own up to
their mistakes and be held accountable for their actions in order to set
matters right and improve themselves. *Mildness* is characterized by a
conciliatory, forgiving attitude towards fellow man, while *Humor* denotes

TABLE 8. Partial Correlational Analysis: Immanent and Ultimate
Justice with Draconian Beliefs and Mildness (289 < N < 304)

| Variable | Order | Variables | | Comparison of correlations | |
		Immanent	Ultimate	z_{emp}	z_{theo}
Draconity 1:	0	.2611**	.2104**	0.83	
Accountability	1a	.1217			
	1b	.1986**			
Mildness	0	−.0368	.0363	1.16	
	1a		.0552		
	1b	−.0555			
Draconity 2:	0	.1368*	−.0783	3.42 > 1.96*	
Refusal of forgiveness	1a	−.1448**			
	1b	.1826**			
Humor	0	.1324*	.1902**	0.92	
	1a		.1517**		
	1b	.0640			

a) Belief in Immanent Justice held constant.
b) Belief in Ultimate Justice held constant.
*p ≤ .05; **p ≤ .01

a friendly and positive disposition in dealing with human error. Conversely, *Draconity 2* expresses a firm and intolerant stance, one that refuses to excuse or reconcile many kinds of error. Immanent justice was assumed to correlate more strongly with both kinds of draconian beliefs, while ultimate justice was assumed to be associated with mildness and humor. These assumptions could only be partially confirmed. Immanent, as well as ultimate justice, showed positive correlations toward the measure of draconian beliefs which emphasized the need for moral accountability. The relationship appears to be somewhat (but not significantly) stronger for immanent justice. This is not so astonishing: accountability as it is demanded in the items of *Draconity 1* includes the possibility of fighting errors and improving life which is compatible with removing injustices and restoring justice as included in the notion of ultimate justice.

There were no significant differences with regards to the *Mildness* scale. Significant differences in the predicted direction were found for the draconian belief measure that emphasized intolerance (*Draconity 2*). While ultimate justice correlated negatively with that intolerance, immanent justice correlated positively with the construct. This becomes plausible when one considers that ultimate justice as well as forgiveness share a certain feature of leaving aside the past and looking at the future positively. Those, however, who relate moral misdemeanors with far-reaching consequences up to severe illness—which is typical for immanent justice—will less be inclined to forgive faults and slips. The positive correlation of immanent justice with *Draconity 2* becomes bigger when ultimate justice is partialled out; vice versa the negative correlation of ultimate justice becomes bigger and significantly negative when immanent justice is partialled out.

Both immanent and ultimate justice showed positive relationships to the humor scale at the bivariate level; however, while the positive relationship disappeared for immanent justice when ultimate justice was partialled out, the relationship between ultimate justice and humor remained stayed significantly positive (at the one-percent level of significance) when immanent justice was held constant.

3.2.4. Immanent Justice, Ultimate Justice, and Adaptive Processes

People who hold the belief that illness is just payment for sins and personal failings is almost certainly anxious about making errors that could predestine them to the sick bed. The belief in immanent justice is thus hardly effective in providing a person with a considerable degree of security. Only persons who are absolutely sure that they have never committed—and never will be able to commit—an error can be sure to lead a life free from cancer. (Of course, this mind-set also implies a certain level of self-serving bias or self-righteousness in one's perception of justice.) The person who believes in immanent justice and nonetheless becomes ill encounters problems even worse. The personal failings or sins that have occasioned the illness must be discovered, and once revealed, must be condemned. In a case such as this, immanent justice would almost certainly be accompanied by rumination and difficulty in adjusting to the new situation. Conversely, the person who looks toward the future (instead of the past) may discover there some kind of resolution to the present difficulty (whatever that may be); with the possibility that presently experienced injustice may be overturned, life can be lived more optimistically. Hence, adaptation to a state of illness is accomplished more quickly and easily. In short, whereas belief in immanent justice might hinder the adaptation to the changed situation, belief in ultimate justice might perform the reverse. Based upon these assumptions, a great number of hypotheses—each based upon a different dependent variable—can be made regarding immanent and ultimate justice. Because the belief that a higher power will dispense justice eventually is a typical one for many religions, one can assume that belief in ultimate justice will be associated with belief in the importance of religion.

Table 9 shows the bivariate and partial correlations with four of the selected variables: the importance of religion, the ability to find meaning in severe illness and mature during the process, the belief that a cure for cancer can be found, and the belief that the cure for cancer might be found very soon. All four variables show the expected significant differences in the strength of their correlation with immanent/ultimate justice.

TABLE 9. Partial Correlational Analysis: Immanent and Ultimate Justice with Religiousness, Finding Meaning, Optimism ($244 < N < 303$)

Variable	Order	Variables		Comparison of correlations	
		Immanent	Ultimate	z_{emp}	z_{theo}
Importance of religion	0	.1315*	.3615**	3.82 > 1.96*	
	1a		.3398**		
	1b	−.0119			
Ability to find meaning	0	.1226*	.2784**	2.53 > 1.96*	
	1a		.2523**		
	1b	.0152			
A cure for cancer can be found	0	.0861	.2087**	1.96 > 1.96*	
	1a		.1909**		
	1b	.0048			
A cure for cancer can be found *soon*	0	.0778	.2201**	2.27 > 1.96*	
	1a		.2068**		
	1b	−.0095			

a) Belief in Immanent Justice held constant
b) Belief in Ultimate Justice held constant
*$p \leq .05$; **$p \leq .01$

Belief in ultimate justice showed positive associations to personal importance of religion, the ability to find meaning in severe illness, and the expectation that a cure is possible and indeed, will be found soon. Immanent justice generally showed no relation to these variables; any positive correlations found disappeared when ultimate justice was partialled out.

Subjects were also surveyed regarding their emotional reactions to the possibility of contracting cancer (see Table 10). Five emotional reactions were regarded: the confidence with which the subject believes he could cope with the illness in that case, feelings of personal invulnerability toward cancer, the sense of danger associated with cancer, hope that one will never suffer from cancer. Finally, and feelings of acceptance toward the cancer (should one ever fall ill).

Assuming that all subjects have experienced personal failure or transgression in their lives, immanent justice would seem to imply a stronger sense of danger, while ultimate justice would lead to greater feelings of hope, more confidence in coping, and invulnerability. Due to the religious resonance inherent to ultimate justice, the latter should also be associated with greater acceptance of fate.

The results were as predicted. With respect to ultimate justice, the significant positive relationships remained constant even when the influence of immanent justice was removed, while the weaker positive relationships associated with immanent justice apparently were based on the shared variance with ultimate justice. The only significant differences

TABLE 10. Partial Correlational Analysis: Immanent and
Ultimate Justice with Emotional Reactions (289 < N < 306)

		Variables		Comparison of correlations	
Variable	Order	Immanent	Ultimate	z_{emp}	z_{theo}
Coping confidence	0	.1564**	.2727**	1.92	
	1a		.2327**		
	1b	.0559			
Invulnerability	0	.2150**	.2468**	0.52	
	1a		.1808**		
	1b	.1327			
Perceived danger	0	.1311*	−.1382*	4.32 > 1.96*	
	1a		−.2079**		
	1b	.2033**			
Acceptance	0	.1234*	.2259**	1.65	
	1a		.1945**		
	1b	.0389			
Hope	0	−.0557	.0537	1.73	
	1a		.0822		
	1b	−.0835			

a) Belief in Immanent Justice held constant.
b) Belief in Ultimate Justice held constant.
*p ≤ .05; **p ≤ .01

at the bivariate level were found for feelings of danger: belief in immanent
justice was associated with stronger feelings of danger, whereas belief in
ultimate justice had just the opposite effect. The positive (negative) correlation with immanent (ultimate) justice increased in strength when the
effects of the opposing belief variant were partialled out.

In later sections of the questionnaire, subjects were presented with
questions of the form, "What would happen if . . . ?" Here, subjects were
asked to describe how they might behave if they had cancer. Table 11 shows
the correlations between just-world beliefs and four such variables. confidence in being able to master cancer competently, the presumption that the
subject would look to role models, people who have already dealt successfully with cancer, for support, self-accusations regarding behavior that
might have brought on the cancer (such as, "What have I done wrong?"),
and self-accusations regarding character traits that might have done the
same ("What kind of person am I?"). Higher correlations between ultimate
justice and confidence in coping competency were expected; the same was
predicted for use of role models: Role models who have coped well with
cancer and for whom justice has apparently been restored are very suitable
to validate belief in ultimate justice and support it through their own
example. Conversely, immanent justice was predicted to correlate more
highly with self-accusations in behavioral and character-related terms.

TABLE 11. Partial Correlational Analysis: Immanent and Ultimate
Justice with Hypothetical Behavior (286 < N < 303)

Variable	Order	Variables Immanent	Variables Ultimate	Comparison of correlations z_{emp}	Comparison of correlations z_{theo}
Confidence in mastery	0	.1033	.2120**	1.74	
	1a		.1875**		
	1b	.0224			
Use of role models	0	.1786**	.3200**	2.32 > 1.96*	
	1a		.2762**		
	1b	.0610			
Behavioral self-blame	0	.3454**	.1844**	2.66 > 1.96*	
	1a		.0568		
	1b	.3020**			
Characterological self-blame	0	.2947**	.2264**	1.13	
	1a		.1261		
	1b	.2299**			

a) Belief in Immanent Justice held constant
b) Belief in Ultimate Justice held constant
*p ≤ .05; **p ≤ .01

All of the correlations observed tended in the expected direction. Use
of role models and behavioral self-accusations demonstrated significant
bivariate correlations to just-world beliefs. Both kinds of self-accusations
showed a slight, positive relationship to ultimate justice, but in both cases,
become insignificant when the shared variance with immanent justice was
partialled out.

3.2.5. Immanent Justice, Ultimate Justice, and Trust

Immanent justice focuses on individual persons with moral shortcomings. Belief in ultimate justice is not only more strongly oriented
toward the future, it is also more strongly oriented toward the environment, because it presupposes the eventual re-establishment of justice
through external means. The precise manner by which restitution occurs
was not specified in the items of this questionnaire; however, one would
expect that, in general, ultimate justice is associated with more trust in
one's fellow human beings and in the environment (at least in those
situations in which persons or the environment can meaningfully contribute to the preservation of justice).

In two separate sections of the questionnaire, subjects were surveyed
regarding which persons or professional groups they trusted to contribute
to the cure of cancer and to the prevention of further illness.

Table 12 shows the relationships between both kinds of just-world
beliefs and trust in nine different categories of people. No hypotheses were

made regarding individual items; instead, there were more global expectations that ultimate justice would be associated with more trust in just
about every instance. Except for doctors (whose scores reflected roughly
equal amounts of trust), this tendency was apparent in all cases. Furthermore, with regards to trust in the cancer patients themselves, families,
friends, pastoral counselors, and nonmedical practitioners, the differences
achieved significance.

Similarly, trust in preventing illness was assessed across 14 different
categories of people. The results can be found in Table 13. Except for
governmental agencies/parties and the media, correlations were generally

TABLE 12. Partial Correlational Analysis: Immanent and Ultimate Justice
with Confidence in Recovery through Various Means (291 < N < 306)

Variable	Order	Variables		Comparison of correlations	
		Immanent	Ultimate	z_{emp}	z_{theo}
Confidence in recovery through:					
Persons afflicted	0	−.0591	.0862	2.29 > 1.96*	
with cancer	1a		.1191		
	1b	−.1013			
Families	0	.0528	.1749**	1.98 > 1.96*	
	1a		.1678**		
	1b	−.0174			
Friends	0	.0622	.1892**	2.02 > 1.96*	
	1a		.1795**		
	1b	−.0132			
Doctors	0	−.0399	−.0499	0.16	
	1a		.0373		
	1b	−.0222			
Caregivers	0	−.0346	.0045	0.63	
	1a		.0197		
	1b	−.039ↄ			
Psychologists	0	−.0211	.0911	1.76	
	1a		.1080		
	1b	−.0620			
Pastoral counselors	0	.0481	.2225**	2.80 > 1.96*	
	1a		.2217**		
	1b	−.0437			
Nonmedical practitioners	0	.0676	.1953**	2.02 > 1.96*	
	1a		.1840**		
	1b	−.0099			
Spiritualists	0	.2219**	.2331**	0.18	
	1a		.1629**		
	1b	.1459**			

a) Belief in Immanent Justice held constant
b) Belief in Ultimate Justice held constant
*p ≤ .05; **p ≤ .01

TABLE 13. Partial Correlational Analysis: Immanent and Ultimate Justice with Confidence in Prevention through Various Means (292 < N < 306)

Variable	Order	Variables		Comparison of correlations	
		Immanent	Ultimate	z_{emp}	z_{theo}
Everyone	0	.2110**	.2584**	0.76	
	1a		.1953**		
	1b	.1235			
Doctors	0	−.0823	.0204	1.60	
	1a		.0574		
	1b	−.0981			
Psychologists	0	.0123	.1418*	2.05 > 1.96*	
	1a		.1489**		
	1b	−.0475			
Pastoral counselors	0	.0972	.2388**	2.28 > 1.96*	
	1a		.2192**		
	1b	.0040			
Nonmedical practitioners	0	.1014	.2066**	1.69	
	1a		.1823**		
	1b	.0227			
Spiritualists	0	.1816**	.2157**	0.55	
	1a		.1598**		
	1b	.1080			
Political parties	0	.0147	−.0198	0.55	
	1a		−.0278		
	1b	.0245			
Media	0	.1277*	.0736	0.85	
	1a		.0258		
	1b	.1077			
Science	0	−.0432	.0468	1.41	
	1a		.0694		
	1b	−.0670			
Industry	0	.0161	.0314	0.23	
	1a		.0273		
	1b	.0041			
Church	0	.1115	.2241**	1.79	
	1a		.1973**		
	1b	.0264			
German Cancer Aid Society	0	.0717	.2346**	2.61 > 1.96*	
	1a		.2251**		
	1b	.0318			
Charitable organizations	0	.0657	.2103**	2.30 > 1.96*	
	1a		.2011**		
	1b	−.0187			
Health insurance companies	0	.0601	.1185*	0.93	
	1a	.1034			
	1b	.0150			

a) Belief in Immanent Justice held constant.
b) Belief in Ultimate Justice held constant.
*p ≤ .05; **p ≤ .01

higher with respect to ultimate justice. These differences achieved significance for psychologists, pastoral counselors, the German Cancer Aid Society, and charitable organizations.

3.2.6. Immanent Justice, Ultimate Justice, and Health Behavior

Finally, the present study examined whether significant differences could be found between beliefs in immanent/ultimate justice and health behavior, expressed either in the decision to forego risky behaviors or participate in early detection examinations. The optimism and confidence reflected by beliefs in ultimate justice would seem to indicate that this form of just-world belief is associated with a greater tendency to forego risky behavior and participate in preventive measures (such as early detection examinations), perhaps because optimism is founded upon low risk-taking behavior or because trust in a just world underscores the rewards associated with low risk-taking behavior, thereby increasing its attractiveness. The pessimism more closely associated with immanent justice might make abstinence from risk behavior or efforts at early prevention appear useless and coalesce into a kind of fatalism. Furthermore, immanent justice appears to associate the existence or nonexistence of illness with a person's moral worth and moral behavior rather than with specific health behavior.

Once again, the design of the present study allowed us to examine various hypotheses. Ultimate justice was expected to more strongly motivate subjects to do without risk-related behavior, to take advantage of early detection examinations, and to train oneself in systematic self-observation techniques for early warning signals. Table 14 shows some of the results of the examination.

The subjects were asked how willing they were to give up alcohol, smoking, coffee, and sunbathing. The subjects' inclination to eliminate unhealthy habits was calculated as the variable Risk Avoidance (alpha = .73). The expected difference was found: The higher the belief in immanent justice, the lower the inclination to do without the unhealthy behaviors described, while the higher the belief in ultimate justice, the greater the inclination to do so.

Why should one give up cigarettes, coffee, and alcohol when it is far more important to be a moral person? When the proportion of variance contributed by ultimate justice is partialled out, the negative correlation between immanent justice and inclination to reduce consumption behavior increases. Likewise, when the effects of immanent justice are held constant, the positive relationship between ultimate justice and inclination to reduce consumption behavior grows stronger. Table 14 also presents a more precise analysis of the corresponding correlations to the four individual variables. Results show a significant correlational differences regarding attitudes towards alcohol and tobacco; conversely attitudes toward drinking coffee and sunbathing failed to reach significance. In fact, regarding the inclination to give up coffee (the least risky of all the health behaviors assessed), there was virtually no difference at all in the correlations observed.

Specific behaviors such as the number of cigarettes smoked daily and the amount of alcohol imbibed weekly were also assessed. The results show a tendency in the expected direction: the higher the belief in ultimate justice, the lower the consumption of alcohol and cigarettes. The differences between immanent and ultimate justice, however, fail to achieve levels of significance. Correlational analysis, of course, cannot explain whether the low levels of alcohol/cigarette consumption allow subjects to entertain the rosy future perspective offered by ultimate justice, or whether

TABLE 14. Partial Correlational Analysis: Immanent and Ultimate Justice with Health Behavior (1)

Variable	Order	Variables		Comparison of correlations	
		Immanent	Ultimate	z_{emp}	z_{theo}
Risk avoidance [N = 72]	0	−.1359	.1257	4.20 > 1.96*	
	1a		.1964		
	1b	−.2029			
Avoidance of risk behavior:					
Less alcohol [N = 295]	0	−.0427	.1204*	2.58 > 1.96*	
	1a		.1492**		
	1b	−.0984			
Less sunbathing [N =158]	0	−.0888	.0134	1.60	
	1a		.0527		
	1b	−.1023			
Less smoking [N = 109]	0	.0710	.2015*	2.09 > 1.96*	
	1a		.1893		
	1b	−.0089			
Less coffee [N = 305]	0	.0263	.0282	0.03	
	1a		.0194		
	1b	.0166			
Consumption of tobacco and alcohol:					
Cigarettes per day	0	−.0578	−.1373*	1.25	
	1a		−.1248		
	1b	−.0044			
Alcohol per week	0	.0086	−.1119	1.91	
	1a		−.1253		
	1b	.0574			

a) Belief in Immanent Justice held constant.
b) Belief in Ultimate Justice held constant.
*p ≤ .05; **p ≤ .01

beliefs in ultimate justice enable them to smoke and drink less (e.g., when confronted with problems).

The subjects were also presented four questions on early detection based on self-observation techniques, namely:

1. whether they believe that one can detect cancer in its early stages by precise and systematic observation;
2. whether they were familiar with the physical changes that require attention;
3. whether they were interested in learning more about these kinds of early warning signs; and
4. whether they were interested in being trained in precision observation and self-examination techniques.

The four questions were incorporated into the variable "Early detection" (alpha = .71). Here too, significant differences were found: Whereas ultimate justice was correlated positively with the inclination towards self-observation, immanent justice correlated negatively with the variable. Each of these relationships became stronger when the variance shared with the opposing just-world belief was partialled out. Table 15 also shows the individual correlations between the four questions and both types of just-world beliefs. Significant differences were found regarding the first two questions, whereas the questions assessing the subjects' inclination to take specific action (questions 3 and 4) did not show any significant differences.

After the questions on self-observation, the subjects were surveyed regarding their participation in prevention and early detection examinations in the following manner:

1. How familiar are you with preventive care examinations?
2. How sensible are preventive care examinations, in your opinion?
3. How unpleasant are preventive care examinations for you?
4. Would you regularly participate in preventive care examinations as soon as you can?

Table 15 shows the bivariate and partial correlations between responses to these four questions and immanent/ultimate justice beliefs. An aggregation of the items was contraindicated due to poor internal consistency (alpha = .55). The pattern of results only tendentially supports the hypothesized relationships; in general, the relationship between such questions and both kinds of just-world beliefs must be viewed as tenuous in the extreme. The only item to show significant differences were ratings regarding the sensefulness of preventive care examinations: subjects with high belief in immanent justice found such examinations to be less sensible than subjects with high belief in ultimate justice. Neither the self-reported familiarity and unpleasantness of the procedures, nor the willingness of subjects to have them, significantly correlated with just-world beliefs.

Altogether, the differences are very small; nevertheless, one might speculate about the different meaning of preventive care examinations for people with high belief in immanent or in ultimate justice. One might suppose that a possible positive diagnosis constitutes no final verdict for people with belief in ultimate justice because they trust in curing and a better future. This may be the reason why they have a more positive attitude toward preventive care examinations than people believing in

TABLE 15. Partial Correlational Analysis: Immanent and Ultimate Justice with Health Behavior (2) (295 < N < 306)

Variable	Order	Variables		Comparison of correlations	
		Immanent	Ultimate	z_{emp}	z_{theo}
Early detection through self observation:					
Early detection	0	−.0472	.1028	2.37 > 1.96*	
	1a		.1320		
	1b	−.0956			
1. Effective in detecting cancer?	0	−.0284	.1732**	3.20 > 1.96*	
	1a		.2004**		
2. Familiar with warning signs?	0	−.0956	.0289	1.97 > 1.96*	
	1a		.0725		
	1b	−.1163			
3. Interested in learning more?	0	−.0618	−.0158	0.72	
	1a		.0091		
	1b	−.0604			
4. Willing to be trained?	0	.0249	.0956	1.12	
	1a		.0934		
	1b	−.0138			
Early detection examinations:					
1. Are you familiar?	0	−.0536	.0498	1.63	
	1a		.0771		
	1b	−.0796			
2. How sensible?	0	−.1542**	−.0111	2.26 > 1.96*	
	1a		.0543		
	1b	−.1629**			
3. How unpleasant?	0	.0123	−.0562	1.07	
	1a		−.0664		
	1b	.0374			
4. Participation?	0	−.0531	.0310	1.32	
	1a		.0564		
	1b	−.0710			

a) Belief in Immanent Justice held constant.

immanent justice. Subjects with high belief in immanent justice must not only cope with the diagnosis but as well with the possible meaning of that diagnosis that is suggested by their belief in immanent justice. They may find such examinations to be more unpleasant than subjects with high belief in ultimate justice, possibly because they equate an examination of their body with an examination of their moral fiber. Hence, somatic symptoms reveal moral deficit. Such questions could not be sufficiently settled in the present study. In view of the high practical relevance and urgency more studies are desirable in order to deal these problems in more detail.

3.2.7. Immanent Justice, Ultimate Justice, and Self-Determinism

One last point: Both kinds of just-world beliefs can be examined as they relate to a vast number of general belief systems. In conclusion, I report on the relationships between just-world beliefs and control beliefs (including notions of personal freedom).

Table 16 presents the correlations between just-world beliefs and the contrasting notions of personal freedom and determinism, respectively. The variable *Free* represents the opinion that human beings are free to choose between alternatives and to act accordingly, whereas *Unfree* reflects the belief that human behavior is determined by a number of internal restrictions and external obstacles. An optimistic viewpoint (which is related to ultimate justice) accords well with belief in free action. Immanent justice underscores the determinism of events much more strongly: If ever an error is made, a sin committed, than punishment is practically inevitable. Immanent justice should thus be associated with beliefs that express the lack of freedom inherent to human behavior. These hypotheses could also be

TABLE 16. Partial Correlational Analysis: Immanent
and Ultimate Justice with Self-Determinism
(Freedom vs. Determinism) $(289 < N < 304)$

Variable	Order	Variables		Comparison of correlations	
		Immanent	Ultimate	z_{emp}	z_{theo}
Unfree	0	.1671**	.0324	2.14 > 1.96*	
	1a		−.0365		
	1b	.1679**			
Free	0	.1264*	.1850**	0.96	
	1a		.1484**		
	1b	.0595			

a) Belief in Immanent Justice held constant.
b) Belief in Ultimate Justice held constant.
*$p \leq .05$; **$p \leq .01$

confirmed. Only immanent justice correlated with deterministic beliefs, whereas the slight positive correlation with ultimate justice changed signs when immanent justice was held constant. Bivariate correlations were significantly different from each other. Beliefs in personal freedom correlated more highly with ultimate than with immanent justice, but the difference between correlations was not significant. In terms of content validity, the assumption of free action is quite compatible—despite a few restrictions—with immanent justice; the person who believes in immanent justice and desires to avoid the portentous outcome associated with human transgression must also believe that life offers different paths to trod. In other words, he or she must concede some degree of actional freedom.

The concrete way in which one avoids cancer, however, may depend a great deal upon whether a person believes in immanent versus ultimate justice. The different methods used to avoid cancer were assessed in the questionnaire using an instrument describing so-called "control channels." Control channels are nothing more than the ways and means used to establish individual control.

Table 17 shows the correlations between just-world beliefs and two such control channels: the belief that abstinence from tobacco, alcohol, etc., can prevent cancer, and conversely the belief that moral behavior can prevent cancer, for example, by "not allowing oneself to be tainted by sin" or by "remaining a respectable human being."

From the perspective of immanent justice, beliefs which state that cancer can be avoided through moral behavior would seem correct, whereas ultimate justice—based upon the results already reported—seems more plausibly associated with the belief that abstinence can help prevent cancer. As expected, highly significant relationships between cancer avoid-

TABLE 17. Partial Correlational Analysis: Immanent and Ultimate Justice with Control Channels (296 < N < 306)

Variable	Order	Variables		Comparison of correlations	
		Immanent	Ultimate	z_{emp}	z_{theo}
Control channels:					
Moral behavior	0	.5305**	.3615**	3.10 > 1.96*	
	1a		.1968**		
	1b	.4533**			
Abstinence	0	.1181*	.1854**	1.07	
	1a		.1523**		
	1b	.0502			

a) Belief in Immanent Justice held constant.
b) Belief in Ultimate Justice held constant.
*p ≤ .05; **p ≤ .01

ance through moral rectitude and just-world beliefs were found. Belief in immanent justice was more strongly correlated with this measure than belief in ultimate justice. The differences concerning abstinence tend in the expected direction but are not significant.

4. SUMMARY

The attempted differentiation between just-world beliefs could be confirmed. Factor analysis differentiated between four different factors: (1) belief in immanent justice, (2) general belief in a just world, (3) belief in ultimate justice, and (4) belief in an unjust world. Item-factor assignment led to highly consistent subscales for belief in immanent (alpha = .83) and ultimate (alpha = .86) justice.

Correlational relationships to a large array of other variables assessed in the questionnaire study on cancer provide evidence for the content validity of this differentiation. Immanent and ultimate justice differentiate significantly with respect to the direction or strength of their relationship to other belief systems (e.g., control beliefs, freedom beliefs) as well as to other cognitive, emotional, and behavioral indices, including the harshness of judgements levied upon victims, perceptual style, illness-related emotions, behavior toward victims and health behavior. The frequently reported relationship between just-world belief and devaluation of the victim (see Montada, 1992) was significantly higher for immanent justice. Conversely, belief in ultimate justice was associated with a more positive impression of the victim. Similar findings were observed with regards to ascription of responsibility. Belief in ultimate justice was clearly less associated with holding the victim responsible than belief in immanent justice; in fact, the relationship disappeared after the proportion of shared variance with immanent justice was partialled out. Only immanent justice was associated with accusations, blame, and acceptance of sanctions against victims, whereas ultimate justice showed absolutely no more even negative correlations. On the other hand, belief in ultimate justice showed clearly positive relationships to adaptive processes such as the ability to find sense and meaning in severe illness, optimism, and confidence in coping with severe illness. The danger posed by cancer was more keenly felt by subjects with beliefs in immanent justice; hence the significant, positive correlation between these two variables. Conversely, the relationship between perceived danger and ultimate justice was significantly negative. Differences between both kinds of just-world beliefs were also found in the support and financing of sociopolitical measures to fight cancer. Whereas belief in ultimate justice corresponded with financing though charitable activities (donations, lotteries, charity organizations), the financial burdening of cancer patients and risk groups was more strongly associated with immanent justice. The belief that justice can be reestablished in the long run appears not only to increase one's willingness to contribute to the preservation of justice, but also to become more health-conscious and abstain from risky behavior.

REFERENCES

Ambrosio, A. L. & Sheehan. S. E. (1991). The just world belief and the AIDS epidemic. Journal of Social Behavior and Personality, 6, 163–170.

Bierhoff, H. W., Klein, R. & Kramp, P. (1991). Evidence for the altruistic personality from data on accident research. Journal of Personality, 59, 263–280.

Bortz, J. (1977). Lehrbuch der Statistik. Für Sozialwissenschaftler. Berlin: Springer.

Bush, A., Krebs, D. L. & Carpendale, J. I. (1993). The structural consistency of moral judgments about AIDS. Journal of Genetic Psychology, 154, 167–175.

Connors, J. & Heaven, P. C. (1990). Belief in a just world and attitudes toward AIDS sufferers. Journal of Social Psychology, 130, 559–560.

Dalbert, C. (1982). Der Glaube an eine gerechte Welt: Zur Güte einer deutschen Version der Skala von Rubin & Peplau. P.I.V.- Bericht Nr .3. (= Berichte aus der Arbeitsgruppe "Verantwortung, Gerechtigkeit, Moral, Nr .10). Trier: Universität Trier, Fachbereich I - Psychologie.

Dalbert, C. & Katona-Sallay, H. (1993). Belief in a Just World in Europe: A Hungarian-German Comparison. University of Tübingen: Unpublished paper.

Dalbert, C., Montada, L. & Schmitt, M. (1987). Glaube an eine gerechte Welt als Motiv: Validierungskorrelate zweier Skalen. Psychologische Beiträge, 29, 596–615.

Furnham, A. (1990). The development of single trait personality theories. Personality and Individual Differences, 11, 923–929.

Glennon, F. & Joseph, S. (1993). Just world beliefs, self esteem, and attitudes towards homosexuals with AIDS. Psychological Reports, 72, 584–586.

Gruman, J. C. & Sloan, R. P. (1983). Disease as justice: Perceptions of victims of physical illness. Basic and Applied Social Psychology, 4, 39–46.

Harper, D. J. & Manasse, P. R. (1992). The Just World and the Third World: British explanations for poverty abroad. Journal of Social Psychology, 132, 783–785.

The Holy Bible and Apocrypha. God. Revised Standard Version. London: Thomas Nelson and Sons, Ltd

Jones, C. & Aronson, E. (1973). Attribution of fault to a rape victim as a function of respectability of the victim. Journal of Personality and Social Psychology, 26, 415–419.

Kerr, N. L. & Kurtz, S. T. (1977). Effects of a victim's suffering and respectability on mock juror judgments: Further evidence on the just world theory. Representative Research in Social Psychology, 8, 42–56.

Kushner, H. S. (1981). When bad things happen to good people. New York: Schocken Books.

Lerner, M. J. (1965). Evaluation of performance as a function of performer's reward and attractiveness. Journal of Personality and Social Psychology, 1, 355–360.

Lerner, M.J. (1970). The desire for justice and reactions to victims. In J. Macaulay & L. Berkowitz (Eds.), Altruism and helping behavior (pp .205–228). New York: Academic Press.

Lerner, M. J. (1980). The belief in a just world. A fundamental delusion. New York: Plenum Press.

Lerner, M. J., Miller, D. & Holmes, J. G. (1976). Deserving and the emergence of forms of justice. In L. Berkowitz (Ed.), Advances in Experimental Social Psychology, Vol. 9, (pp. 133- 162). New York: Academic Press.

MacLean, M. J. & Chown, S. M. (1988). Just world beliefs and attitudes toward helping elderly people: A comparison of British and Canadian university students. International Journal of Aging and Human Development, 26, 249–260.

Maes, J. (1992). Konstruktion und Analyse eines mehrdimensionalen Gerechte-Welt-Fragebogens.(Berichte aus der Arbeitsgruppe "Verantwortung, Gerechtigkeit, Moral," Nr. 64). Trier: Universität Trier, Fachbereich I - Psychologie.

Maes, J. (1994). Drakonität als Personmerkmal: Entwicklung und erste Erprobung eines Fragebogens zur Erfassung von Urteilsstrenge (Drakonität) versus Milde. (Berichte aus der Arbeitsgruppe "Verantwortung, Gerechtigkeit, Moral" Nr .78). Trier: Universität Trier, Fachbereich I - Psychologie.,

Miller, D. T. (1977). Altruism and threat to a belief in a just world. Journal of Eperimental Social Psychology, 13, 113–124.

Montada, L. (1992). Attribution of responsibility for losses and perceived injustice. In L. Montada, S.-H. Filipp & M.J. Lerner (Eds.), Life Crises and the Experience of Loss in Adulthood, (pp. 133–161). Hillsdale, N.J.: Lawrence Erlbaum.

Montada, L. & Schneider, A. (1989). Justice and emotional reactions to the disadvantaged. Social Justice Research, 3, 313–344.

Montada, L. & Schneider, A. (1991). Justice and prosocial commitments. In: L. Montada & H. W. Bierhoff (Eds.), Altruism in social systems, (pp. 58–81). Göttingen: Hogrefe.

Murphy-Berman, V. & Berman, J. J. (1990). The Effect of Respondents' Just World Beliefs and Target Person's Social Worth and Awareness-of-Risk on Perceptions of a Person with AIDS. Social Justice Research, 4, 215–228.

Olkin, I. (1967). Correlations revisited. In J. C. Stanley (Ed), Improving experimental design and statistical analysis. Chicago: Rand McNally.

O'Quin, K. & Vogler, C. C. (1990). Use of the Just World Scale with prison inmates: A methodological note. Perceptual and Motor Skills, 70, 395–400.

Piaget, J. (1932). Le jugement moral chez l'enfant. Paris: Alcan.

Rubin, Z. & Peplau, L. A. (1973). Belief in a just world and reactions to another's lot: A study of participants in the National Draft Lottery. Journal of Social Issues, 29(4), 73–93.

Rubin, Z. & Peplau, L. A. (1975). Who believes in a just world? Journal of Social Issues, 31(3), 65–89.

Schmitt, M., Kilders, M., Mosle, A., Müller, L., Pfrengle, A., Rabenberg, H., Schott, F., Stolz, J., Suda, U., Williams, M. & Zimmermann, G.. (1991). Gerechte-Welt-Glaube, Gewinn und Verlust: Rechtfertigung oder ausgleichende Gerechtigkeit. Zeitschrift für Sozialpsychologie, 22, 37–45.

Schneider, A. (1988). Glaube an die gerechte Welt: Replikation der Validierungskorrelate zweier Skalen. (Berichte aus der Arbeitsgruppe "Verantwortung, Gerechtigkeit, Moral" Nr. 40). Trier: Universität Trier, Fachbereich I - Psychologie.

Sherman, M. F., Smith, R. & Cooper, R. (1982). Reactions toward the dying: The effects of a patient's illness and respondents' belief in a just world. Omega Journal of Death and Dying, 13, 173–189.

Sloan, R. P.& Gruman, J. C. (1983). Beliefs about cancer, heart disease, and their victims. Psychological Reports, 52, 415- 424.

Thornton, B., Ryckman, R. M. & Robbins, M. A. (1982). The relationships of observer characteristics to beliefs in the causal responsibility of victims of sexual assaults. Human Relations, 35, 321–330.

Weir, J. A. & Wrightsman, L. S. (1990). The determinants of mock jurors' verdicts in a rape case. Journal of Applied Social Psychology, 20, 901–919.

Zucker, G. S. & Weiner, B. (1993). Conservatism and perceptions of poverty: An attributional analysis. Journal of Applied Social Psychology, 23, 925–943.

Zuckerman, M., Gerbasi, K. C., Kravitz, R. I. & Wheeler, L. (1975). The belief in a just world and reactions to innocent victims. Catalog of Selected Documents in Psychology, 5, 326.

Chapter 3

BJW and Self-Efficacy in Coping with Observed Victimization
RESULTS FROM A STUDY ABOUT UNEMPLOYMENT

CHANGIZ MOHIYEDDINI and LEO MONTADA

With the theory of "Belief in a Just World" (BJW), Lerner (1970, 1980) has given an explanation as to why people blame innocent victims for self-infliction of their fate and why they derogate innocent victims. They do so to deny injustices, respectively, to defend their belief in a just world. BJW in its most general form implies the conviction that everybody gets what he or she justly deserves. The other side of the coin is that everybody deserves what happens to him or her. When oneself or others enjoy advantages or suffer disadvantages, we care about justice. BJW motivates the search for legitimate reasons. Deservingness is the most legitimate reason for many people.

Providing compensations for the victims are another way one can avoid viewing the world as unjust. Innocent victims deserve support and compensation. People may consider to grant or to claim support for the victims as long as the costs of help are not too high. When people cannot help innocent victims—and thus cannot remedy the injustice in reality—or if they decide not to help because help is too costly, they tend to downgrade the victims or to blame them for self-infliction, and then tend to even more

CHANGIZ MOHIYEDDINI • Psychologisches Institut, Universität Mainz (FB 12), Staudingerweg 9, D-55099 Mainz, Germany. LEO MONTADA • Department of Psychology, Universität Trier, D-54286 Trier, Germany.

Responses to Victimizations and Belief in a Just World, edited by Montada and Lerner. Plenum Press, New York, 1998.

so the more victims are suffering. These forms of defending one's BJW can, of course, be considered a secondary victimization of victims. Although most empirical investigations support Melvin Lerner's hypotheses about the impact of BJW on the tendency to blame victims for their hardships, some studies are published which do not. Several studies have observed that the victims were not derogated (Kerr & Kurtz, 1977; Gruman & Sloan, 1983) and in some quasiexperimental surveys referring to game situations the victims were even upgraded and the winners were derogated (see also Schmitt in this volume).

Thinking about possible reasons for these inconsistent results has led us to hypothesize about varying subjective meanings of measured BJW, respectively, about variants of world views implying justice. In this chapter, two variants are introduced: Hope for a Just World (HJW), and Self-Efficacy to Promote Justice in the World (SEJW). The construct SEJW implies that injustices do occur but that they can be corrected, at least reduced; moreover, that the subject him-/herself can contribute to correct or to reduce occurring injustice. SEJW is a precondition for considering a just world as a subjective "action goal." To contribute to a just world can mean, for example, that innocent victims are upgraded, that sympathy for them is expressed, and thereby, they are a bit compensated for their suffered injustices. Other efforts to reduce injustice may be supporting victims and claiming help for victims in the political arena. SEJW serves as a plausible (post hoc) hypothesis to explain findings that victims have been upgraded.

Which relationships between SEJW and BJW are expected? BJW and SEJW are conceived of as conceptual independent constructs. A low score on a BJW measure implies that the current existing world of an individual is not evaluated as a just one. This does neither preclude nor imply high scores on a measure of SEJW. A high score on a BJW measure may also be associated with high and with low SEJW scores.

How do BJW and SEJW interact in responding to cases of victimization? In the case of a high BJW, subjects scoring low on SEJW should tend to defend or to restore justice subjectively by blaming the victims. This is the only way they have to save their BJW. What is with subjects scoring high on SEJW? Most likely, it will depend on the kind of victimization and the means to restore justice. If subjects have the necessary means at costs that are not too high, they might be willing to help. On the average, across many cases, subjects who score high on SEJW are expected to blame victims less than low scoring subjects because some of them at least have means to restore justice in reality by helping the victims.

What is in the case of a low BJW? On the average, subjects who score high on SEJW can be expected to help victims or to claim help for victims a bit more. (A positive evaluation of victims can be considered a means of help.) However, it is expected that this tendency to help is mediated by subjects' motivation to help, or maybe by their justice motive,[1] their empathy, or their altruism. Subjects who do not care much about justice may not be motivated to help victims for reasons of justice even if they feel able to give help. Subjects who score low on SEJW (as well as on BJW) are neither motivated to blame the victim nor to help them. Upgrading or derogating of victims might occur in this case but will be based on another motivation as justice, e.g., sympathy or social prejudices.

The Hope for a Just World (HJW) differs from BJW in that occurring injustices are not incompatible with this world view. HJW will not be threatened by observed injustices but will be evoked. HJW and Immanent BJW are not compatible in a strict sense, but belief that the world is a just one as it is without any exceptions and at every point in time would be a perfectly unrealistic view and is probably not held by any reasonable person at all. For all who believe that the world is, in general, a just one, HJW may function as a supportive view. Therefore, HJW and BJW are not incompatible. Nevertheless, we consider HJW as an independent construct because we expect that a lot of people who doubt that the world is a just one at present do hope for a just world in the future. Others, however, might not even hope for justice, still others do not care about justice at all. For these reasons we do not have a rational hypotheses about the correlations between BJW and HJW.

HJW is not conceived of to be perfectly independent from SEJW: The self-efficient intervention in order to make the world more just presupposes in a sense the hope that the world will be just or more just in the future. However, HJW does not imply SEJW. Even subjects scoring low on SEJW may score high on HJW when they believe in powerful others or deities to care for future justice.

In order to examine these different facets, two scales were developed: the SEJW scale and the HJW scale. These two scales were combined and factor analyzed together with the GBJW scale (Dalbert, Montada, & Schmitt, 1987). It was expected that GBJW, HJW, and SEJW items are loading on three orthogonal factors. The correlations of the resulting scales were expected to be weak on the basis of the arguments given above.

1. HYPOTHESES

1. *Main effects of SEJW:* It was expected that SEJW will be correlated with the readiness to remove the objective injustice by adequate intervention (e.g., political protest, individual help). Moreover, it

---

[1] This hypothesis presupposes that BJW does not represent the justice motive in a pure form but that BJW is a hybrid of the justice motive and self-interest (cf. Montada in this volume).

is expected that with increasing SEJW, the probability of becoming a member of sociopolitical organizations (which are frequently concerned with justice) also increases. No such hypotheses are formulated for HJW.

2. *Interactions of BJW and SEJW:* It was expected that the influence of BJW and blaming victims was moderated by SEJW. With higher BJW and lower SEJW, more derogating and blaming of victims was expected. The same hypothesis is derived for sympathy for (or pity with) the victims: With higher BJW and lower SEJW, less sympathy was expected. Contrastingly, we expected that with decreasing BJW and increasing SEJW, the extent of blaming victims decreases and feelings of sympathy with the victims increases. These hypotheses were tested in a study that examined causes and consequences of unemployment as well as responses to unemployment from the perspective of justice psychology (Montada & Mohiyeddini, 1995).

2. METHODS

2.1. Subjects and Procedure

A random sample was drawn from two urban areas in Germany. From the entire sample, a subsample of 143 subjects (42% female) who were in permanent employment was selected. The results presented in this chapter were computed from the responses given by this subsample. This subsample was selected because the subjects were privileged compared to the unemployed, who are the focused "victims" in this study. Age ranged from 21 to 63 years, with a mean of 45 years (SD = 15 years).

2.2. Justice Related Scales

1. *General Belief in a Just World (GBJW):* To measure GBJW, the Dalbert, Montada, & Schmitt (1987) scale was used.
2. *Self-Efficacy (SEJW)* in contributing to justice: This scale was newly developed. It consists of nine items, examples are "I can contribute to give more people in the world what they justly deserve." "I can contribute to make the world more just." Subjects were asked to rate these statements on a six-point rating scale ranging from 1 = "not right at all" to 6 = "absolutely right."
3. *Hope for a Just World (HJW):* This scale, too, was newly developed. It consists of eight items. Examples are the following ones: "I hope for a world which is generally just." "I hope for a world in which more people get what they justly deserve."

2.3. Factor and Reliability Analysis of the Scales to Measure BJW, SEJW, and HJW

The 22 items of the three scales BJW, SEJW, and HJW were entered simultaneously into a principle axes analysis. The eigenvalue plot suggested three common factors.

After varimax rotation of the first three principle axes to simple structure, a loading pattern emerged which corresponded perfectly to the a priori structure. All SEJW items loaded on one factor, all HJW items loaded on a second factor, and all BJW items loaded on a third factor. Together, the three factors explained 54.1% of the total variance of the items.

In a second step, the items of each scale were submitted separately to principle axes analysis. The eigenvalue plots indicated clearly that the items of each scale had only one factor in common. Consequently, each scale measures a one-dimensional construct. The reliability turned out to be very high for each scale. The internal consistency coefficients alpha was .94 for SEJW, .89 for HJW, and .76 for the BJW scales, respectively. Table 1 shows the distributions of items.

TABLE 1. Loading Pattern, Communality (h^2),
Item Total Correlation (r_{it}), Mean (M), and
Standard Deviation (SD) of the Variables

Variable	l_1	l_2	l_3	h^2	r_{it}	M	SD
SEJW1	.89	.13	−.01	.80	.84	3.18	1.54
SEJW2	.83	.11	.07	.71	.79	3.28	1.52
SEJW3	.78	.17	.02	.64	.73	3.74	1.48
SEJW4	.78	.23	.05	.66	.75	4.21	1.39
SEJW5	.77	.22	.16	.67	.75	3.52	1.48
SEJW6	.76	.13	.22	.64	.71	3.42	1.44
SEJW7	.76	−.01	−.11	.59	.65	3.12	1.38
SEJW8	.71	.15	.17	.55	.66	3.95	1.45
SEJW9	.67	−.05	.02	.45	.57	3.59	1.47
HJW1	.08	.84	−.05	.71	.72	1.85	1.25
HJW2	.05	.82	−.01	.68	.71	1.87	1.07
HJW3	.12	.75	−.04	.58	.66	1.93	1.21
HJW4	.04	.75	.00	.56	.62	2.21	1.18
HJW5	.15	.69	.01	.49	.58	1.88	1.03
HJW6	.19	.63	.02	.43	.56	1.92	1.12
HJW7	.03	.51	.10	.27	.39	1.91	1.17
HJW8	.25	.50	−.02	.31	.42	1.87	1.05
BJW1	.18	−.03	.79	.66	.59	5.08	1.09
BJW2	−.02	.05	.77	.60	.53	4.53	1.26
BJW3	.11	.10	.59	.37	.42	4.26	1.42
BJW4	.02	−.00	.58	.34	.43	4.52	1.45
BJW5	−.02	.02	.54	.29	.37	4.30	1.45
BJW6	.15	−.38	.52	.44	.40	3.41	1.48

2.4. Prosocial and "Antisocial" Responses to Victims

From a comprehensive questionnaire, some prosocial and antisocial variables were selected to test the hypotheses outlined before. The following variables were selected:

1. *Sympathy with the unemployed (SYMP):* Subjects rated their sympathy with the unemployed on a six-point rating scale form 1 = "no sympathy at all" to 6 = "strong sympathy."
2. *Negative statements about the unemployed:* Subjects were asked to rate the following statements on a six-point rating scale ranging from 1 = "not right at all" to 6 = "absolutely right."

   a. Insufficient qualification of the unemployed is the reason for their unemployment.
   b. Unemployment is normally the consequence of the unemployed's own faults.
   c. Many long-term unemployed do not want to work.
   d. Everybody who really wants to work will find a job sooner or later.
   e. Most long-term unemployed do not have any usable qualifications.

3. *Willingness to fight against unemployment:* Two kinds of willingness to fight against unemployment were measured by means of financial help (WFI) and by political activities (WPO).

   a. WFI was measured by the following questions:

      i. Would you be willing to support a production facility of unemployed people by buying their products even if they were more expensive than normal?
      ii. Would you be willing to give donations for the establishment of some new jobs?
      iii. Would you be willing to buy lottery tickets in favor of unemployed people?

   b. WPO was measured by the following questions:

      i. Would you be willing to write to politicians asking them to improve their measures against unemployment?
      ii. Would you be willing to sign your name on a petition demanding additional measures against unemployment?
      iii. Would you be willing to join a demonstration in order to make the unemployeds' rights, concerns, and interests heard?

   These statements were rated on a six-point rating scale from 1 = "No, definitely not" to 6 = "Yes, definitely."

4. *Membership in a social or political organization (MSPO):* We have also included membership in a social or political organization as a global indicator for prosocial orientations. MSPO is not restricted to organizations concerned with unemployment. The variable is coded either 0 (= no membership) or 1 (= membership).

2.5. Factor and Reliability Analysis of the Measures for BVSI, WFI, and WPO

Blaming "victims" for self-infliction of their fate (BVSI): According to the eigenvalue plot, the items measure only one common factor. The internal consistency of the scale was $\alpha = .70$.

The willingness to fight against unemployment by means of financial help (WFI) and on a political level (WPO): The six items of the two scales WFI and WPO were entered simultaneously into a principle axes analysis. The eigenvalue plot suggested two common factors. All WFI items loaded on one factor and all WPO items loaded on a second factor. Together, the three factors explained 68.5% of the total variance of the items. The internal consistency coefficients were $\alpha = .74$ for WFI and $\alpha = .76$ for the WPO scales.

3. RESULTS

3.1. Correlations between BJW, HJW, and SEJW

As can be seen from Table 2, BJW and HJW do not correlate. Since HJW (as a vision) takes at least some injustices in the existing world for granted, this result is not inconsistent with the expectations outlined before. SEJW and BJW turned out to be positively correlated ($r = .29$): BJW does not exclude the possibility that people see themselves as effective in securing justice in the world, or in helping to create more justice. SEJW and HJW have a correlation of $r = .25$. This makes sense assuming that it would be a failing effort to fight for justice in a world when it is not expected that justice will prosper.

3.2. Intercorrelations between GBJW, HJW, and SEJW and BVSI, WFI, WPO, and SYMP

GBJW is correlated with *Blaming the Victims for Self-Infliction* (BVSI, $r = .25$) as was expected by Lerner's theory. This, however, is not all about GBJW: there is a small correlation with *Willingness to financially support* unemployed people a bit (WFI, $r = .15$), but a negative correlation with *Willingness to politically support* them (WPO, $r = -.16$). BJW is uncorrelated with BVSI, and positively correlated with *Sympathy for the Unemployed*

TABLE 2. Correlation among the Variables

	GBJW	SEJW	HJW	WFI	WPO	BVSI	SYMP
GBJW	1.00						
SEJW	.22*	1.00					
HJW	−.02	.32**	1.00				
WFI	.15	.20*	.19*	1.00			
WPO	−.16	.18*	.18*	.42**	1.00		
BVSI	.25**	−.02	.02	−.21**	−.29**	1.00	
SYMP	−.02	.14	.24**	.27**	.25**	−.17*	1.00

*p < .05; **p < .01

(SYMP, r = .24) and both forms of support for them (WFI, r = .19; WPO, r = .18). SEJW is correlated with both forms of support of the unemployed (WFU, r = .20) WPO, r = .18). SEJW is not correlated with BVSI, but positively though not significantly with SYMP.

3.3. Two-Way Interactions of GBJW and SEJW in Predicting Sympathy (SYMP), BVSI, and Willingness to Help the Victims (WFI, WPO)

In a next step of analyses, the expected two-way interactions of GBJW and SEJW were tested for *Sympathy* and BVSI without including any additional variables. Interaction effects were found for both *Sympathy* (SYMP) and *Blaming the Victims for Self-Infliction of their Fate* (BVSI). The conditional means are given in Figures 1 and 2, respectively.

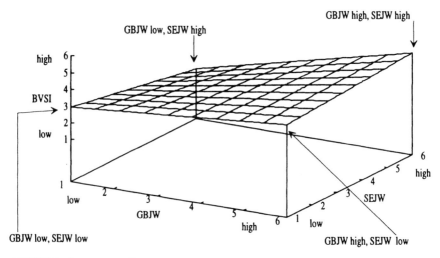

FIGURE 1. Interaction effects of General Belief in a Just World (GBJW) and Self-Efficacy to Promote Justice in the World (SEJW) on Blaming the Victims for Self-Infliction (BVSI).

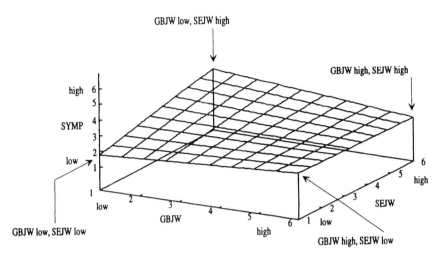

FIGURE 2. Interactions effects of General Belief in a Just World (GBJW) and Self-Efficacy to Promote Justice in the World (SEJW) on Sympathy for the Unemployed (SYMP).

Both effects are consistent with the hypotheses. As can be seen from Figures 1 and 2, a strong BJW motivates (a) blaming the victims (BVSI) and (b) interferes with sympathy (SYMP) for the unemployed but it does so only when SEJW is low. These effects decrease with decreasing BJW and increasing SEJW. The lowest score on BVSI and the highest scores for SYMP with the unemployed result when SEJW is high and BJW is low.

Similar interaction effects were found (see Figures 3 and 4) for the two variables assessing subjects' willingness to support the unemployed financially (WFI) or politically (WPO). Most willingness to support exists for subjects scoring high on GBJW and scoring low on SEJW.

In summary, we can say that GBJW is associated with low sympathy for the victims, with blaming them for self-infliction, and with low willingness to support them, especially with subjects who score low on SEJW. High SEJW buffers these effects of GBJW significantly.

3.4. Estimation of Unique Effects of GBJW, SEJW, and HJW

In order to test and estimate the unique contributions of the predictor terms GBJW, SEJW, and HJW, the three predictor terms were entered simultaneously in multiple regression analyses for each dependent variable (BVSI, SYMP) and the two willingness to support variables (WFI, WPO). All significant effects are summarized as a path model in Figure 5.

The standardized path coefficients show that BVSI could be predicted significantly by the GBJW scale: The stronger the BJW, the higher BVSI will be.

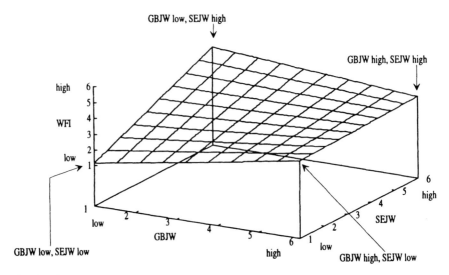

FIGURE 3. Interaction effects of General Belief in a Just World (BGJW) and Self-Efficacy to Promote Justice in the World (SEJW) on Willingness to Fight Unemployment by Means of Financial Help (WFI).

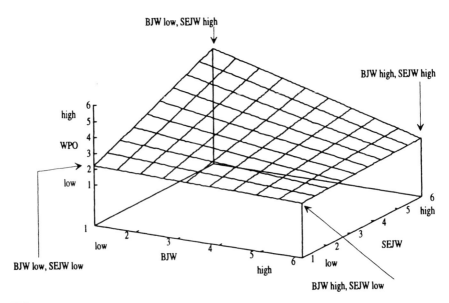

FIGURE 4. Interaction effects of General Belief in a Just World (BGJW) and Self-Efficacy to Promote Justice in the World (SEJW) on Willingness to Fight Unemployment on a Political Level (WPO).

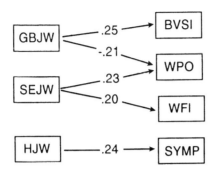

FIGURE 5.   Main effects of justice variables on the criteria BVSI, WPO, WFI, SYMP.

GBJW and HJW do not help to predict the willingness for financial support (WFI). This willingness to support variable depends exclusively on SEJW. (The second willingness to support variable (WPO) depends on increasing SEJW and decreasing GBJW: The higher the willingness to fight against unemployment politically (WPO), the higher SEJW and the lower GBJW).

Sympathy for the unemployed (SYMP) is only predicted by HJW which does not have an independent effect on any other variable considered here.

3.5. Membership in a Social or Political Organization (MSPO)

Using logistic regression analysis it was examined whether MSPO could be predicted by the three predictors (Fig. 6).

As can be seen from Figure 6, the probability for membership rises with increasing SEJW, and falls with increasing HJW. GBJW does not

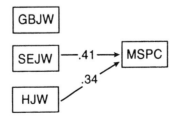

FIGURE 6.   Main effects of justice variables on the criterion MSPO.

contribute to the prediction of membership. With this model, more than 70% of all cases could be identified correctly.

4. DISCUSSION

The results suggest that the new constructs SEJW and HJW portray dispositions which we consider useful supplementations to Lerner's Belief in a Just World theory.

According to Lerner and Miller (1978), a strong BJW will motivate blaming or derogating victims when a restoration of justice is, in reality, impossible or costly.

Psychologically, what is impossible or costly depends on persons' views of the world, their own perceived abilities, and their resources. Therefore, when people consider themselves unable to restore justice, it is more likely that they consider a restoration of justice impossible or costly. High scores on SEJW imply that respondents feel able to reduce injustices. Moreover, high scores on SEJW imply a motivation to care for justice.

Therefore, we have hypothesized that GBJW and SEJW will interact in a person's tendency to derogate or to blame innocent victims in order to maintain their belief in a just world. The blaming of victims was expected to decrease significantly with increasing SEJW, and this should happen across all levels of BJW. The results we obtained corroborate this hypothesis. An analogue hypothesis can be formulated for sympathy with the victims (SYMP). Our results corroborate this hypothesis, too: sympathy for the unemployed is the least with subjects who score high on GBJW and low on SEJW. Analogue hypotheses were tested for the respondents' willingness (WFI, WPO) to support victims. The willingness is the least when GBJW is high and SEJW is low.

The interaction effects of GBJW and SEJW are especially enlightening for the relationship between the two constructs: The effects of GBJW on sympathy for the victims, on willingness to help them, and on the tendency to blame them for self-infliction are significantly moderated by SEJW, which acts as a buffer of the "antisocial" effects of GBJW. With these consistent results, we are able to postulate a hypothesis for the explanation of the inconsistent results we found for BJW effects on derogating and blaming victims: In studies where SEJW was not controlled for, it is possible that a larger proportion of respondents had high levels of SEJW that buffered the expected effects of BJW.

These results allow an explication of the psychological meaning of SEJW. The construct SEJW entails two components: self-efficacy and concern for justice. The combination of both components represents the conviction that one is able to make the world a more just one. Incidences of injustice mean another challenge for respondents who score high on SEJW than for subjects who score high on BJW. More respondents who score high on SEJW should think about taking efforts to restore justice in reality than respondents who score high on BJW. For the latter it does not matter whether justice is restored either in reality or cognitively by reappraising the case. For the respondent with high scores on SEJW, cognitive reappraisal is not a satisfactory way to deal with injustices given their self-concept of abilities and resourcefulness.

This is clearly demonstrated in the present study by looking at the main effects in multiple regression analyses (Fig. 5 and Fig. 6). SEJW is the only positive predictor of willingness to support victims (WFI, WPO), whereas GBJW is the sole predictor of BVSI, and HJW is the sole predictor of SYMP. (The bivariate correlational patterns are less informative because of the existing correlations between the justice variables, e.g., between SEJW and HJW and between GBJW and SEJW, which are masking the "pure" relationships.)

The expected effect of SEJW and HJW on the membership in a social organization serve as first evidence of the new scales' validity, respectively, the new constructs' psychological meaning. People who perceive themselves as efficient in creating (more) justice in the world are involved in a social organization in order to help the victims. People who cultivate their hope in a just world do not have to make an effort in restoring justice.

Based on these results, it seems worthwhile to consider these differential effects in future research. Longitudinal studies are necessary in order to examine the course of these effects as well as their stability. On the basis of peer ratings and similar objective data (e.g., the assessment of actual donation behavior rather than the assessment of the willingness to donate to a cause) the proposed scales can be validated. In experimental studies—for example, in game situations—the observation was made if the loser was valued positively in dependency from SEJW or HJW. More criteria group comparisons could certainly be used for the validation of these new scales. Nevertheless, at the time being, SEJW seems to be a variable that measures a construct which interacts with BJW in a very meaningful way. It is to consider in the face of inconsistent results as well as in the effort to clarify the psychological meaning of every scale designed to assess the "latent" variable BJW.

REFERENCES

Dalbert, C., Montada, L. & Schmitt, M. (1987). Glaube an eine gerechte Welt als Motiv: Validierungskorrelate zweier Skalen. Psychologische Beiträge, 29, 596–615.

Gruman, J.C. & Sloan, R.P. (1983).. Disease as justice: perceptions of victims of physical illness. Basic and Applied Social Psychology, 4, 39–46.

Kerr, K.L. & Kurtz, S.T. (1977). Effects of a victim's suffering and respectability on mock juror judgements: Further evidence on the just world theory. Representative Research in Social Psychology, 8, 42–56.

Lerner, M.J. (1970). The desire for justice and reactions to victims. In J. Macaulay & L. Berkowitz (Eds.), Altruism and helping behavior (pp. 205–228). New York: Academic Press.

Lerner, M.J. (1980). The Belief in a Just World: A fundamental delusion. New York: Plenum Press.

Lerner, M.J. & Miller, D.T. (1978). Just world research and the attribution process: Looking back and ahead. Psychological Bulletin, 85, 1030–1050.

Montada, L. & Mohiyeddini, C. (1995). Arbeitslosigkeit und Gerechtigkeit. (Berichte aus der Arbeitsgruppe "Verantwortung, Gerechtigkeit, Moral" Nr. 87). Trier: Universität Trier, FbI–Psychologie.

Chapter 4

How Do Observers of Victimization Preserve Their Belief in a Just World Cognitively or Actionally?

FINDINGS FROM A LONGITUDINAL STUDY

BARBARA REICHLE, ANGELA SCHNEIDER, and
LEO MONTADA

1. RESEARCH QUESTIONS

Individuals have a need to believe that they live in a world where people generally get what they deserve. The belief that the world is just enables the individual to confront his physical and social environment as though they were stable and orderly. Without such a belief it would be difficult for the individual to commit himself to the pursuit of long-range goals or even to the socially regulated behavior of day-to-day life. Since the belief that the world is just serves such an important adaptive function for the individual, people are very reluctant to give up this belief, and they can be greatly troubled if they encounter evidence that suggest that the world is not really just or orderly after all" (Lerner & Miller, 1978, pp. 1030–1031).

It is assumed that the justice motive leads the person who observes an injustice to attempt to restore justice. The restoration of justice can be accomplished in different ways: One can compensate the victim or one can

BARBARA REICHLE, ANGELA SCHNEIDER, and LEO MONTADA • Department of Psychology, Universität Trier, D-54286 Trier, Germany.

Responses to Victimizations and Belief in a Just World, edited by Montada and Lerner. Plenum Press, New York, 1998.

persuade oneself that the victim deserves to suffer because of a bad character or because of engaging in bad acts (e.g. Lerner, 1970, 1975, 1980; Lerner & Miller, 1978). Although not stated explicitly, Lerner seems to assume that the Belief in a Just World is universal (see also Furnham in this volume). Universality is not incompatible with the existence of interindividual differences in strength nor is it incompatible with intraindividual variation depending upon characteristics of the victim and characteristics of the situation. Rubin and Peplau (1973) were the first researchers to publish a self-report measure that assumed to assess Belief in a Just World as a trait-like, generalized, and stable interindividually varying world view (for a summary, see Furnham & Procter, 1989).

Conceptualizing Belief in a Just World as a motivational disposition to view the world, with interindividual as well as intraindividual variation, allows the specification of the basic hypothesis: The stronger a person's Belief in a Just World, the more threatening observed or experienced injustices will be, and consequently, the stronger a person's motivation to defend his or her Belief in a Just World either by attempts to restore justice or by attempts to deny injustice by appropriate (re)appraisals of the case.

We tested this hypothesis in a study where relatively well suited subjects (well suited in terms of living conditions, social security, education) were confronted with problems and needs of less fortunate persons: the poor living in developing countries, Turkish guest workers in Germany, and the unemployed. The problems and needs of these people were vividly described in scenarios that left to varying views about deservedness and (in)justices open, therefore allowing interindividually varying responses.

In this study, we assessed not only the interindividual variation of Belief in a Just World but the domain specificity of Belief in a Just World as well. When asked about justice in the world, subjects may think of more or less specific sections of the world. Some may think of their own worlds (their family, their neighborhood, their country) or of one of these. Others may think of broader sections of the world. We do not know what subjects are focusing on when they are asked unless we specify the section of the world in question which we chose to do in this study. A scale to measure the general, unspecified Belief in a Just World (GBJW) was used and, in addition, three specific scales (SPBJW) for assessing the respondents' views about the (1) justice of developing countries in the so-called Third World, (2) justice concerns of the unemployed in Germany, and (3) justice concerns of Turkish migrant workers in Germany.

The longitudinal study was designed with two waves of assessment to obtain information about the stability and change of BJW as well as information about predictors of stability and change. Thus, we were able to assess the stability of BJW as well as to identify predictors of change. Our hypothesis was that both strategies of defending BJW—restoration of justice (e.g., by means of prosocial commitments for less fortunate persons or groups) or denial of injustice (e.g., by blaming the less fortunate for self-infliction or by denying their state of need)—should result in the maintenance, i.e., the stability of BJW. While other results from this study were published (Montada, Reichle & Schneider, 1988; Montada & Schneider, 1989, 1991) the data analyses for this hypothesis were done for the present chapter and are published for the first time.

2. REACTIONS TO THE DISADVANTAGED: COMPENSATION VERSUS COGNITIVE RESTORATION TO MAINTAIN THE BELIEF IN A JUST WORLD

These theoretical conjectures lead to the following hypotheses: (1) If the awareness of the unjust suffering of another person threatens one's BJW, the strength of that threat should be a function of the strength of the belief—the stronger the belief, the more threat is experienced. The more threat a person feels, the stronger she or he should react—the extent of the reaction should be a function of the extent of the BJW. Consequently, the stronger the BJW, the more efforts to compensate victims should be expected. We therefore expect respondents with a strong BJW to express more (a) responsibility to help the needy, and (b) more readiness to prosocial actions in favor of the needy than respondents who rate their own BJW as rather low.

As was outlined above, another means to restore one's threatened BJW is to persuade oneself that the victim deserves to suffer because of the victim's own faulty actions, or omissions, or a bad character. Alternatively, the observer could downplay the suffering of the other, i.e., minimize or even derogate the bad situation of the victim. Justifying the observer's own privileged situation could function as another strategy. Again, the extent of all these reactions should be a function of the extent of the individual's Belief in a Just World. Hypothesis (2) states that the stronger an observer's BJW, the more he or she will blame the victim, downplay the severity of the injustice, and justify his or her own privileged situation.

All these reactions—compensation, blaming the victim, downplaying, and justification—are thought to be instigated by a threat to an observer's BJW, and that finally, preserve his or her BJW. This is to say that (3) over time, compensating actions, victim blaming cognitions, and derogatory thoughts should have positive effects on a person's Belief in a Just World.

3. THE STUDY

In two consecutive projects, reactions to the suffering of others were studied correlationally (Montada, Schmitt, & Dalbert, 1986) and longitudinally by the authors (Schneider, Reichle, & Montada, 1986; Montada & Schneider, 1990; Montada, Dalbert, & Schneider, 1990). The suffering others were poor people living in the Third World, Turkish migrants in Germany, and unemployed persons in Germany.

This longitudinal study on reactions to the disadvantaged was conducted in 1985 and 1986. Questionnaires were administered twice with a time difference of five months between the two waves (Schneider, Reichle, & Montada, 1986).

3.1. Subjects

The original sample consists of n = 865 West Germans who responded in the first wave, with n=434 of these who responded in both waves. The mean age was 36 years, with a minimum of 18 and a maximum of 86 years. Fifty-nine percent of the sample was male. The first half of the sample was recruited randomly from the adult population of a relatively privileged neighborhood of a middle sized West German city. The second half of the sample consisted of university students of various disciplines (38%) and two criterion groups with maximal job security, respectively, without job security.

3.2. Instruments

The material for the entire study consisted of a set of 14 questionnaires covering a broad palette of variables. These were administered twice, with a time interval of five months between the two waves. Each wave consisted of four packs of questionnaires that were sent to the subjects consecutively (Schneider, Reichle, & Montada, 1986).

For the present chapter new analyses were done using the following selected variables: General BJW, Specific BJWs assessed with the Just World Inventory, three cognitive appraisals of the disadvantages of others (blaming victims for self-infliction, minimization of their disadvantages and hardships, justification of own advantages) were assessed with the Existential Guilt Inventory, and willingness to various prosocial activities in favor of the disadvantaged with the Prosocial Actions-Inventory (cf. Schneider, Reichle, & Montada, 1986). Most of these variables were newly developed and have adequate scale qualities. The General BJW was taken from a previous study (Dalbert, Montada, & Schmitt, 1987). Moreover, a scale to assess the tendency to social desirability was used (Lück & Timaeus, 1969).

3.3. Just World Scales

This inventory consists of two parts: the first part is a six-item scale aimed at measuring a *General Belief in a Just World* (GBJW) constructed by Dalbert, Montada, & Schmitt (1987; cf. also Montada in this volume). The second part is a nine-item scale constructed to measure *Specific Beliefs in a Just World* (SPBJW) in three domains with three items each:, the domain of poor people in Third World countries, the domain of Turkish migrant workers in West Germany, and the domain of unemployed persons in West Germany. This domain-specific scale is an extension and modification by the present authors (Schneider, Reichle, & Montada, 1986) of a scale constructed by Dalbert et al. (1987). Both parts, the general as well as the specific, have been successfully tested for validity and reliability (Dalbert et al., 1987; Dalbert & Schneider, 1995; Schneider, Montada, Reichle, & Meissner, 1986; Schneider, 1988).

3.4. Existential Guilt Inventory

This questionnaire samples cognitive, emotional, and actional reactions to the problems of disadvantaged persons. The original version was constructed by Montada et al. (1986). The version used in the study described here was modified by the present authors (Reichle, Montada, & Schneider, 1985). It consists of a total of nine scenarios describing disadvantages of Turkish migrant workers in Germany (three scenarios), of unemployed Germans (three scenarios), and of poor people in the Third World (three scenarios). The disadvantages that are described include financial problems, insecurity concerning the future, poor working conditions, underpayment, insufficient medical care, poor housing, loss of status.

Only three of the cognitive appraisals that are rated on six-point scales were used for the present analyses: *Perception of the Disadvantage as Self-Inflicted* (e.g., "Many unemployed have caused their fate themselves"), *Minimization of the Disadvantage* (e.g., "One cannot generalize—many unemployed manage their situation pretty well"), *Justification of Own Advantages* (e.g., "It is not just because of luck that I am better off, I really deserve what I have").

3.5. Willingness to Act Prosocially Inventory

This questionnaire asked respondents to rate their own willingness to act prosocially for Turkish migrant workers in Germany, unemployed persons in Germany, poor people in Third World countries, handicapped persons, and environmental concerns. For each target group, two different actions had to be rated that could be reached by spending money, another two to be reached by the signing of a petition, another two to be reached by participating in a march or demonstration, and another two to be reached by joining a group of activists (Schneider, Reichle, & Montada, 1986). As in the other instruments described, the ratings were on six-point scales.

4. RESULTS

The first hypothesis refers to compensation as a means to defend one's BJW. Table 1 depicts the correlations between BJW measures (GBJW, SPBJW) and the two action variables *Responsibility to Help the Needy* and *Willingness to Act Prosocially.*

As can be seen from Table 1, there is no correlation between a GBJW and the aggregated two actional variables Responsibility to Help the Needy and Willingness to Prosocial Action (the aggregated score here is the mean score in Responsibility to Help and Willingness to prosocial action favor of each group of victims). There are, however, substantial and significant correlations between the SPBJW measures in all three domains—Migrants, the Poor in Third World countries, and Unemployed persons in Germany—and the domain specific action variables. All these correlations are negative. This is to say that respondents scoring higher on SPBJW indicate a lower Willingness to act prosocially in favor of the needy and a lower Responsibility to Help the Needy. It should be mentioned, however, that this negative correlation is cancelled or even reversed into a positive one, when the tendency to blame victims for self infliction and the preference for the equity principle—both variables are correlated with SPBJW—are partialled out in multiple regression analyses (cf. Montada in this volume).

TABLE 1. Correlations between Belief in a Just World (BJW) and Compensating Actions (Willingness to Act Prosocially) (822 ≤ n ≤ 823)

	GBJW	SPBJW Migrants	3rd World	Unemployed
Responsibility to Help the Needy				
Aggregated	−.07			
Migrants		−.34**		
3rd World			−.36**	
Unemployed				−.20**
Willingness to Act Prosocially				
Aggregated	−.04			
Migrants		−.20**		
Unemployed			−.25**	
3rd World				−.18**

**$p < .01$.

Hypothesis 2 states that respondents could restore their BJW by denying injustices, either by blaming the victim for self-infliction of their needs, or by downplaying these needs, or by justifying the own advantages. We consequently expected significant correlations between BJW measures and these variables. Table 2 depicts the respective correlations.

As can be seen, strategies of cognitive restoration of justice are substantially correlated with a GBJW as well as with a SPBJW, with the latter correlations being consistently higher. Here, the signs of the correlations are all in accord with the hypotheses.

Hypothesis 3 is the crucial one we wanted to test: The impact of actional efforts versus cognitive reappraisals on BJW over time. This hypothesis was tested in a longitudinal study with two assessments (t_1 and, five months later, t_2). By multiple regression analysis, we tested the effects of strategies of cognitive restoration and of strategies of actional restoration at t_1 on BJW at t_2, including the autoregressors (BJW scores t_1), and a control for Social Desirability. Since the three strategies of cognitive restoration are highly intercorrelated (with coefficients ranging from $r = .65$ to $r = .86$), an aggregate variable "Cognitive Strategies" was computed by aggregating the three cognitive strategies of minimization, blaming the victims for self-infliction, and justification. Strategies of actional restoration were operationalized as before, i.e., a respondent's mean Willingness to Act Prosocially in reaction to each group of victims. As the previous results clearly point toward a domain specificity of BJW, this analysis was con-

TABLE 2. Correlations between BJW and Strategies
of Cognitive Restoration (823 < n < 822)

| | GBJW | SPBJW | | |
		Migrants	3rd World	Unemployed
Self-Infliction				
Aggregated	.39**			
Migrants		.56**		
3rd World			.57**	
Unemployed				.53**
Minimization				
Aggregated	.44**			
Migrants		.58**		
3rd World			.58**	
Unemployed				.62**
Justification				
Aggregated	.42**			
Migrants		.57**		
3rd World			.58**	
Unemployed				.52**

**p < .01.

ducted repeatedly with the specific constructs for each group of disadvantaged. The results are shown in Table 3.

As can be seen from Table 3, the use of cognitive restoration strategies at t_1 has significant and substantial effects on SPBJW at t_2 in each of the three domains, over and above the autoregressors. In the domain of unemployment, there is also a small effect of Social Desirability. That means, the use of cognitive reappraisals which deny the existence of injustice in fact strengthens SPBJW which was measured a couple of months later. The strong effects of the autoregressors reflect the stability of BJW measures over time. In all three domains, there were no significant effects of the actional variable of *Willingness to Act Prosocially*. This is not to say that compensating actions were never effective. Rather, these strategies were not employed by subjects scoring high on BJW.

From what was stated before, we conclude that the stability and change of SPBJW in all three domains (unemployment, Turkish migrant workers in Germany, the poor in Third World countries) depend on how subjects cope with observations or information that increase their doubts about the justness of the world.

Finally, differences in correlations by level of specificity have to be noted. Correlations increase with level of specificity measured and are maximal if constructs on the same level of specificity are correlated. Aggregation across the same level of specificity leads to even higher intercorrelations. This phenomenon is well known from research conducted during the consistency debate in personality (cf. Schmitt & Borkenau, 1992, for an explication and discussion).

5. DISCUSSION

The data analyses selected for this chapter fit Lerner's BJW theory of blaming the victim phenomena nicely. We will discuss three results.

TABLE 3. Prediction of SPBJW at t_2 as a Function of the Actional Variable *Willingness to Act Prosocially* and the Aggregated Cognitive Strategies Variable at t_1 Controlling for Social Desirability and the Autoregressor SPBJW at t_1 (413 < n < 414)

Dependent	Predictors	beta	t	sig t	R2
t_2 SPBJW-Migrants	t_1 SPBJW-Migrants	.58	15.90	.00	
	t_1 Cognitive Strategies	.31	8.42	.00	.65
t_2 SPBJW-3rd World	t_1 SPBJW-3rd World	.61	15.45	.00	
	t_1 Cognitive Strategies	.24	6.03	.00	.61
t_2 SPBJW-Unemployed	t_1 SPBJW-Unemployed	.48	11.36	.00	
	t_1 Cognitive Strategies	.32	7.71	.00	
	t_1 Social Desirability	.07	2.08	.04	.57

1. The correlations between BJW measures and various cognitive (re-)appraisals of significant social inequalities (between the respondents and the three categories of less fortunate people) corroborate the theoretical expectations. When confronted with needy people suffering hardships, BJW motivates respondents to deny the injustices. Three kinds of (re-)appraisals were used in this study: (a) blaming the needy for self-infliction, (b) cognitive minimization of the existing needs, (c) justification of own advantages. The pattern of correlations is consistent with the hypothesis that cognitive denial of injustices is used as a strategy to defend BJW.

2. The actional restoration of justice might be considered as the primary strategy to defend BJW. We assessed respondents' felt responsibility to act in favor of the disadvantaged, and their readiness to help restore justice by own sharing or caring as well as by claiming support from powerful others (e.g., governments). These variables were not related to GBJW and were negatively related to SPBJW. How does this result fit with Lerner's theory? Prosocial activities are expected only in cases when efficient help seems possible and not too costly. The categories of needs and disadvantaged persons addressed in this study are very large. Efficient help would be impossible for many if not most respondents, with maybe the exception of a participation in political activities to claim support for the disadvantaged. In such events, challenges to one's BJW cannot be overcome by engaging in prosocial actions. Therefore, the negative correlation is consistent with the theory.

3. The theory claims that challenges to BJW are responded to by efforts either to restore justice in reality or to deny injustice by adequate (re-)appraisals of the challenging events. The correlations between BJW and cognitive (re-)appraisals measured at one point in time are not a definitive proof of the BJW protecting function of appraisals which deny injustices. Such denial may well be motivated to defend BJW, but at one and the same point in time it cannot be shown that such a defense is successful.

To answer this question a follow-up study is required and was carried out in the present context. The follow up of SPBJW clearly demonstrates that the use of injustice denying appraisals has positive effects on the level of SPBJW measured later in time. These positive effects may either be in stabilizing the initial level of BJW, or in preventing a drop in BJW, or in raising BJW even above the initial level. These positive effects are not spurious ones but rather substantial ones, and they are consistent over three categories of disadvantaged. Insofar, the results are a valid support of Lerner's theory.

ACKNOWLEDGMENTS

This research was supported by a grant from the Deutsche For-
schungsgemeinschaft (German Research Foundation).

REFERENCES

Dalbert, C., Montada, L., & Schmitt, M. (1987). Glaube an eine gerechte Welt als Motiv:
    Validierungskorrelate zweier Skalen. Psychologische Beiträge, 4, 596–615.
Dalbert, C., & Schneider, A. (1995). Die Allgemeine Gerechte-Welt-Skala: Dimensionalität,
    Stabilität und Fremdurteiler-Validität (Berichte aus der Arbeitsgruppe "Verantwor-
    tung, Gerechtigkeit, Moral" Nr. 86). Trier: Universität Trier, Fachbereich I - Psychologie.
Furnham, A., & Procter, E. (1989). Belief in a just world: Review and critique of the individual
    difference literature. British Journal of Social Psychology, 28, 365–384.
Lerner, M.J. (1970). The justice motive: Some hypotheses as to its origins and forms. Journal
    of Personality, 45, 1–52.
Lerner, M.J. (1975). The justice motive in social behavior. Journal of Social Issues, 31, 1–19.
Lerner, M.J. (1980). The belief in a just world: A fundamental delusion. New York:
    Plenum.
Lerner, M.J., & Miller, D.T. (1978). Just world research and the attribution process: Looking
    back and ahead. Psychological Bulletin, 85, 1030–1151.
Lück, H.E., & Timaeus, E. (1969). Skalen zur Messung Manifester Angst (MAS) und sozialer
    Wünschbarkeit (SES-E und SDS-CM). Diagnostica, 15, 134–141.
Montada, L., Dalbert, C., & Schneider, A. (1990). Coping mit Problemen sozial Schwacher:
    Annotierte Ergebnistabellen (Berichte aus der Arbeitsgruppe "Verantwortung, Gere-
    chtigkeit, Moral" Nr. 53). Trier: Universität Trier. Fachbereich I - Psychologie.
Montada, L., Schmitt, M., & Dalbert, C. (1986). Thinking about justice and dealing with one's
    own privileges: A study of existential guilt. In H.W. Bierhoff, R. Cohen, & J. Greenberg
    (Eds.), Justice in social relations (pp. 125–142). New York: Plenum.
Montada, L., & Schneider, A. (1990). Justice and emotional reactions to the disadvantaged.
    Social Justice Research, 3, 313–344.
Reichle, B., Montada, L., & Schneider, A. (1985). Existentielle Schuld: Differenzierung eines
    Konstruktes. (Berichte aus der Arbeitsgruppe "Verantwortung, Gerechtigkeit, Moral"
    Nr. 35). Trier: Universität Trier, Fachbereich I - Psychologie.
Rubin, Z., & Peplau, L.A. (1973). Belief in a just world and reactions to another's lot: A study
    of participants in the National Draft Lottery. Journal of Social Issues, 29, 73–93.
Schmitt, M., & Borkenau, P. (1992). The consistency of personality. In G.-V. Caprara & G.L.
    Van Heck (Eds.), Modern personality psychology. Critical reviews and new directions
    (pp. 29–55). New York: Harvester-Wheatsheaf.
Schneider, A. (1988). Glaube an die gerechte Welt: Replikation der Validierungskorrelate
    zweier Skalen (Berichte aus der Arbeitsgruppe "Verantwortung, Gerechtigkeit,
    Moral" Nr. 44). Trier: Universität Trier, Fachbereich I - Psychologie.
Schneider, A., Montada, L., Reichle, B., & Meissner, A. (1986). Auseinandersetzung mit
    Privilegunterschieden und existentieller Schuld: Item- und Skalenanalysen I (Berichte
    aus der Arbeitsgruppe "Verantwortung, Gerechtigkeit, Moral" Nr. 37) Trier: Univer-
    sität Trier, Fachbereich I - Psychologie.
Schneider, A., Reichle, B., & Montada, L. (1986). Existentielle Schuld: Stichprobenrekru-
    tierung, Erhebungsinstrumente und Untersuchungsplan (Berichte aus der Ar-
    beitsgruppe "Verantwortung, Gerechtigkeit, Moral" Nr. 36). Trier: Universität Trier,
    Fachbereich I - Psychologie.

Chapter 5

Individual Differences in the Belief in a Just World and Responses to Personal Misfortune

CAROLYN L. HAFER and JAMES M. OLSON

According to just world theory (Lerner, 1977, 1980; Lerner, Miller, & Holmes, 1976), people have a basic need to believe that the world is a just place—a place where individuals get what they deserve and deserve what they get. The belief in a just world provides an explanation for people's responses to the suffering of others, especially their tendency to blame innocent victims for their fate (see Lerner & Miller, 1978, for a review). Rubin and Peplau (1975) proposed that individuals differ in the extent to which they actually believe the world is a just place. Studies investigating the relationship between individual differences in just world beliefs and attitudes toward suffering generally show that strong believers in a just world have a greater tendency to blame victims for their misfortune and a greater acceptance of general social inequalities than do weak believers (e.g., Clyman, Roth, Sniderman, & Charrier, 1980; Dalbert, Fisch, & Montada, 1992; Furnham, 1985; Furnham & Gunter, 1984; Glennon & Joseph, 1993; Smith, 1985; Wagstaff, 1983; Zuckerman, Gerbasi, Kravitz, & Wheeler, 1975; see Furnham & Procter, 1989, for a review).

CAROLYN L. HAFER • Department of Psychology, Brock University, St. Catharines, Ontario, Canada L2S 3A1. JAMES M. OLSON • Department of Psychology, University of Western Ontario, London, Ontario, Canada N6A 5C2.

Responses to Victimizations and Belief in a Just World, edited by Montada and Lerner. Plenum Press, New York, 1998.

A relatively new area of just world research examines the role of individual differences in just world beliefs and responses to one's *own* negative outcomes, rather than the negative outcomes of others. The present chapter will discuss this recent development with reference to our own research on the belief in a just world. We will first describe a theoretical rationale for expecting specific associations between individual differences in beliefs in a just world and responses to personal misfortune. This will be followed by a statement of the four research questions that have guided our work in this area. Next, we will discuss three studies we have conducted that address one or more of these questions. Finally, we give a summary of the findings across the three studies and suggest some avenues for future work in this area.

1. BELIEFS IN A JUST WORLD AND RESPONSES TO MISFORTUNE

We expected that individual differences in beliefs in a just world would influence responses to personal misfortune through similar mechanisms to those presumably underlying the relation between just world beliefs and responses to other's misfortune. Thus, we will first outline our perspective on the mechanisms accounting for reactions to the suffering of others, and then show how these processes can be extended to responses to one's own negative outcomes.

According to just world theory, undeserved suffering in others threatens the belief in a just world by providing evidence to the contrary. This threat leads to discomfort, similar to Festinger's (1957) dissonance, that the individual is motivated to reduce (Lerner, 1970, 1977). Given that there is a basic need to maintain the belief in a just world (without it, we would have little trust in our own futures), individuals may be more likely to reduce the discomfort by altering the situation so it becomes "fair," rather than by changing their beliefs in the fairness of the world. According to Lerner (1980), fairness can be created out of others' suffering through "rational" strategies such as compensating victims or through "defensive" or psychological strategies such as blaming victims for their fate. These latter strategies may be preferred because they are often less costly (Walster, Berscheid, & Walster, 1976).

Individuals with a particularly strong belief in a just world should experience more discomfort in the face of contradictory evidence than individuals with weak just world beliefs, because of the greater discrepancy between their beliefs and the witnessed suffering. Thus, these individuals may be more motivated to reduce the discrepancy, often through some psychological strategy, than weak believers. This process would result in strong believers in a just world perceiving others' negative outcomes as more fair than weak believers. This logic is consistent with the previously mentioned findings that strong believers in a just world have a greater tendency than weak believers to blame victims for their misfortune and to accept social inequalities.

Lerner (1980), Hafer and Olson (1989, 1993) and others have proposed that individual differences in the belief in a just world are related to how people respond to their *own* misfortune as well as the misfortune of others. Personal misfortune that is undeserved should pose a threat to the belief in a just world, just as an innocently suffering other poses a threat to this belief. As with the suffering of others, the motivation to reduce the discrepancy between current events and the belief in a just world should be greater for those who believe very strongly that the world is a fair place. This more intense motivation along with a preference for reducing these discrepancies through psychological means should lead to a tendency for strong believers in a just world to perceive their own negative outcomes as more fair than weak believers. Studies 1 and 3 presented in this chapter investigate how the perceived fairness of personal misfortune varies as a function of beliefs in a just world. To our knowledge, this is the only research that directly addresses this issue.

As well as investigating differences in perceived fairness, we have also been interested in other responses to personal misfortune as a function of beliefs in a just world. Relative deprivation theorists have proposed that a sense of unfairness or injustice is associated with emotions such as anger, outrage, and resentment (e.g., Crosby, 1976; Folger, 1984). This form of emotional response has been referred to as affective relative deprivation (e.g., Birt & Dion, 1987; Guimond & Dubé-Simard, 1983; Olson & Hafer, in press; Petta & Walker, 1992) or discontent (e.g., Hafer & Olson, 1993). If strong believers in a just world perceive their own misfortune as more fair than do weak believers, we might also expect them to experience less discontent (i.e., anger, resentment, outrage, etc.) than weak believers. All three studies presented in this chapter address this hypothesis. Again, we know of no other research directly addressing this question.

We are also interested in how beliefs in a just world might relate to emotional responses to personal misfortune other than discontent. For example, do individual differences in just world beliefs predict happy, anxious, or depressive emotions? There is mixed evidence about whether strong believers in a just world experience more positive emotion or less negative emotion in the face of personal adversity than do weak believers. Bulman and Wortman (1977) found that victims of spinal cord injuries who held a strong belief in a just world reported more happiness than those holding a weaker belief in a just world. Similarly, in a study of East-German women, Dalbert (1992) found significant relations between strong just world beliefs and positive mood, and between strong just world beliefs and life satisfaction. These relations remained after controlling for self-esteem. The relation between just world beliefs and positive mood remained after controlling for dispositional well-being. There was no association between just world beliefs and negative mood. Ritter, Benson, and Snyder (1990), in a survey of Northern Ireland residents, reported that strong beliefs in a just world were associated with *lower* scores on a measure of depressed mood. However, within the same sample, Benson and Ritter (1990) reported that strong beliefs in a just world intensified the effect of job loss on depression such that strong believers in a just world who had recently suffered job loss showed significantly higher levels of depression than strong believers who had not recently lost their jobs; weak believers in a just world did not differ in their levels of depression as a function of job loss.

It is not entirely clear, then, how individual differences in just world beliefs are linked to various emotional responses to personal misfortune, especially negative emotions. It is possible, for example, that these emotional responses will be determined in part by the specific strategy with which an individual reduces the discrepancy between the negative event and his/her belief in justice (e.g., blaming one's character, blaming one's behaviour, reinterpreting the meaning of the event, etc.). Study 3 of this chapter tests the relation between beliefs in a just world and various emotional responses to one's own negative outcomes; no a priori predictions were made for emotions other than discontent.

Finally, Studies 2 and 3 in this chapter investigate whether individual differences in beliefs in a just world predict behavioural responses to one's own negative outcomes. To our knowledge, no other researchers have examined this question. The social action literature has shown that perceived fairness and discontent predicts behavioural attempts to change negative outcomes or assertive actions (see Olson & Hafer, in press, for a review). Thus, because we expected strong believers in a just world to perceive less unfairness and to experience less discontent when confronted with negative outcomes than weak believers, we hypothesized that strong just world beliefs would be associated with fewer attempts at assertive action.

2. SUMMARY OF GUIDING RESEARCH QUESTIONS

The previous discussion of individual differences in the belief in a just world and responses to personal misfortune highlighted four research questions. These questions will provide the framework for reviewing the research presented in the rest of this chapter.

Research Question 1 is, do strong believers in a just world perceive their own negative outcomes as less unfair than weak believers? Based on the logic articulated above, we predicted that strong believers *would* see their outcomes as more fair. Our second research question is, do strong believers in a just world experience less discontent (i.e., emotions related to a sense of injustice, such as anger and resentment) than weak believers? Again, based on our previously stated logic, we predicted that strong believers in a just world *would* experience and report less discontent. Research Question 3 is, are beliefs in a just world predictive of other affective responses to personal misfortune? Finally, our fourth question is, are individual differences in the belief in a just world associated with particular behavioural reactions to one's own negative outcomes? We hypothesized that strong believers in a just world would be less likely to engage in behavioural attempts to change their negative outcomes than would weak believers. In the next three sections, we describe three studies examining one or more of these issues in very different contexts.

2.1. Study 1: Beliefs in a Just World and Responses to a Laboratory-Induced Deprivation

Hafer and Olson (1989) conducted two laboratory experiments designed to investigate the relation between individual differences in the belief in a just world and reactions to one's own negative outcomes. In each experiment, university students completed Rubin and Peplau's (1975) Just World Scale, and were then given false failure feedback on a computer task. This failure, and its resultant loss of reward, constituted the negative outcome.

In the first study, 83 male and 72 female undergraduates were shown two computer tasks, both of which they were told they would perform for points. These points were valuable because the greater number of points they gained, the less time they would have to remain in the experiment. (It was made apparent to participants that the experiment could involve performing several rather boring tasks for an indefinite amount of time, thus heightening their desire to leave.) Participants were told that, if they scored high enough on the first task they performed, they would earn some "bonus" points toward their score on the second task, thereby increasing their chances of leaving early.

We manipulated how much personal choice participants had in the task they performed for these bonus points. In one condition, participants chose for themselves which task they performed for the bonus points (the choice condition); in another condition, the experimenter randomly assigned them to a bonus points task (the assigned condition). After performing the bonus points task, all participants were told that they failed to earn the extra points and, therefore, probably would not gain enough points on the next task to leave the experiment early. The experimenter then manipulated the extent to which participants could easily imagine better alternative outcomes having occurred (i.e., Folger's [1986] concept of "referent outcomes"). As this variable was not expected to interact with beliefs in a just world (and did not), it will not be discussed further in this chapter.

After the manipulations were completed, participants anonymously filled out a questionnaire assessing their opinions and feelings about the experiment so far. There were four dependent measures. First, participants rated how *fair* they thought the experiment had been. This was done on a 7-point scale, where 1 was labelled "very unfair," and 7 was labelled "very fair." Participants also rated the extent to which they felt unjustly deprived, angry, and resentful. These ratings were completed on 7-point scales, where 1 was labelled "not at all," and 7 was labelled "very." These three emotions were highly intercorrelated and were summed to yield an overall measure of discontent. The questionnaire also included manipulation checks. After completing the questionnaire, participants were told that the experiment was in fact over, and they were thoroughly debriefed.

Consistent with our prediction for Research Question 1, we expected that strong believers in a just world would perceive their misfortune (i.e., their low probability of leaving early) as more fair than would weak believers. We predicted that this relation between beliefs in a just world and perceived fairness would be especially powerful in the choice condition, when participants chose the task that led to their negative outcomes. This is because the choice condition gave participants a salient cue for self-blame and, therefore, provided an easy way for strong believers in a just world to interpret negative outcomes as deserved (and therefore fair). When cues for self-blame were not made salient, namely in the assigned condition, we thought that strong believers in a just world would have more difficulty perceiving their misfortune as fair, although there would still be some tendency for strong believers to perceive less unfairness than weak believers.

A regression analysis was conducted with perceived fairness as the criterion, in which the main effects for individual differences in the belief in a just world (a continuous variable) and the two manipulations (dichotomous variables) were entered first, followed by the two-way interactions, then the three-way interaction. This analysis produced the hypothesized main effect for beliefs in a just world, $F(1, 130) = 8.53, p < .04$, such that strong believers in a just world perceived the experimental situation to be more fair than did weak believers, $r(132) = .25$. This main effect was subsumed by an interaction between the choice manipulation and beliefs in a just world, $F(1, 127) = 4.35$, $p < .04$. As predicted for this experiment, in the choice condition, beliefs in a just world and perceived fairness were positively correlated, $r(67) = .39$. In the assigned condition, however, there was no relation between beliefs in a just world and perceived fairness, $r(63) = .00$ (whereas we had expected simply a weaker correlation).

A similar regression analysis predicting discontent (the composite measure of unjust deprivation, resentment, and anger) revealed a marginal interaction between beliefs in a just world and the choice manipulation, $F(1, 128) = 3.39$, $p < .07$, which followed the same pattern as the interaction for the fairness measure. In the choice condition, strong believers in a just world reported less discontent than did weak believers, $r(68) = -.22$, whereas in the assigned condition, there was no relation between beliefs in a just world and discontent, $r(63) = .11$.

The pattern of results in the choice condition supports our expectations presented in the previous section of this chapter with regards to perceived fairness and discontent. In accordance with our predictions for both the first and second research questions, strong believers in a just world reported greater perceptions of fairness and weaker feelings of discontent than did weak believers. Strong believers may have used the fact that they had personally chosen the task leading to their misfortune as a way to rationalize that the deprivation was deserved, leading to less perceived unfairness and weaker emotions associated with a sense of injustice.

The major purpose of the second study in Hafer and Olson (1989) was to explore the reason for finding no correlation between beliefs in a just world and perceived fairness or discontent in the assigned condition (where we had expected a weaker, but still reliable, correlation between the variables). This study replicated the overall correlation between strong beliefs in a just world and perceived fairness from Study 1. Findings also suggested that the nonsignificant relation between variables in the assigned condition of the first study may have been due to the fact that random assignment seemed unbiased and thus prevented even weak believers in a just world from reporting perceived unfairness or discontent.

In summary, Hafer and Olson (1989) provided the first direct evidence that individual differences in the belief in a just world are predictive of responses to one's own deprivation. When faced with potentially unjust outcomes, strong believers in a just world perceived more fairness and experienced less discontent than did weak believers. Hafer and Olson (1989), therefore, primarily addressed Research Questions 1 and 2. The next section will describe a study addressing Research Questions 2 and 4; that is, the role of just world beliefs in discontent, as well as in behavioural responses to negative outcomes.

2.2. Study 2: Beliefs in a Just World and Women's Responses to Their Job Situation

Our success with the laboratory experiments prompted us to conduct a field study examining the relation between beliefs in a just world and responses to personal misfortune (Hafer & Olson, 1993).[1]

We surveyed 70 women working full-time outside the home in London, Ontario, Canada. These women represented a wide range of occupations, salary levels, ages, and education levels. Our sample conformed relatively well to the 1986 London census breakdown of occupations for women working full-time (see Hafer & Olson, 1993, Table 1).

In an initial survey, the women were given Rubin and Peplau's (1975) Just World Scale. Also, among other items, the survey included four questions assessing these women's discontent with their job situation. Specifically, the respondents were asked how satisfied they were with their present job situation, how satisfied they were with their present job situation compared to the job situations of other women in the workforce, how satisfied they were with their jobs compared to men in the workforce, and, finally, how resentful they were about their present job situation. We included satisfaction items with different referents (i.e., men vs. women) because Martin (1986) suggests that respondents will give different answers to questions regarding deprivation and discontent depending on whether or not a particular standard is provided and, if one is provided, the nature of the standard (see Olson, Roese, Meen, & Robertson, in press, for an empirical example of the effects of using different referents). These items were answered on 7-point scales, where 1 indicated low levels of satisfaction/resentment, and 7 indicated high levels of satisfaction/resentment.

Approximately one month later, a second survey was distributed. This survey consisted of a list of several behaviours that are possible reactions to job dissatisfaction. The items relevant to this chapter were 20 actions aimed at improving one's own job situation. Respondents placed a check mark beside any behaviour that they had performed over the past month.

Measures of emotional and behavioural responses were created from the two surveys. The four ratings of discontent were significantly intercorrelated and a composite measure of personal discontent was created for each respondent by summing her responses to the four items. The satis-

---

[1] We also examined beliefs in a just world, discontent, and behaviour within the context of these women's perceptions of their group as a whole (i.e., working women). This chapter is only concerned with responses to one's *personal* outcomes, not the outcomes of one's group; therefore, assessment of and analyses including the group level variables will not be covered here (see Hafer & Olson, 1993, for a complete account of these data).

faction questions were reverse-keyed before summing so that high values on the composite measure of discontent meant high levels of *dis*satisfaction and resentment.

Five measures of behavioural response or assertive action were created from the 20 behaviours relevant to one's own job situation. Originally, one overall measure of "self-directed" behaviour was created for each respondent by summing the number of checkmarks for the 20 actions. In light of the research presented in the next section of this chapter, we later created measures for five subtypes of self-directed behaviour. The 20 behaviours were first divided into three main categories—self-improvement behaviours, system-directed behaviours, and leaving the situation. Seven behaviours were categorized as self-improvement. These involved any attempt to better one's job situation through improving the quality or quantity of one's output (e.g., practising job skills away from work to improve performance, receiving formal extra training to improve job qualifications). Nine behaviours were classified as system-directed. These behaviours were directed toward the structure of the job situation rather than aimed at improving oneself in some way. System-directed behaviours were further broken down into change versus protest behaviours. Change behaviours (three in total) were those directly aimed at changing the job situation such as making a written suggestion to a supervisor about how one would like to see one's job improved. Protest behaviours (six in total) involved complaining about the structure of the job situation. Examples of protest behaviours included decreasing the quality of one's work to show dissatisfaction with the job, and refusing to comply with an unfair request. Finally, four behaviours involved attempting to leave the current job (e.g., looking for another job, obtaining information from a professional about how to get a better job); these were classified as leaving the situation. The 20 self-directed behaviours were assigned to the behavioural categories by two independent judges. The judges agreed on all of the behaviour assignments. The behaviour categories are similar to ones suggested by relative deprivation theorists interested in predictors of behavioural responses to felt injustice (e.g., Crosby, 1976; Mark & Folger, 1984; see Olson & Hafer, in press, for a review).

Assigning respondents scores for each of the five subtypes of behaviour based on the number of checkmarks they had placed within each category resulted in continuous measures with extremely skewed distributions (few participants checked off more than one behaviour within a given category). Therefore, we decided to make these behavioural measures dichotomous, such that participants who engaged in at least one of the behaviours in a given category were assigned a "1" for that category; participants indicating that they had engaged in none of the behaviours within a category were assigned a "0."

In summary, there was one composite measure of emotional response to potential misfortune (discontent) and six measures of behavioural response: five dichotomous measures of particular types of behaviour (self-improvement, system-directed, change, protest, and leaving the situation) and one continuous measure of overall assertive action.

Table 1 presents the endorsement frequencies for the dichotomous behaviour measures. Self-improvement was engaged in more frequently (78.6%) than system-directed behaviour (50%) and leaving the situation (54.3%), which were endorsed about equally often. Change and protest behaviours were reported for 40% and 30% of the women, respectively. All measures showed sufficient variability to be retained for statistical analyses (Rummel, 1970).

The first column of Table 2 presents the correlations between discontent and the various behavioural responses. The overall measure of behaviour was significantly related to discontent. It would seem that much of this relation can be accounted for by the association of discontent with attempts to leave one's job. The positive correlation between discontent and behaviour in general is consistent with the literature on predictors of social action. Emotions such as anger and resentment have been shown to predict behavioural and attitudinal responses to deprivation (Olson & Hafer, in press).

TABLE 1. Endorsement Frequencies and Percentages
for the Five Categories of Behavioural Response

Category	Frequency	Percent
Self-improvement	55	78.6
System-directed	35	50
Change	28	40
Protest	21	30
Leaving the situation	38	54.3

Note. N = 70.

TABLE 2. Correlations between Discontent and
Just World Beliefs and Behavioural Responses

	Discontent	Just world beliefs
Self-improvement	−.03	−.19
System-directed	.26*	−.36**
Change	.10	−.24*
Protest	.26*	−.36**
Leaving the situation	.45***	−.12
Total behaviour	.30**	−.32**

Note. Correlations involving discontent are based on $N = 69$. For all other correlations, $N = 70$.
*$p < .05$; **$p < .01$; ***$p < .001$

Individual differences in beliefs in a just world were not significantly correlated with discontent, $r(67) = -.01$, n.s. This finding was surprising, as we had expected strong beliefs in a just world to be related to weaker feelings of discontent, in accordance with our predictions for the second research question presented above.

The second column of Table 2 presents the correlations between beliefs in a just world and behavioural responses. Overall, stronger just world beliefs were associated with a tendency to engage in fewer assertive actions. It appears that it is mainly system-directed behaviours (both protest and change behaviours) that are related to just world beliefs here. Strong believers in a just world are less willing to attack the structure of their job situation itself, especially through protest, than are weak believers.[2]

One way to interpret these data is as follows. A negative job situation that is undeserved threatens the belief in a just world, especially for those who hold that belief fairly strongly. Strong believers would be especially motivated, then, to engage in strategies to protect this belief. One such strategy is to hold oneself partly responsible for the negative outcome. If one holds oneself responsible, there is little reason (or motivation) to alter the job situation itself (i.e., to engage in system-directed action). Thus, strong believers in a just world may be less likely to engage in system-directed behaviour than weak believers.

If it is the case that strong believers are, in fact, holding themselves more responsible for their negative job situation, we might expect that they would engage in more self-improvement than weak believers. Yet, if anything, beliefs in a just world in this study were associated with a tendency *not* to engage in self-improvement. However, self-blame can take many forms, some of which would not motivate self-improvement behaviours. For example, a negative job situation could be attributed to poor performance as the result of temporary external pressures (e.g., family troubles) or an inherent lack of ability. In these cases, feelings of personal responsibility would result in a tendency *not* to engage in self-improvement (because of a belief that everything will right itself soon, or because of a sense of helplessness [Weiner, 1985; Weiner, Russell, & Lerman, 1979]).

In summary, this study of working women again showed that individual differences in the belief in a just world play a role in responses to

---

[2] We conducted the same correlational analyses shown in Table 2, controlling for age, salary, and education. The relation between discontent and system-directed behaviour and the relation between beliefs in a just world and change became nonsignificant after controlling for these demographic variables, $r(55) = .12$ and $r(55) = -.17$, respectively; otherwise, all the significant correlations in Table 2 remained so, as did all the nonsignificant correlations. The correlation between beliefs in a just world and discontent did not change substantially when controlling for demographics.

personal outcomes. Although findings were not supportive of our hypothesis for Research Question 2 (the relation between beliefs in a just world and discontent), the study did find support for a relation between beliefs in a just world and behavioural responses (Research Question 4), such that strong beliefs in a just world were related to fewer behavioural responses.

The study described in the next section of this chapter was an attempt to address simultaneously Research Questions 1, 2, 3, and 4. Another goal of this study was to assess affective and behavioural reactions to misfortune in a more open-ended fashion than in the previously described research. We hoped that this would increase the ecological validity of our findings, as well as providing more varied measures of affect than in our previous work.

2.3. Study 3: Beliefs in a Just World and Student's Responses to Grades

In a recent study conducted with L. Jesik, we investigated beliefs in a just world and university students' responses to receiving a poor grade. In past research by Olson (see Olson, 1986), almost 100% of students, when asked, reported that they have received a grade with which they were dissatisfied. These poor grades were often seen as an unjust deprivation. Thus, unsatisfactory grades seemed a viable context within which to test the effects of beliefs in a just world.

Sixty-seven undergraduate psychology students (55 women and 12 men) completed the two sessions of the study. In both sessions, participants were tested in small groups.

In the first session, the students completed several individual difference questionnaires in randomized order, including the Just World Scale (Rubin & Peplau, 1975) and Paulhus's Spheres of Control subscales (Paulhus, 1983). We included the latter individual difference measure because the Just World Scale has been criticized for its tendency to correlate with an internal locus of control (e.g., Furnham & Karani, 1985; Hafer & Olson, 1989; Lerner, 1978; Zuckerman & Gerbasi, 1975). We hoped to show that any relations between beliefs in a just world and responses to personal misfortune would remain significant even after controlling for locus of control.

In the second session, approximately one month later, participants were asked to think about a grade they had received with which they were dissatisfied. They then provided a written response to the following questions: "How did you react when you found out about this mark?" and "Did you do anything about this situation? If so, what did you do?" Three students could not think of an unsatisfactory grade and were thus deleted from the sample.

Answers to the open-ended questions were coded for emotional and behavioural responses to the poor grade. The majority of the emotion words mentioned by participants were coded according to Shaver, Schwartz, Kirson, and O'Connor's (1987) hierarchical cluster analysis of 135 emotion words, which determined how people organize these emotions in terms of similarity. Through this procedure, Shaver et al. arrived at six "basic" emotions, which can be further divided into 25 subcategories of emotion. The six basic emotions are Love, Joy, Surprise, Anger, Sadness, and Fear. We created an additional response category that reflected our interest in assessing a sense of unfairness as well as in more prototypical emotional states. This category was labelled Unfairness and included responses such as feeling betrayed or cheated, and feeling that the grade was unfair or unjust (none of these words are mentioned in the Shaver et al. taxonomy). A few emotion words were neither mentioned by Shaver et al. nor were relevant to unfairness. If possible, these remaining words were coded according to Higgins's (1987) work on the emotional concomitants of self-discrepancies (Higgins's categorization is almost identical to Shaver et al.'s, though not as comprehensive); otherwise, they were classified into the seven categories (the six basic emotions plus unfairness) by two judges who independently agreed on 88% (7/8) of the assignments.

For each category of emotional response and for Unfairness, participants received a "1" if they used one or more words belonging to the category; otherwise, they were assigned a "0" for that category. Not surprisingly, there was little variability in the scores for Love and Joy (due to a preponderance of "0"s). Somewhat less expected was the lack of variability in surprise-related emotions (merely 10.9% of the participants reported feeling surprised, astonished, or disbelieving). Only Anger, Sadness, Fear, and Unfairness demonstrated sufficient variability to be retained for statistical analyses (see Rummel, 1970). Sadness was renamed Disappointment, and Fear was renamed Anxiety to more accurately reflect the specific emotions reported by our participants.

Three behavioural scores were also created for each participant. First, an overall behaviour score was created by assigning participants a "1" if they had engaged in *any* action directed toward changing the current outcome (i.e., the poor grade) or preventing similar negative outcomes in the future, and a "0" if they reported doing nothing. Second, behaviours were classified as either self-improvement (e.g., working longer hours, improving test-taking skills, etc.) or as system-directed (e.g., attempting to get the current mark changed, attempting to change the format of future tests or assignments). Only one individual reported leaving the situation as a response, and it was difficult to divide system-directed behaviours into protest or change; thus, the three other categories of behavioural response used in the study with working women were not retained here. The first author and another judge independently agreed on 89% of the behaviour classifications. Participants received a

"1" for a particular category of behaviour if they had engaged in at least one behaviour belonging to the category; otherwise, they received a "0."

In summary, coding of participants' open-ended responses led to three measures of emotional response (anger, disappointment, anxiety) plus unfairness and three measures of behavioural response (overall behaviour, self-improvement, and system-directed behaviour). All measures were dichotomous.

The frequency and percentage of participants who gave responses belonging to each of the response categories is presented in Table 3. The most frequently mentioned emotions were those related to anger, followed by disappointment. Unfairness and anxiety were endorsed about 27% and 20% of the time respectively. Self-improvement behaviours were endorsed more frequently (59.4%) than system-directed behaviours (20.3)%.

Table 4 shows the correlations among the response categories. A few of these results deserve comment. The positive correlation between anger and system-directed behaviour conforms to research demonstrating an association between emotions such as anger and resentment and social action (note also that unfairness is positively correlated with system-directed behaviour, although this finding is nonsignificant; see Olson & Hafer, in press, for a review). Analyses revealed negative correlations between unfairness and self-improvement and between anger and self-improvement, and a positive correlation between disappointment and self-improvement. Differential attributions may explain this overall pattern of findings. A poor grade attributed to a controllable, external cause (e.g., an inadequate marking scheme or an overly difficult exam) is likely to lead to a sense of unfairness and anger (Weiner, 1985; Weiner, Graham, & Chandler, 1982), which may motivate attempts to change the system rather than to improve oneself. A poor grade attributed to an internal, controllable cause (e.g., inadequate preparation) may be more likely to lead to disappointment and attempts to improve one's own perceived inadequa-

TABLE 3. Endorsement Frequencies and Percentages
for the Six Response Categories

Category	Frequency	Percent
Unfairness	17	26.6
Anger	41	64.1
Disappointment	30	46.9
Anxiety	13	20.3
Self-improvement	38	59.4
System-directed	13	20.3
Overall behaviour	49	76.7

Note. N = 64.

TABLE 4. Correlation among the Response Measures

	Unfairness	Anger	Disapp.	Anxiety	Self-imp.	System
Anger	.16					
Disapp.	−.35**	−.41***				
Anxiety	−.04	−.03	−.01			
Self-imp.	−.29**	−.29**	.27*	.02		
System	.14	.30**	−.01	−.06	−.37**	
Behaviour	−.17	−.03	.22*	−.09	.67***	.28**

Note. $N = 64$. Disapp. = Disappointment. Self-imp. = Self-improvement behaviour. System = System-directed behaviour. Behaviour = Overall behaviour.
*$p < .05$; **$p < .01$; ***$p < .001$

cies (Weiner, 1985). We did not measure attributions in this study, so testing these hypotheses must await further research.

The first column of Table 5 shows the correlations between scores on the Just World Scale and endorsement of the response categories. As mentioned above, the Just World Scale has been criticized for sharing variance with measures of locus of control. We found that scores on the Just World Scale were *not* significantly correlated with total scores on Paulhus's measure of locus of control, $r(65) = .09$; however, beliefs in a just world were marginally associated with scores on the personal efficacy subscale, $r(65) = .19$, $p = .06$ (there was no reliable association between just world beliefs and scores on the sociopolitical or interpersonal subscales of Paulhus's measure). Therefore, we decided to compute the correlations between beliefs in a just world and the responses measures, controlling for overall locus of control and for personal efficacy. These partial correlations are shown in the second and third columns of Table 5, respectively.

In accordance with the prediction for our first research question, strong believers in a just world were less likely to report unfairness in

TABLE 5. Correlations between Beliefs in a Just World and Response Categories: Bivariate and Controlling for Locus of Control Measures

Response	BJW	BJW/LOC	BJW/Efficacy
Unfairness	−.24**	−.24**	−.25**
Anger	−.23**	−.23**	−.25**
Disappointment	.23**	.23**	.27**
Anxiety	.23**	.20*	.21**
Self-improvement	.12	.13	.15
System-directed	−.09	−.09	−.08
Behaviour	−.00	.00	.04

Note. $N = 64$. BJW = Beliefs in a just world. BJW/LOC = Beliefs in a just world, controlling for locus of control. BJW/Efficacy = Beliefs in a just world, controlling for personal efficacy. Behaviour = Overall behaviour.
*$p = .05$; **$p < .05$

response to their poor grade than were weak believers. This relation held even after controlling for locus of control and personal efficacy.

Our hypothesis for Research Question 2 was also supported. Strong believers in a just world were less likely to report anger than were weak believers, even after controlling for locus of control and personal efficacy.

To investigate Research Question 3, we examined the relation between beliefs in a just world and emotional responses other than those typically associated with injustice and discontent. Strong believers in a just world, although less likely to report anger and unfairness than weak believers, were *more* likely to report disappointment and anxiety than were weak believers in a just world, even after partialling out the control measures.

Our fourth research direction was to examine how beliefs in a just world were related to behavioural reactions to personal misfortune. Neither of the correlations between just world beliefs and the behaviour measures were significant, even when the control measures were partialled out.[3]

In light of our reasoning presented at the beginning of this chapter, this pattern of results can be interpreted in the following manner. The receipt of an undeserved poor grade (previous work by Olson [1986] suggests that students often perceive low grades as undeserved) poses a threat to the belief in a just world, especially to students with strong beliefs in this domain. Strong believers in a just world will therefore be motivated to reduce the discrepancy between this negative event and their beliefs, for example by reinterpreting the event to create an appearance of fairness. Thus, as we found, strong believers should be less likely than weak believers to report that the poor grade was unfair, and should also be less likely to report emotions that have been associated with unfairness in past research, such as anger. The positive correlations between beliefs in a just world and disappointment and anxiety are again consistent with the hypothesis that strong believers blamed themselves for their poor grade, which produced disappointment and anxiety rather than discontent (see Weiner, Graham, & Chandler, 1982).

The fact that there was no relation between beliefs in a just world and behavioural responses may reflect the operation of other important variables. Similar to our interpretation of the results in the working women

---

[3] We also conducted zero-order correlations between participants' total locus of control scores, their personal efficacy scores, and the response categories. Only two of these correlations were reliable. Total locus of control was negatively correlated with anxiety, $r(62) = -.24$, $p < .05$, and personal efficacy was negatively correlated with overall behaviour, $r(62) = -.25$, $p < .05$. We also conducted logistic regression analyses to investigate the possibility that beliefs in a just world and locus of control or personal efficacy interacted to influence responses to negative outcomes. No significant interactions emerged from these analyses.

study, beliefs in a just world may not be significantly related to self-improvement behaviours here because self-blame can take many forms. For example, blaming a poor grade on a stable lack of ability will discourage attempts at self-improvement.

We also found no relation between beliefs in a just world and system-directed behaviours. One might expect this correlation to be significant and negative, given the results of the working women study. However, it is likely that system-directed change or protest (i.e., attempting to have the grade or the marking scheme changed) did not seem like a particularly viable option to these students (note the low percentage of participants endorsing this behavioural category), given the power structure between instructors and students in the university setting.

In summary, our hypotheses for Research Questions 1 and 2 were supported in that strong believers in a just world were less likely to perceive their misfortune as unfair and less likely to report anger-related emotions than were weak believers. With respect to Research Questions 3 and 4, we found that strong just world beliefs were associated with greater reports of disappointment and anxiety; however, there was no relation between beliefs in a just world and behavioural responses to personal misfortune.

3. CONCLUSIONS AND SUGGESTIONS FOR FUTURE RESEARCH

In this final section, we integrate the results of our three studies with respect to our original research questions regarding the role of just world beliefs in responses to personal misfortune. Future research directions are also suggested.

3.1. Do Strong Believers in a Just World Perceive Their Own Negative Outcomes as Less Unfair Than Weak Believers?

We proposed that strong believers in a just world would feel more threatened than weak believers by undeserved negative outcomes, and therefore would be highly motivated to resolve the contradiction between their misfortune and their beliefs, typically through some form of rationalization. Whatever the particular strategy used to reduce the discrepancy, the result should be a tendency to see the negative outcome as less unfair (compared to weak believers). Both studies addressing this question supported the prediction that strong believers in a just world would perceive their own misfortune as less unfair than weak believers. This pattern was obtained twice, once in the context of responses to a laboratory-induced negative outcome (i.e., losing the chance to leave an experiment early) and once in the context of responses to a naturally occurring misfortune (i.e., a poor grade). Thus, this effect appears to be quite robust.

3.2. Do Strong Believers in a Just World Experience Less Discontent (i.e., Emotions Related to a Sense of Injustice Such as Anger and Resentment) When Confronted with Personal Misfortune Than Weak Believers?

If strong believers in a just world perceive their misfortunes as less unfair than weak believers, one might also expect strong believers to report less discontent. All three studies addressed this issue. Strong believers in a just world did report less discontent than weak believers in Study 3, when the negative outcome was a poor grade, and in the choice condition of Study 1, when the negative outcome was having to spend more time in an experimental situation. No such relation was found for working women's responses to their job situations. Perhaps job situations are different from the "negative" settings in the other studies, in that participants have been experiencing them for a long time and have been forced to come to terms with any discontent they feel. Also, perhaps all women, even those who are weak believers in a just world, accept some responsibility for their job situation, which might reduce variation in discontent across participants. Evidence for this logic comes from Crosby (1982), who has demonstrated that women generally report little personal deprivation with respect to their jobs, perhaps as a result of denial (Crosby, 1984; Crosby, Pufall, Snyder, O'Connell, & Whalen, 1989). At any rate, the relation between beliefs in a just world and discontent was replicable across two settings, although it did not always appear.

Future research on this question should distinguish between discontent and other emotional responses such as disappointment and anxiety. Allowing participants to give their spontaneous emotional responses to misfortune and then coding these according to an accepted classification scheme, as in Study 3, is one way of pursuing this goal in the future. Another approach would be to supply participants with a relatively exhaustive list of relevant emotions, each of which could be rated for intensity on continuous response scales. Emotions theoretically belonging together could be grouped, and some form of composite scores calculated.

3.3. Are Beliefs in a Just World Predictive of Other Emotional Responses to Personal Misfortune?

Study 3 demonstrated that strong believers in a just world were more likely to respond to personal misfortune (i.e., a poor grade) with disappointment and anxiety than were weak believers. We propose that such emotional responses are dependent, in part, on the manner in which individuals choose to reduce the discrepancy between undeserved outcomes and beliefs about fairness. For example, protecting one's belief in a just world by attributing negative outcomes to one's own lack of effort might produce disappointment, whereas protecting one's belief in a just world by denying that an outcome was negative would not produce disappointment. Thus, we do not expect that the associations found in Study 3 will necessarily generalize to other research. In fact, there is already some inconsistency in the research on just world beliefs and emotional responses to personal misfortune (noted earlier in this chapter). Theories of the emotional consequences of various attributions in achievement settings (Weiner, 1985; 1986) and of individual differences in attributional styles (Abramson, Seligman, & Teasdale, 1978) might help to shed light on these issues in future research.

3.4. Are Individual Differences in the Belief in a Just World Associated with Particular Behavioural Reactions to One's Own Negative Outcomes?

Studies 2 and 3 addressed this issue. For working women, strong believers in a just world were less likely to modify their present job situation (i.e., system-directed action) and less likely to take steps toward leaving their current job situation than weak believers. For students responding to a poor grade, there was no relation between just world beliefs and assertive behaviour.

We suggest that these inconsistent findings are due to other variables that are important predictors of behaviour. First, the particular method of dealing with the discrepancy between undeserved outcomes and justice beliefs will, in part, determine behavioural responses (e.g., blaming one's lack of effort might stimulate self-improvement, whereas blaming one's ability might induce apathy and helplessness). Again, attribution theories would help to inform future research on this topic. Second, situational constraints (actual or perceived) will limit the range of behaviours deemed feasible by individuals. Research on the relation between attitudes and behaviour (see Eagly & Chaiken, 1993; Olson & Zanna, 1993) and on the importance of resources in instituting social action (Martin, Brickman, & Murray, 1984; McCarthy & Zald, 1977) should be incorporated into future research.

4. CONCLUSION

In conclusion, our studies show that individual differences in beliefs in a just world are relevant to responses to personal misfortune, and not just the misfortune of others. Individuals who strongly believe in a just world typically perceive less unfairness in personal misfortune and experience less discontent than weak believers. The strategy used to deal with the threat of undeserved outcomes may determine other emotional responses. Behavioural responses may also be influenced by these strategies, as well as by perceived or actual constraints against certain forms of action.

In the future, researchers should propose more complex models of the role of just world beliefs in responses to negative outcomes. These models should take into account a variety of emotional and behavioural responses, various strategies for reducing the discrepancy between misfortune and justice beliefs, and the role of perceived or actual limitations on various types of action.

REFERENCES

Abramson, L. Y., Seligman, M. E. P., & Teasdale, J. D. (1978). Learned helplessness in humans: Critique and reformulation. Journal of Abnormal Psychology, 87, 49–74.

Benson, D. E., & Ritter, C. (1990). Belief in a just world, job loss, and depression. Sociological Focus, 23, 49–61.

Birt, C. M., & Dion, K. L. (1987). Relative deprivation theory and responses to discrimination is a gay male and lesbian sample. British Journal of Social Psychology, 26, 139–145.

Bulman, R. J., & Wortman, C. B. (1977). Attributions of blame and coping in the "real world": Severe accident victims react to their lot. Journal of Personality and Social Psychology, 35, 351–363.

Clyman, R. I., Roth, R. S., Sniderman, S. H., & Charrier, J. (1980). Does a belief in a "just world" affect health care providers' reactions to perinatal illness? Journal of Medical Education, 55, 538–539.

Crosby, F. (1976). A model of egoistical relative deprivation. Psychological Review, 83, 85–113.

Crosby, F. J. (1982). Relative deprivation and working women (pp. x-x): New York: Oxford University Press.

Crosby, F. (1984). The denial of personal discrimination. American Behavioral Scientist, 27, 371–386.

Crosby, F. J., Pufall, A., Snyder, R. C., O'Connell, M., & Whalen, P. (1989). The denial of personal disadvantage among you, me, and all the other ostriches. In M. Crawford & M. Gentry (Eds.), Gender and thought: Psychological perspectives (pp. 79–99). New York: Springer-Verlag.

Dalbert, C. (July, 1992). Gefährdung des Wohlbefindens durch Arbeitsplatzunsicherheit: Eine Analyse der Einflußfaktoren Selbstwert und Gerechte-Welt-Glaube. Paper presented at the 25th meeting of the International Congress of Psychology, Brussels.

Dalbert, C., Fisch, U., & Montada, L. (1992). Is inequality unjust? Evaluating women's career chances. Revue Européenne de Psychologie Appliquée, 42, 11–17.

Eagly, A. H., & Chaiken, S. (1993). The psychology of attitudes. Fort Worth, TX: Harcourt Brace Jovanovich.

Festinger, L. (1957). A theory of cognitive dissonance. Stanford University: Stanford University Press.

Folger, R. (1984). The sense of injustice: Social psychological perspectives. New York: Plenum.

Folger, R. (1986). A referent cognitions theory of relative deprivation. In J. M. Olson, C. P. Herman, & M. P. Zanna (Eds.), Relative deprivation and social comparison: The Ontario symposium (Vol. 4, pp. 33–55). Hillsdale, NJ: Erlbaum.

Furnham, A. (1985). Just world beliefs in an unjust society: A cross cultural comparison. European Journal of Social Psychology, 15, 363–366.

Furnham, A., & Gunter, B. (1984). Just world beliefs and attitudes towards the poor. British Journal of Social Psychology, 15, 265–269.

Furnham, A., & Karani, R. (1985). A cross-cultural study of attitudes to women, just world, and locus of control beliefs. Psychologia: An International Journal of Research in the Orient, 28, 11–20.

Furnham, A., & Procter, E. (1989). Belief in a just world: Review and critique of the individual difference literature. British Journal of Social Psychology, 28, 365–384.

Glennon, F., & Joseph, S. (1993). Just world beliefs, self-esteem, and attitudes towards homosexuals with AIDS. Psychological Reports, 72, 584–585.

Guimond, S., & Dubé-Simard, L. (1983). Relative deprivation theory and the Quebec nationalist movement: The cognition-emotion distinction and the personal-group deprivation issue. Journal of Personality and Social Psychology, 44, 526–535.

Hafer, C. L., & Olson, J. M. (1989). Beliefs in a just world and reactions to personal deprivation. Journal of Personality, 57, 799–823.

Hafer, C. L., & Olson, J. M. (1993). Beliefs in a just world, discontent, and assertive actions by working women. Personality and Social Psychology Bulletin, 19, 30–38.

Higgins, E. T. (1987). Self-discrepancy: A theory relating self and affect. Psychological Review, 94, 319–340.

Lerner, M. J. (1970). The desire for justice and reactions to victims. In J. Macaulay & L. Berkowitz (Eds.), Altruism and helping behavior (pp. 205–229). New York: Academic Press.

Lerner, M. J. (1977). The justice motive: Some hypotheses as to its origins and forms. Journal of Personality, 45, 1–52.

Lerner, M. J. (1978). "Belief in a just world" versus the "authoritarian" syndrome...but nobody liked the Indians. Ethnicity, 5, 229–237.

Lerner, M. J. (1980). The belief in a just world: A fundamental delusion. New York: Plenum.

Lerner, M. J., & Miller, D. T. (1978). Just world research and the attribution process. Looking back and ahead. Psychological Bulletin, 85, 1030–1051.

Lerner, M. J., Miller, D. T., & Holmes, J. G. (1976). Deserving and the emergence of forms of justice. In L. Berkowitz & E. Walster, Advances in experimental social psychology (Vol. 9, pp. 134–162). New York: Academic Press.

Mark, M. M., & Folger, R. (1984). Responses to relative deprivation. A conceptual framework. In P. Shaver (Ed.), Review of personality and social psychology (Vol. 5, pp. 192–218). Beverly Hills, CA: Sage.

Martin, J. (1986). The tolerance of injustice. In J. M. Olson, C. P. Herman, & M. P. Zanna (Eds.), Relative deprivation and social comparion: The Ontario symposium (Vol. 4, pp. 217–242). Hillsdale, NJ: Erlbaum.

Martin, J., Brickman, P., & Murray, A. (1984). Moral outrage and pragmatism: Explanations for collective action. Journal of Experimental and Social Psychology, 20, 484–496.

McCarthy, J. D., & Zald, M. N. (1977). Resource mobilization and social movement: A partial theory. American Journal of Sociology, 82, 1212–1241.

Olson, J. M. (1986). Resentment about deprivation: Entitlement and hopefulness as mediators of the effects of qualifications. In J. M. Olson, C. P. Herman, & M. P. Zanna (Eds.), Relative deprivation and social comparison: The Ontario symposium (Vol. 4, pp. 57–77). Hillsdale, NJ: Erlbaum.

Olson, J. M., & Hafer, C. L. (in press). Affect, motivation, and cognition in relative deprivation research. In R. M. Sorrentino & E. T. Higgins (Eds.), Handbook of motivation and cognition (Vol. 3). New York: Guilford.

Olson, J. M., & Zanna, M. P. (1993). Attitudes and attitude change. Annual Review of Psychology, 44, 117–154.

Olson, J. M., Roese, N. J., Meen, J., & Robertson, D. J. (in press). The preconditions and consequences of relative deprivation: Two field studies. Journal of Applied Social Psychology.

Paulhus, D. (1983). Sphere-specific measures of perceived control. Journal of Personality and Social Psychology, 44, 1253–1265.

Petta, G., & Walker, I. (1992). Relative deprivation and ethnic identity. British Journal of Social Psychology, 31, 285–293.

Ritter, C., Benson, D. E., & Snyder, C. (1990). Belief in a just world and depression. Sociological Perspectives, 33, 235–252.

Rubin, Z., & Peplau, L. A. (1975). Who believes in a just world? Journal of Social Issues, 31, 65–89.

Rummel, R. J. (1970). Applied factor analysis. Evanston, IL: Northwestern University Press.

Shaver, P., Schwartz, J., Kirson, D., & O'Connor, C. (1987). Emotion knowledge: Further exploration of a prototype approach. Journal of Personality and Social Psychology, 52, 1061–1086.

Smith, K. B. (1985). Seeing justice in poverty: The belief in a just world and ideas about inequalities. Sociological Spectrum, 5, 17–29.

Wagstaff, G. F. (1983). Correlates of the just world in Britain. Journal of Social Psychology, 12, 145–146.

Walster, E., Berscheid, E., & Walster, G. W. (1976). New directions in equity research. In L. Berkowitz & E. Walster (Eds.), Advances in experimental social psychology (Vol. 9, pp. 1–42). New York: Academic Press.

Weiner, B. (1985). An attributional theory of achievement motivation and emotion. Psychological Review, 92, 548–573.

Weiner, B. (1986). An attributional theory of motivation and emotion. New York: Springer-Verlag.

Weiner, B., Graham, S., & Chandler, C. (1982). Causal antecendents of pity, anger, and guilt. Personality and Social Psychology Bulletin, 8, 226–232.

Weiner, B., Russell, D., & Lerman, D. (1979). The cognition-emotion process in achievement-related contexts. Journal of Personality and Social Psychology, 37, 1211–1220.

Zuckerman, M., & Gerbasi, K. C. (1975). Belief in internal control or belief in a just world: The use and misuse of the I-E scale in prediction of attitudes and behavior. Journal of Personality, 45, 356–378.

Zuckerman, M., Gerbasi, K. C., Kravitz, R. I., & Wheeler, I. (1975). The belief in a just world and reactions to innocent victims. JSAS Catalog of Selected Documents in Psychology, 5, 326.

Chapter 6

Belief in a Just World, Well-Being, and Coping with an Unjust Fate

CLAUDIA DALBERT

People ordinarily operate on the basis of unquestioned assumptions about the self, the world and the future. These cognitive schemata describe the benign world or optimism about the future, the meaningful world and the self as worthy (cf., Epstein, 1990; Janoff-Bulman, 1979; Weinstein, 1980). They do not comprise exact descriptions of reality but rather positive misperceptions; therefore they are named by Taylor (e.g., 1989) as positive illusions. Taylor and Brown (1988) showed that this kind of illusions seems to be adaptive for mental health and well-being.

In my opinion one important positive illusion indicating the belief in a meaningful world is the belief in a just world (cf., Lerner, 1965). The just world hypothesis states that people are motivated to believe that they live in a world where people generally get what they deserve. The just world belief indicates the interindividually varying strength of this justice motive, which enables people to confront their physical and social environment as though it were stable and orderly (cf., Lerner & Miller, 1987).

My research was guided by the assumption that this justice motive is central for human development in several ways:

CLAUDIA DALBERT • Department of Psychology, University of Kaiserslautern, D-67653 Kaiserslautern, Germany.

Responses to Victimizations and Belief in a Just World, edited by Montada and Lerner. Plenum Press, New York, 1998.

1. It influences the reconstruction and perception of one's life course. Injustices and discriminations will be denied more strongly in one's own group than in other groups (e.g., Dalbert & Yamauchi, 1994; Taylor, Wright, Moghaddam, & Lalonde, 1990); and one tends to believe more strongly in a personal than in a general just world (cf., Dalbert & Lerner, in prep; Lipkus, Dalbert, & Siegler, in press); and the belief to be fairly treated in one's childhood is even stronger (Dalbert & Goch, 1995).

2. The justice motive guides social interactions. In situations with broad social and political unfairness just world belief fosters the denial of the observed injustice (cf., for an review, Furnham and Procter, 1989). But when confronted with specific prosocial situations, in which substantial help is possible, just world belief and prosocial commitment are positively related. For example, subjects helping an accident victim more strongly believed in a just world than non-helpers (cf., Bierhoff, Klein, & Kramp, 1991). Finally, just world belief leads one to expect a good fate as reward for one's own good actions (cf., Zuckerman, 1975).

3. The belief in a world which is stable and just enables people to cope more easily with their daily hassles. For instance, Ritter, Benson, and Snyder (1990) reported a negative relationship between just world belief and depressive symptoms for a representative sample of adults from Northern Ireland. Direct evidence for this positive impact of just world belief on coping with day-to-day stress was recently given by an experiment of Tomaka and Blascovich (1994). When confronted with a potentially stressful laboratory task just world belief served as a stress buffer. Subjects high in just world belief compared to those low in just world belief appraised the task more as challenge, rated the task as less stressful post hoc, outperformed subjects low in just world belief and differed in their physiological reactions (cf., Tomaka & Blascovich, 1994).

4. First evidence that just world belief is as well adaptive for victims of an unjust fate can be found by Bulman and Wortman (1977): Severe accident victims were happier the more they believed in a just world. Recently, Lerner and Somers (1992) showed that workers anticipating plant closure showed a better well-being the better their personal beliefs were; just world belief was part of the personal belief construct. On the contrary for a sample of burn patients Kiecolt-Glaser and Williams (1987) found no relationship between just world belief and different indicators of psychological adjustment.

Taken collectively, the belief in a just world seems to serve an important adaptive function. In line with this considerations my basic hypothesis states that belief in a just world and psychic well-being should be positively related. The aim of this chapter is a closer look on this relationship. In the first part the direct link between both will be described and differentiations due to different populations and different well-being dimensions will be tested. In the second part the indirect relationship between just world belief and well-being will be investigated. More precisely, important coping reactions for victims of an unjust fate will be described as mediators of the relationship between just world belief and actual well-being.

1. JUST WORLD BELIEF AND WELL-BEING: THE DIRECT RELATIONSHIP

The overall result pattern leads to the hypothesis that just world belief and well-being should be positively related for people normally engaged in their day-to-day activities as well as for subjects threatened by an unjust fate. A direct comparison of this relationship for threatened and unthreatened samples was done by Benson and Ritter (1990). They split the sample from Northern Ireland (cf., Ritter, Benson, & Snyder, 1990) into groups of unemployed and employed people and showed that the negative relationship between just world belief and depressive symptoms was only true for the employed subjects. For the unemployed the opposite was true; just world belief and depressive symptoms were positively related. This result is in contrast to the aforementioned results describing a positive relationship between just world belief and well-being. A systematic comparison of different threatened and unthreatened samples is needed to reveal a more convincing answer whether the hypothesized adaptive relationship is equally true for threatened and unthreatened samples.

Additionally, another theoretical weakness must be addressed. Psychic well-being consists of different dimensions. An emotional dimension could be differentiated from a cognitive dimension (cf., Diener, 1984); the emotional dimension could be called mood level and the cognitive dimension is best described as satisfaction with one's life. These two dimensions together describe the more stable, trait-like part of the subjective well-being (cf., Dalbert 1992). Trait well-being should be differentiated from the actual or state-like well-being (cf., Becker, 1991; Dalbert, 1992). Mood states or depressive symptoms are for example part of the actual well-being.

Therefore, the question arises whether just world belief is equally related to different well-being dimensions. Different studies showed that just world belief mainly influence the cognitive reactions towards a situation (e.g., Montada, Dalbert, Reichle, & Schmitt, 1986). This may result in a stronger relationship between just world belief and life satisfaction compared to other well-being dimensions. Bulman and Wortman (1977) described a positive relationship between actual positive mood and just world belief. For depressive symptoms or depressive mood the results were mixed (Benson & Ritter, 1990; Kiecolt-Glaser & Williams, 1987; Ritter, Benson, & Snyder, 1990).

In different samples just world belief and several well-being dimensions were measured to clarify in as much the hypothesized general adaptive relationship between just world belief and psychic well-being should be differentiated. Beside student samples from East (n = 61) and West Germany (n = 135), which serve as samples of unthreatened subjects, two samples of subjects coping with an unjust fate were investigated. These were unemployed East German workers (n = 53) and mothers (mostly West German) with a disabled child (n = 94). All subjects (n = 343) were female; 57% (n = 196) were unthreatened and 43% (n = 147) were coping with an unjust fate.

In all samples four well-being dimensions were measured. The Trait Well-Being Scale (cf., Dalbert, 1992) was applied which consists of a German version of Underwood and Froming's mood level scale (1980: cf., Dalbert, 1992; 6 items, e.g., I consider myself a happy person)—measuring the emotional dimension of the trait well-being—and the German Life Satisfaction Scale (cf., Dalbert, Montada, Schmitt, & Schneider, 1984; 7 items, e.g., I am satisfied with my life)—measuring the cognitive dimension of the trait well-being. In addition actual positive and negative mood—dimensions of the state subjective well-being—were measured with a German version of the Profile of Mood States (McNair, Lorr, & Doppleman, 1971; cf., Dalbert, 1992; 14 adjective measuring negative and 6 adjectives measuring positive mood "in the last week"). For both victim samples *depressive symptoms* were measured as another indicator of state subjective well-being. This was done with the German short version (cf., Hautzinger & Bailer, 1993) of the Center of Epidemiological Studies Depression Scale (Radloff, 1977; 15 items, e.g., In the last week everything was exhausting for me). Belief in a just world was measured with the German *General Just World Scale* (cf., Dalbert, Montada & Schmitt, 1987; 6 items, e.g.: I think basically the world is a just place). For all scales a high value reflects a strong construct.

Table 1 depicts the bivariate correlations between just world belief and the five well-being dimensions for the total sample as well as for each subsample separately. For the total sample just world belief correlated significantly in the expected direction with four of the five well-being variables. Only depressive symptoms and just world belief were uncorrelated. But this result pattern has to be differentiated when comparing the subsamples' results. Life satisfaction was the only variable

TABLE 1. Correlations between Just World Belief and
Different Well-Being Dimensions (n = 343; All Female)

	Trait well-being		Actual well-being		
Samples	Life satisfaction	Mood level	Positive mood	Negative mood	Depressive symptoms
Non-victims					
Students (East)	.28[b]	.15	.16	−.13	—
Students (West)	.34[d]	.23[c]	—	−.20[b]	—
Victims					
Mothers of a disabled child	.43[d]	.39[d]	.28[c]	−.20[a]	−.10
Unemployed workers	.53[d]	.30[b]	.19	−.21	.05
Total	.29[d]	.26[d]	.17[b]	−.18[c]	−.04

Note: — means 'not measured in this sample.' [a]$p \le .10$; [b]$p \le .05$; [c]$p \le .01$; [d]$p \le .001$

significantly correlated with just world belief within all four groups. All subjects were more satisfied with their life in general, the more they believed in a just world. The positive correlation between just world belief and mood level for the total sample was as strong as the correlation of life satisfaction with just world belief, but this correlation was significant only in three out of the four subsamples. For all subjects except the East German students the mood level was more positive, the more they believed in a just world. Although both actual mood dimensions were significantly correlated with just world belief for the total sample, within the subsamples there was only one significant correlation for each actual mood dimension. In line with this observations, depressive symptoms were as well uncorrelated with just world belief in both victim samples.

In a next step it was investigated whether just world belief and well-being was equally strong correlated for victims and non-victims. The interaction of just world belief and the dichotomous victim-factor was tested by multiple regression analyses for the four well-being dimensions measured in victim- and non-victim samples. The victim-factor was entered in the first and just world belief was entered in the second step, their product was entered finally. The interaction term was not significant for mood level and actual positive and negative mood (all: $p > .20$), but it was significant for life satisfaction ($p = .033$; $F_{total} = 19.158$, $p < .001$). Victim status alone did not explain one's life satisfaction ($p = .186$), just world belief explained 13% and the interaction term explained one additional percent of the life satisfaction's variance. The positive relationship between just world belief and life satisfaction was significantly stronger for the victims ($b = .47$) than for the non-victims ($b = .26$).

In a next step it was tested which of the two relationships between just world belief and trait well-being was most typical. Therefore, multiple regression analyses were done from each trait well-being dimension on the other trait well-being dimension in the first and just world belief in the second step. When mood level was controlled for life satisfaction just world belief could no longer predict mood level ($p = .13$). But when life satisfaction was controlled for mood level just world belief could still predict life satisfaction ($p = .002$; beta $= .13$). If mood level and the interaction of just world belief with the victim-factor were combined, the interaction term lost some of its power ($p = .080$). Mood level explained 47% of the life satisfaction variance, the victim-factor explained again no variance, just world belief explained additional 3%, and the interaction term only 0.5%. The positive relationship between just world belief and life satisfaction was marginally stronger for the victims ($b = .24$) than for the non-victims ($b = .11$), when controlled for mood level.

To predict more precisely actual positive and negative mood which are highly correlated with the trait well-being dimensions, especially mood level, multiple regression analyses were done. Each state well-being dimension was regressed on mood level in the first step and just world belief in the second step. Just world belief could neither predict the actual positive nor the actual negative mood's state residuum, which is the actual mood controlled for mood level. This was true for each subsample as well as for the total sample (all: $p > .20$).

The results for depressive symptoms were somewhat different. For the sample of mothers with a disabled child just world belief was as well unrelated ($p > .20$) to the depressive symptoms' state residuum, which is depressive symptoms controlled for mood level. For the unemployed workers this relationship was marginally significant ($p = .055$). When aggregated over both victim samples the relationship between just world belief and the depressive symptoms' state residuum became significant ($p = .032$). But contrary to my expectations those relationships were positive (workers: beta $= .24$; total: beta $= .16$). When controlled for mood level, the probability of depressive symptoms were higher, the more especially the unemployed workers believed in a just world. So far it is not clear whether this unexpected result is due to chance, because it was only one marginally significant result out of nine regression analyses done in the subsamples. I will come back to this point later.

The results so far are very clear in one point. For all subjects, victims and non-victims, just world belief and life satisfaction were positively related. This was not only true for all samples, but also the pattern remained stable when controlled for mood level, the other trait well-being dimension. This means, just world belief and life satisfaction had something specific in common which could not be explained by mood level. On the other hand this stable result pattern could only be observed for life satisfaction and for no other well-being dimension. Therefore, I would like to conclude that the adaptive relationship between just world belief and life satisfaction is the most typical in this field. Further research is needed to clarify, whether in addition to the just world's main effect a buffering effect could be observed as well. In this study the interaction term was not as stable as the main effect. Therefore it remains unclear whether the relationship between just world belief and life satisfaction is somewhat stronger for victims than for non-victims.

Another result could be retained as well. Just world belief and actual positive or negative mood showed no direct relationship. This was not only true for five out of seven bivariate relationships tested in the sub-samples. It was revealed unambiguously when actual mood was controlled for mood level. In each case the state specific residuum was unrelated the just world belief. The relationship between just world belief and actual mood consisted of nothing specific which could not be explained by mood level. This result pattern seems to be in contrast to a positive relationship observed by other authors (Bulman & Wortman, 1977; Lerner & Somers, 1992). Beside differences between samples and measurement methods, the discrepancy may be traced back to the missing control of trait well-being in the other studies. Therefore, it could not be differentiated whether there was really found a just world's relationship which was specific for actual mood or whether the observed relationships were confounded by trait well-being.

Depressive symptoms are more than actual negative mood. Concentration problems, sleeping disorders, and problems in social relationships are included in the symptoms list. This broader description of the last week's well-being was measured only in the victim samples. The results were mixed. Both bivariate correlations are not significant. For the unemployed workers but not for the mothers with a disabled child just world belief was marginally positively related to the state-specific depressive residuum. This maladaptive relationship was not expected, but it is somewhat in line with Benson and Ritter's result (1990), that just world belief and depressive symptoms were positively correlated for unemployed people from Northern Ireland. Maybe this positive relationship is typical for unemployed people. But also for the unemployment studies the results were not totally consistent: In contrast to Benson and Ritter (1990) in my study the direct link between depression and just world belief was not significant.

The overall results can give some support to the hypothesis that just world belief and life satisfaction are in an adaptive relationship, whether people are facing an unjust fate or not. The more one believes to live in a just world, in which everybody gets what he/she deserves, the more one is satisfied with one's life in general. This supports the interpretation of just world belief as a coping resource rather than a coping product. The poor and unexpected relationships between just world belief and actual well-being, namely depressive symptoms, turns us back to the coping question. If just world belief is a coping resource, which directs and maybe enables people to cope with an unjust fate, than the just world's effect on actual well-being should be mediated by the subjects' coping efforts. This maybe especially true for depressive symptoms as the mixed results of my study suggest. In a next step, the indirect link between just world belief and depressive symptoms, or more specifically the depressive symptoms' state residuum, will be closely examined.

2. JUST WORLD BELIEF AND WELL-BEING: THE INDIRECT RELATIONSHIP

When people are confronted with an unjust fate like having a disabled child or becoming unemployed due to plant closure or broader socio-economic changes they are urged to defend their just world belief. The more they believe in a just world, the more they will restore justice cognitively, because real compensation is not possible in the near future. At least three coping mechanisms can be discussed here. Victims can reappraise their fate as self inflicted or they can reevaluate their fate as more positive as seen at first sight. A positive fate or a self-inflicted aversive fate is no longer unjust. Therefore, these cognitions may help to defend the belief in a just world. Focussing on the positive is a well known adaptive coping reaction; the results about causal self-attributions and psychological adaption when facing a life threat are much more mixed (cf., Dalbert, 1996). On the opposite, the more victims of an unjust fate ruminate about the "why me?"-question, the more their just world belief should be threatened. Believing in a just world means to believe in a meaningful world. But the "why me?"-question reveals existential doubts about the meaningfulness of the world. Subjects believing in a just world and at the same time ruminating about the "why me?"-question must be despairing.

If the relationship between just world belief and actual well-being is mediated by these coping reactions, two direct relationships must be carefully examined: the one between just world belief and coping as well as the one between coping and well-being. This was done for both victim samples mentioned above. Results are described elsewhere in detail (Dalbert, 1996). Here will be given a short overview of the results related (a) to causal self-attributions which are often discussed in this context, and (b) to the "why me?"-question which seems to be important under specific circumstances. Positive reappraisals seem to be less clearly related to the just world belief than expected. Results are therefore not discussed in this section.

2.1. Causal Self-Attributions

The hypothesis that just world belief fosters causal self-attributions which should be adaptive for the actual well-being was carefully examined in the study with the mothers of disabled children. Only one victim study directly investigated the relationship between just world belief and causal self-attributions of the victimizing event; the more burn patients believed in a just world, the more they blamed themselves for the accident (Kiecolt-Glaser & Williams, 1987). But self-blame seemed to be maladaptive for the burn patients; it was positively correlated with depression and pain behavior and it was negatively correlated with compliance.

These last findings were contrary to the hypothesis that self-attributions should be adaptive because they defend the just world belief and foster the belief in personal control. In four studies of mothers with risk children the hypothesized positive relationship between psychic adaption and causal self-attributions of 'the child's medical problem' was tested, but it was found in only one study (Affleck, McGrade, Allen, & McQueeney, 1985). In the other studies a non-significant relationship was observed (Affleck, Allen, McGrade, & McQuenney, 1982; Affleck, Allen, Tennen, McGrade, & Ratzan, 1985; Tennen, Affleck, & Gershman, 1986). Dalbert and Warndorf (1995) argued that it must be differentiated between the causal attributions of the child's disability—for example its mental retardation—and the causal attributions of the child's concrete problem—that the child do not eat for example. In most cases the child's disability will not significantly change in the future, but the concrete problem can often dramatically change. Therefore, only self-attributions of the concrete problem may enhance the mother's feelings of control. In line with this considerations only the causal self-attributions of the concrete problem seemed to be adaptive; they were negatively related to the depressive symptoms' state residuum. But this was not true for the self-attributions of the disability, which were positively related to the depressive symptoms' state residuum (Dalbert & Warndorf, 1995).

Within this mothers sample just world belief was neither directly related to depressive symptoms nor to its state residuum, which is again depressive symptoms controlled for mood level. But the question arise whether just world belief showed an indirect relationship to the state residuum, mediated by the self-attribution of the child's concrete problem. The idea was that two kinds of self-attributions should be differentiated. There are more realistic attributions describing how the mother had really contributed to the concrete problem. Beside this realistic attributions there are self-attributions motivated to protect one's just world belief. These attributions are some kind of motivated reappraisals and should be much less realistic.

The mothers rated whether (a) their behavior and (b) themselves as a person (cf., Janoff-Bulman, 1979) did cause the child's concrete problem. Both ratings were highly correlated; therefore their mean was used as self-attribution variable. Just world belief and the maternal self-attributions were uncorrelated ($p > .20$). In addition experts were asked whether they assume, that the parent's behavior had contributed to the development of the child's concrete problem. The study was done in a pediatric clinic in southern Germany during the child's stay in the clinic; experts were the psychologist who treated the child. Their rating was used as an indicator of the attribution's realism. Mothers' and experts' ratings were positively correlated ($r = .37$; $p = .001$).

The moderated regression analyses, which tested the hypothesized interaction of just world belief and the experts' ratings was significant ($Ftotal = 5.920$; $p = .001$). In addition to the experts' ratings, which explained 14% of the variance, and in addition to just world belief which did not explain any variance, the interaction term explained 5% of the variance ($T = -2.239$; $p = .028$) in the maternal self-attributions.

The lower the mothers' just world belief was, the stronger their self-attributions were related to the experts' ratings. If for example the just world belief was low (M – SD) than the experts' ratings were strongly related to the maternal attributions ($b = .42$). If on the other hand the just world belief was high (M + SD) than the experts' ratings were unrelated to the maternal attributions ($b = .07$). This relationship is depicted in Figure 1. Given a strong just world belief reality as indicated by the

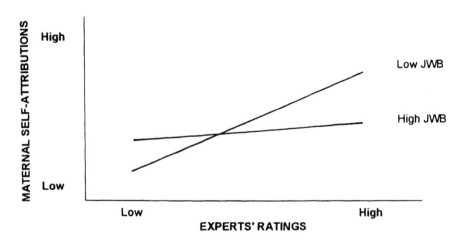

FIGURE 1. The mothers' self-attributions of the disabled child's concrete problem predicted by the experts' attributions of the disabled child's concrete problem to the parent's behavior and the mothers' just world belief (JWB).

experts' ratings did not predict the maternal attributions; but the lower the just world belief was, the more the maternal attributions seemed to depict what really happened. The just world belief did foster maternal self-attributions only under the condition of low experts' ratings.

The result pattern could be summed up as follows: The more the mothers believed in a just world, the more they made unrealistic causal self-attributions. Only those not believing in a just world made realistic self-attributions. This was as expected. There seem to be two kinds of self-attributions, the one which are motivated by the belief in a just world and others which are more exact descriptions of reality. This raised the further question whether these two kinds of attributions are differently related to the mothers' well-being. The question of realism is so far not discussed in the attributional context. But for control appraisals it was claimed that it is not adaptive to perceive control in uncontrollable situations (cf., Cohen & Lazarus, 1983). When confronted with reality, illusions of control based on unrealistic attributions will collapse. Helgeson (1992) for example showed that only realistic vicarious control appraisals were adaptive for a sample of first cardiac event patients.

Overall, it was shown by Dalbert and Warndorf (1995) that specific causal self-attributions were negatively related with the depressive symptoms' state residuum: The more the mothers saw their child's concrete problem at least partly as self inflicted, the smaller their probability of depressive symptoms was, when controlled for mood level. But when differentiating between realistic and unrealistic self-attributions only the realistic ones can at least in the long run enhance feelings of control and thereby enhance one's well-being.

To test this hypothesis a multiple regression analysis was done from the mothers' depressive symptoms on mood level, their self-attributions, experts' ratings and the product of maternal and experts' attributions. The interaction term was marginally significant ($T = -1.740$; $p = .086$), explaining 3% of the variance in addition to 26% percent explained by mood level and 3% explained by the maternal self-attributions' main effect. When controlled for additional predictors of the mothers' depressive symptoms, this interaction became more pronounced ($p < .001$; cf., Dalbert, 1996). This suggests that the interaction is important for explaining the mothers' actual well-being, although it is only marginally significant when tested isolated. The meaning of the interaction term is in line with the expectations. The more realistic the causal attributions were, the stronger was the negative relationship between the maternal attributions and the depressive symptoms' state residuum. If the experts strongly attributed the child's concrete problem to the parent's behavior ($M + SD$), than maternal self-attributions were negatively related to depression ($b = -.18$). This relationship became weaker the less the experts rated the parents' behavior as a cause of the child's concrete problem. If the experts did not see the parent's behavior as a cause $(M - SD)$, than the maternal attributions were slightly positively related to depression $(b = .06)$. Only realistic self-attributions seemed to protect the mothers' actual well-being.

Putting the puzzle together we can state, that the just world belief seems to enhance unrealistic self-attributions of the child's concrete problem, and this unrealistic attributions are at best unrelated to the actual well-being. The results suggest that unrealistic self-attributions may in fact promote depressive symptoms. There was a slight positive relationship between the unrealistic attributions and the depressive symptoms' state residuum, and this maladaptive relationship became more pronounced when other significant predictors of depression were controlled additionally (cf., Dalbert, 1996). Only realistic maternal attributions were connected with a low probability of depressive symptoms. Although the just world belief was not directly related to the mothers' depressive symptoms or its state residuum, just world belief was indirectly, but positively related to the depressive symptoms; this relationship was mediated through unrealistic self-attributions. Thus far we can see that the just world belief is important for explaining coping reactions. Contrary to our expectations but in line with Kiecolt-Glaser and Williams' results (1987) its indirect effect on the mothers' actual well-being was slightly maladaptive.

In the case of structural unemployment typically causal self-attribution of the job loss is unrealistic and an unusual coping reaction (cf., Bergman, 1992; Lerner, 1993). This may be true not only because of its unrealism. Other coping reactions as for example positive reevaluations are as well seldom (cf., Dalbert, in print). Victims of structural unemployment seem to wait for the end of their aversive situation, at least in the first time after job loss. In the unemployment study already mentioned above only 4 out of the 53 unemployed workers saw in their own behavior at least partly a cause of the job loss. Although only few self-attributions were observed, these behavioral attributions were positively correlated with the workers' just world belief $(r = .27; p = .062)$, but unrelated to depressive symptoms or its state residuum. These results are in line with the results of the mothers study. Taken collectively, the just world belief leads victims of an unjust fate to engage in unrealistic causal self-attributions, and these attributions are not adaptive for the victims psychic adaption.

2.2. Why Me?

In the frequency of asking the "why me?"-question the unemployed workers did not differ from other victims of a serious life stroke (e.g., Affleck et al., 1985; Bulman & Wortman, 1977; Gotay, 1985; Silver, Boon, & Stone, 1983). Ten workers had never asked themselves this question; 29 women asked themselves the "why me?"-question but did not find an answer; and 13 workers asked the question but found an answer. In line with our expectations just world belief and the "why me?"-question were negatively correlated $(r = -.30; p = .030)$; those not asking the "why me?"-question stronger believed in a just world than those not ruminating about it. This result was especially true for the half of the sample who were unemployed for less than a half year $(p = .023)$; and the relationship could not be observed for those women who lost their job more than a half year ago $(p > .20)$. Finding an answer or not was unrelated to the just world belief.

It was already shown in the first part of the chapter that just world belief and the depressive symptoms' state residuum were positively related in this sample. It was hypothesized that this maladaptive relationship should be especially strong for those ruminating about the "why me?"-question. This hypothesis was tested with a moderated regression on the interaction of just world belief and dummy variables for "asking the question" and "finding an answer". In addition to mood level and length of unemployment which together explained 62% of the depressive symptoms' variance, and in addition to the three non-significant main effects, the interaction of just world belief with "asking the question" explained 9% and the just world's interaction with "finding an answer" explained 5% additionally. The interaction worked in line with the theoretical considerations. For those not asking the "why me?"-question just world belief was negatively related to the depressive state residuum $(b = -.32)$; for those asking the question without finding an answer the relationship was positive $(b = .26)$; finding an answer seemed to be compensating, for those workers just world belief was unrelated to the state residuum $(b = -.03)$. Because a majority was ruminating about the "why me?"-question without finding an answer, this moderated relationship between just world belief and depressive symptoms' state residuum seemed to be positive when tested aggregated over the three groups.

For the mothers of a disabled child the "why me?"-question was not important for explaining their actual well-being. But just world belief was similarly correlated to the "why me?"-question as in the unemployment study. For the half of the sample with a child disabled less than 55 month, just world belief was marginally positively related to asking the "why me?"-question or not $(p = .087)$. The more the mothers believed in a just world the lower the probability of asking the "why me?"-question was. For the other half of the sample just world belief and the "why me?"-question were not correlated $(p > .20)$.

The results can be summed up as follows. The just world belief seems to protect victims of an unjust fate from ruminating about the "why me?"-question. This was true at least for the first time after the aversive experience. Whether the just world belief is adaptive or not varies with the victims' coping reactions. Only for those not asking themselves the "why me?"-question, the just world belief can protect the actual well-being. Serious doubts about the world's meaningfulness as indicated by an unanswered "why me?"-question threatens the just world belief and seems to raise the probability of depressive symptoms. This seems to be especially true, if victims avoid other cognitive coping reactions.

3. DISCUSSION

The present studies showed that the just world belief should be regarded when explaining coping reactions of victims facing a serious life stroke. Results in both victim samples were predominantly consistent to this point. Much less clear is the answer whether just world belief is adaptive or not. There is no direct link between the belief to live in a just world and the actual well-being. The indirect link seems to differ in dependency of the kind of life stroke and the coping reactions shown by the subject.

Very clear is the relationship between just world belief and different well-being dimensions. Just world belief is typically positively correlated with one's life satisfaction. This is true for victims and non-victims and when controlled for other trait well-being dimensions as shown above or when controlled for other coping resources like for example self-worth (cf., Dalbert, 1993). On the basis of these results and in connection with the results describing the relationship between just world belief and different coping reactions I would prefer to interpret just world belief as a personal coping resource.

In line with this interpretation in most research just world belief is treated as a personal disposition or basic schema (cf., Cantor, 1990; Epstein, 1990) which cannot easily be altered by experience. This addresses the just world belief's stability. Experimental tests of the assumed stability should be on the agenda of the near future. First experiments indicate relative stability of the general just world belief (cf., Dalbert & Lerner, in prep.).

Although just world belief is not directly related to actual state well-being of victims or non-victims, it can explain how people react when confronted with an unjust fate. Obviously, just world belief motivates people to unrealistically attribute their fate to themselves. This relationship between just world belief and unrealistic causal self-attributions was observed in both victim studies mentioned above. But only realistic self-attributions can protect the psychic adaption. Unrealistic self-attributions are at best unrelated to the victims' actual well-being. Therefore, when focussing on self-attributions just world belief seems to be systematically related to this coping reaction but unrelated or negatively related to one's actual well-being. It must be added that this is only true for self-attributions of changeable problems like unemployment or the child's concrete problem. For causal self-attributions of a stable state the opposite seems to be true. The more realistic causal self-attributions of the child's disability were, the worse the mothers' actual well-being was, and this kind of self-attributions were unrelated to just world belief (cf., Dalbert, 1996).

Correspondingly in both victim samples just world belief seems to protect from ruminating about the "why me?"-question at least in the first time after the victimizing experience. Only for the unemployed workers in East Germany just world belief and its interaction with the "why me?"-question were most important in explaining the women's actual well-being. For those not struggling with the cognitive dissonance of believing in a just world and at the same time doubting about one's fate, the probability of depressive symptoms was low. But for those believing in a just world but simultaneously ruminating about the "why me?"-question the probability of depressive symptoms was high. Finding an answer can compensate the ruminating's maladaptive effect; for this subsample just world belief and depressive symptoms were unrelated. The described results were observed when controlled for mood level and length of unemployment which typically raises the depressive symptoms' probability.

As clear as the result pattern was for the unemployment sample this interactive relationship was the single one observed only in one of both victim samples. One can only speculate why this happened. It can be due to chance. But the consistently observed negative relation between just world belief and actual well-being for unemployed people (cf., in addition Benson & Ritter, 1990) suggests that this is a systematic result. An interpretation would be that the "why me?"-question became important because reappraisals like self-attributions were untypical for the unemployed. Further research is needed to systematically test whether the "why me?"-question's importance for predicting the actual well-being varies in dependency of the frequency and importance of other more reappraising coping reactions.

Believing in a just world is a powerful personal resource influencing the coping process in different ways. This basic assumption was supported through several results. But the studies described here testing different hypotheses derived from this assumption can be characterized by some short comings. First of all, all studies were cross-sectional questionnaire studies. Causal influences and adaptiveness can be proofed only in experimental or longitudinal studies. Controlling the trait well-being is one technique to more clearly relate predictors to the actual mood state. This is a more conservative test of the hypothesized relationships and gives more certainty about identifying important predictors. But it is still no compensation for longitudinal testing. Consequently, the question of long-term adaptiveness is as well left unanswered. It can turn out for a coping reaction which is adaptive in the short run to be maladaptive in the long run. We do not know for example whether avoiding the "why me?"-question is adaptive if the worker is still unemployed after years. Avoiding senseless and endless ruminating should be adaptive, but evading a constructive exposition with one's fate may turn out as awkward.

The discussion was constrained to self-attribution processes and to the "why me?"-question. The relationship of just world belief and positive reevaluations are discussed elsewhere (cf., Dalbert, 1996). But there are still other important coping reactions not yet discussed. Tomaka and Blascovich (1994) showed that the just world belief predicts the primary appraisal of a daily stressor as challenge or stress. It should be worthwhile to test whether this finding could be generalized to more serious stressors like existential loss experiences for example. The relationship between just world belief and seeking for social support can be discussed too. Maybe that under specific circumstances receiving important help from others can be interpreted as some kind of compensation for an unjust fate? We still do not know anything about this relationship. In addition, social comparison processes are normally discussed within a self-concept framework. But it can be speculated that especially upward comparisons and just world belief are negatively related. Is it a just world in which other people are better off than I am?

As we can see a lot of questions are still unanswered. But I hope to have shown the necessity to look at the belief in a just world to gain a full understanding of the coping process. There is no doubt that the just world belief heavily influences how victims will cope with their unjust fate. For some of them and under specific conditions the just world belief promotes adaptive coping reactions, for others the justice motivated coping reactions turn out to be maladaptive. But for all of them it does matter whether they believe in a just world or not.

This is true for non-victims engaging in their daily activities as well. The more they believe in a just world, the more positive their look at their lives is. Just world belief enables people to experience daily hassles as less stressful, to see the personal life course as guided by justice and to expect reward for good deeds. As a consequence just world belief fosters satisfaction with one's life. I would therefore like to end with the argument that the need to believe in a just world is an existential guiding line for all of us.

REFERENCES

Affleck, G., Allen, D.A., McGrade, B.J., & McQueeney, M. (1982). Maternal causal attributions at hospital discharge of high-risk infants. American Journal of Mental Deficiency, 86, 575–580.

Affleck, G., Allen, D.A., Tennen, H., McGrade, B.J., & Ratzan, S. (1985). Causal and control cognitions in parent coping with a chronically ill child. Journal of Social and Clinical Psychology, 3, 369–379.

Affleck, G., McGrade, B.J., Allen, D., & McQueeney, M. (1985). Mothers' beliefs about behavioral causes for their developmentally disabled infant's condition: What do they signify? Journal of Pediatric Psychology, 10, 293–303.

Becker, P. (1991). Theoretische Grundlagen. In A. Abele, & P. Becker (Eds.), Wohlbefinden (Well-being) (pp. 13–49). Weinheim: Juventa.

Benson, D.E. & Ritter, C. (1990). Belief in a just world, job loss and depression. Sociological Focus, 23, 49–63.

Bergmann, B. (1992). Erleben und Bew„ltigen von Arbeitsunsicherheit - Eine Studie aus dem Raum Dresden (Experience of and coping with job uncertainty - A study in the area of Dresden). Dresden, Technische Universität, unveröffentlichtes Manuskript.

Bierhoff, H.W., Klein, R., & Kramp, P. (1991). Evidence for the altruistic personality from data on accident research. Journal of Personality, 59, 263–280.

Bulman, R.J. & Wortman, C.B. (1977). Attributions of blame and coping in the "real world": Severe accident victims react to their lot. Journal of Personality and Social Psychology, 35, 351–363.

Cantor, N. (1990). From thought to behavior. American Psychologist, 45, 735–750.

Cohen, F. & Lazarus, R.S. (1983). Coping and adaption in health and illness. In D. Mechanic (Ed.), Handbook of health, health care, and the health professions (pp. 608–631). New York: Free Press.

Dalbert, C. (1992). Subjektives Wohlbefinden junger Erwachsener: Theoretische und empirische Analysen der Struktur und Stabilität (Young adults' subjective well-being: Theoretical and empirical analyses of its structure and stability). Zeitschrift für Differentielle und Diagnostische Psychologie, 13, 207–220.

Dalbert, C. (1993). Gefährdung des Wohlbefindens durch Arbeitsplatzunsicherheit: Eine Analyse der Einflußfaktoren Selbstwert und Gerechte-Welt-Glaube (Well-being's jeopardy by job insecurity: An analysis of self-worth and just world belief). Zeitschrift für Gesundheitspsychologie, 1, 235–253.

Dalbert, C. (in print). Über den Umgang mit Ungerechtigkeit (On dealing with injustice). Bern: Huber

Dalbert, C. & Goch, I. (1995). Child rearing practices, family climate, perceived familial justice, and the belief in a just world. Unpublished data.

Dalbert, C. & Lerner, M.J. (in prep.). General and personal just world belief: Situational constructions or personal dispostions?

Dalbert, C., Montada, L., & Schmitt, M. (1987). Glaube an eine gerechte Welt als Motiv: Validierungskorrelate zweier Skalen (Belief in a just world: Validation correlation of two scales). Psychologische Beiträge, 29, 596–615.

Dalbert, C., Montada, L., Schmitt, M., & Schneider, A. (1984). Existentielle Schuld: Ergebnisse der Item- und Skalenanalysen (Existential guilt: Results of item and scale analyses) (= Berichte aus der Arbeitsgruppe "Verantwortung, Gerechtigkeit, Moral" Nr. 24). Trier: Universität Trier, FB I - Psychologie.

Dalbert, C. & Warndorf, P. K., (1995). Informationsverarbeitung und depressive Symptome bei Müttern behinderter Kinder: Die Bedeutung von Ungewissheitstoleranz, Selbstzuschreibungen und Heilungsprognosen (Information processing and depressive symptoms of mothers with a disabled child: The meaning of uncertainty tolerance, self-attributions and healing prognoses). Zeitschrift für Klinische Psychologie, 24, 328–336.

Dalbert, C. & Yamauchi, L. (1994). Belief in a just world and attitudes toward immigrants and foreign workers: A cultural comparison between Hawaii and Germany. Journal of Applied Social Psychology, 24, 1612–1626.

Diener, E. (1984). Subjective well-being. Psychological Bulletin, 95, 542–575.

Epstein, S. (1990). Cognitive-experiential self-theory. In L.A. Pervin (Ed.), Handbook of Personality. Theory and Research (pp. 165–192). New York: Guilford Press.

Furnham, A. & Procter, E. (1989). Belief in a just world: Review and critique of the individual difference literature. British Journal of Social Psychology, 28, 365–384.

Gotay, C.C. (1985). Why me? Attributions and adjustment by cancer patients and their mates at two stages in the disease process. Social Science and Medicine, 20, 825–831.

Hautzinger, M. & Bailer, M. (1993). Allgemeine Depressionsskala (ADS) (General depression scale). Weinheim: Beltz-Test.

Helgeson, V.S. (1992). Moderators of the relation between perceived control and adjustment to chronic illness. Journal of Personality and Social Psychology, 63, 656–666.

Janoff-Bulman, R. (1979). Characterological versus behavioural self-blame: Inquiries into depression and rape. Journal of Personality and Social Psychology, 37, 1798–1809.

Kiecolt-Glaser, J.K. & Williams, D.A. (1987). Self-blame, compliance, and distress among burn patients. Journal of Personality and Social Psychology, 53, 187–193.

Lerner, M.J. (1965). Evaluation of performance as a function of performer's reward and attractiveness. Journal of Personality and Social Psychology, 1, 355–360.

Lerner, M.J. (1993). Coping with contemporary economic realities: Social-Psychological consequences of plant closures, down-sizing, and employment insecurity. Paper given at the 4th International Conference on Social Justice Research in Trier.

Lerner, M.J. & Miller, D.T. (1978). Just world research and the attribution process: Looking back and ahead. Psychological Bulletin, 85, 1030–1051.

Lerner, M.J. & Somers, D.G. (1992). Employees' reactions to an anticipated plant closure: The influence of positive illusions. In L. Montada & S. H. Filipp (Eds.), Life crises and experiences of loss in adulthood (pp. 229–254). Hillsdale, N.J.: LEA.

Lipkus, I.M., Dalbert, C. & Siegler, I.C. (in press). The importance of distinguishing the belief in a just world for self versus others. Personality and Social Psychology Bulletin.

Montada, L., Dalbert, C., Reichle, B., & Schmitt, M. (1986). Urteile über Gerechtigkeit, "existentielle Schuld" und Strategien der Schuldabwehr (Justice judgements, "existential guilt", and guilt reducing strategies). In F. Oser, W. Althof & D. Garz (Eds.), Moralische Zugänge zum Menschen - Zugänge zum moralischen Menschen (pp. 205–225). München: Kindler.

Radloff, L.S. (1977). The CES-D Scale: A self-report depression scale for research in the general population. Applied Psychological Measurement, 1, 385–401.

Ritter, C., Benson, D.E., & Snyder, C. (1990). Belief in a just world and depression. Sociological Perspectives, 33, 235–252.

Silver, R.L., Boon, C., & Stones, M.H. (1983). Searching for meaning in misfortune making sense of incest. Journal of Social Issues, 39(2), 81–102.

Taylor, D.M., Wright, G.C., Moghaddam, F.M., & Lalonde, R.N. (1990). The personal/group discrimination discrepancy: Perceiving my group, but not myself, to be a target for discrimination. Personality and Social Psychology Bulletin, 16, 254–262.

Taylor, S.E. (1989). Positive Illusions. New York: Basic Books.

Taylor, S.E. & Brown, G. (1988). Illusion and well-being: A social psychological perspective on mental health. Psychological Bulletin, 103, 193–210.

Tennen, H., Affleck, G., & Gershman, K. (1986). Self-blame among parents of infants with perinatal complications: The role of self-protective motives. Journal of Personality and Social Psychology, 50, 690–696.

Tomaka, J. & Blascovich, J. (1994). Effects of justice beliefs on cognitive appraisals of and subjective, physiological, and behavioral responses to potential stress. Journal of Personality and Social Psychology, 67, 732–740.

Underwood, B. & Froming, W.J. (1980). The mood survey: A personality measure of happy and sad moods. Journal of Personality Assessment, 44, 404–414.

Weinstein, N.D. (1980). Unrealistic optimism about future life events. Journal of Personality and Social Psychology, 39, 806–820.
Zuckerman, M. (1975). Belief in a just world and altruistic behaviour. Journal of Personality and Social Psychology, 31, 972–976.

Chapter 7

Belief in a Just World and Right-Wing Authoritarianism as Moderators of Perceived Risk

ALAN J. LAMBERT, THOMAS BURROUGHS, and
ALISON L. CHASTEEN

We live in a world filled with risk. Nearly every day, we face the prospect of many different types of threats ranging from relatively common, everyday risks (e.g., of losing one's wallet) to the most serious personal calamities (e.g., getting hit by a car, dying of AIDS). From a psychological standpoint, understanding how people form subjective estimates of risk, and the factors that influence such perceptions, is of critical importance. In particular, it seems likely that one's subjective sense of well-being may depend on whether one feels personally vulnerable to these threats or not. Thus, understanding when and why people feel vulnerable to life's many risks should offer more general insights into the factors mediating mental health. Perceptions of risk also seem likely to play a role in mediating many sorts of decisions and behaviors (cf. Johnson & Tversky, 1983, for a related discussion). For example, such simple acts as driving a car probably involve the implicit or explicit assessment of different sorts of risks (e.g.,

ALAN J. LAMBERT, THOMAS BURROUGHS, and ALISON L. CHASTEEN • Department of Psychology, Washington University, 1 Brookings Drive/Box 1125, St. Louis, Missouri 63130-4899.

Responses to Victimizations and Belief in a Just World, edited by Montada and Lerner. Plenum Press, New York, 1998.

the probability of getting in an accident) and these perceptions may strongly determine many of the choices we make (e.g., how fast to drive on a stormy night).

In light of these considerations, it is hardly surprising that psychologists have generated a great deal of research on perceptions of risk and why people might feel more or less vulnerable under certain conditions. For one thing, social and clinical psychologists have long sought to understand how people maintain illusions of invulnerability, even when such beliefs are not well justified (for a review, see Taylor & Brown, 1988). Relatedly, work by Weinstein (1980, 1982) has demonstrated the well-known "above average" effect, namely, the tendency for most people to believe that they are more likely to experience positive outcomes compared to the average person. Researchers have also sought to understand the precise cognitive and affective processes that mediate perceptions of risk as well as examine such perceptions within a larger framework of decision theory or other conceptual models (e.g., Johnson & Tversky, 1983; Kahneman & Tversky, 1979, 1984; Slovic, 1987; Slovic, Fischoff, & Lichtenstein, 1978).

Much of the work in this area has been nomothetic, that is, has examined how most people, on the average, go about forming risk perceptions and the processes that mediate these perceptions. (For a notable exception, see Scheier & Carver, 1987). Although this approach has yielded many important insights, little work has examined the possibility that there might be relatively stable, individual differences in perceptions of vulnerability. For example, most of us know (or have heard about) people who seem to live in constant fear that something bad might happen to them or, alternatively, people who seem to believe that they are relatively invulnerable to these risks. To the extent that these stable differences indeed exist, it becomes important to understand (a) what sorts of psychological variables might be useful in predicting who does, and does not, feel vulnerable and (b) the psychological mechanisms that underlie these differences across individuals.

When we began our exploration of this "individual difference" issue in our own laboratory, we anticipated that at least two kinds of personality variables might play key roles in mediating perceptions of risk, namely, (a) belief in a just world (Lerner, 1980) and (b) right-wing authoritarianism (Adorno et al., 1950; Altemeyer, 1988). Why did we focus on these particular personality constructs? As we shall discuss in more detail shortly, careful consideration of the theoretical tenets of models of belief in a just world (BJW) and right wing authoritarianism (RWA) suggested that both constructs could play important roles in the perceptions of risk. Nevertheless, despite the plausible theoretical links between perceived risk and these constructs, we could find very little work that has examined these issues empirically. A major goal of our work, therefore, has been to address this theoretical gap and, in so doing, gain greater insight into the role of BJW and RWA in moderating perceptions of risk and personal vulnerability. One provocative aspect of our work, which forms the centerpiece of the present chapter, is that individual differences in BJW and RWA appear to have *interactive*, rather than independent, effects on perceived risk. That is, although both variables play important roles in moderating these perceptions, we have found that neither variable is *in itself* a reliable predictor of perceptions of risk. Thus, by examining both variables in combination with each other, we have been able to predict with much greater success differences in perceived vulnerability across people than if either variable is examined in isolation.

The present chapter is organized into three main sections. In the first section, we briefly consider the main theoretical tenets of BJW and RWA, with particular emphasis on the role that each might play in perceptions of risk. In the second section, we describe some of the findings we have recently obtained in our laboratory and, in light of these results, present a working theoretical framework that specifies the role of BJW and RWA in perceptions of vulnerability and articulates the psychological processes underlying these effects. Finally, given the focus of the present volume on just world beliefs, we consider the broader implications of our results for current research and theory on just world, and the kinds of future directions that might be taken to address some of the issues raised by the findings we present here.

1. BELIEF IN A JUST WORLD AND PERCEPTIONS OF RISK

Because the basic assumptions underlying current models of BJW have been covered elsewhere in this volume, we shall only briefly summarize these here. The " just world hypothesis " (Lerner, 1965) was proposed, in part, to explain why people might blame victims (e.g., of rape) for their own misfortunes. In postulating this theory, Lerner has argued that "individuals have a need to believe that they live in a world where people generally get what they deserve" (Lerner & Miller, 1978; pp. 1030). According to this perspective, derogating the victim ("she deserved to be raped") serves to maintain one's underlying sense of justice by attributing negative qualities to the victim, thus bolstering a belief system in which favorable events happen to good people and unfavorable events happen to bad people. If one assumes that most people think of themselves in relatively favorable terms, BJW may be thought of as a kind of "psychological buffer", shielding the self (and other good people) from the potentially threatening elements in the environment.

To the extent that there are individual differences in people's tendencies to personally believe in a just world, the degree to which these "buffering " effects arise should presumably depend on whether people are high or low in BJW. In fact, a growing body of research has shown that people who believe in a just world are (a) more likely to derogate victims, (b) have higher levels of subjective well being and positive affect, and (c) cope more effectively with stressful events than people who do not believe in a just world (e.g., Bullman & Wortman, 1977; Dalbert, 1993; Lerner & Somers, 1992; Tomaka & Blascovich, 1994). It is important to note that there is currently some disagreement over the (multi)dimensionality of BJW and researchers have proposed different instruments designed to measure such beliefs (Rubin & Peplau, 1975; Dalbert & Yamauchi, 1994; Lipkus, 1991, Lipkus & Siegler,1995; Lipkus, Dalbert, & Siegler, 1996; for a related discussion, see Lipkus, this volume). In the research we describe in the present chapter, we have used the older Rubin and Peplau (1975) scale as well as a more recent instrument derived from a recent scale developed by Dalbert and her colleagues (Dalbert & Yamauchi, 1994; Lipkus, Dalbert, & Siegler (1996). Although there are some important differences that distinguish these measures of BJW from one another (cf. Lipkus et al., 1996 for a relevant discussion), we find in our own work, at least, that both scales reveal essentially similar findings in regards to perceived risk. However, because we find that the newer scale by Dalbert and her colleagues yields consistently higher reliabilities than the Rubin and Peplau (1975) scale, we restrict our attention in this chapter to the former measure.

If it is true that belief in a just world serves the general sort of "buffering" role articulated above, then it may also be the case that perceptions of risk are generally lower for people who believe in a just world compared to people who do not. Thus, for example, when individuals are asked to estimate the probability that something bad will happen to the self (e.g., get hit by lightning) people who are high in BJW should, all else being equal, feel less at risk compared to people who are low. Somewhat surprisingly, however, we were unable to find any research that has examined this possibility directly.

Although the relation between BJW and perceptions of vulnerability to negative events has yet to be explored empirically, a recent study by Tomaka & Blascovich (1994) generated some support for this notion. Briefly, these researchers found that when participants were asked to perform a potentially stressful laboratory task, persons high in BJW experienced less stressful reactions than persons low in BJW, and this was true with respect to self-report as well as physiological measures. It is important to note that the Tomaka and Blascovich (1994) investigation (which was concerned with responses to a stressful task) is rather different than the present article, which is concerned with the subjective likelihood of negative events happening to the self. Nevertheless, such findings are consistent with our general assumption that BJW acts as a kind of psychological buffer for the self and, hence, bolstered our confidence in the idea that this construct might moderate perceptions of risk and subjective vulnerability to general threats from the environment.

2. RIGHT-WING AUTHORITARIANISM AND PERCEPTIONS OF RISK

The construct of authoritarianism was originally developed by Adorno et al. (1950) in order to explain why certain people might be more prejudiced than others. At the core of Adorno's argument was the idea that some types of persons tend to view their world with a certain moral rigidity, rewarding those who uphold old-fashioned, conventional behavior and punishing others who are perceived as violating these norms. Although the concept of authoritarianism received a great deal of attention among social and personality psychologists, the original measure of authoritarianism (the F scale) has been strongly criticized on a number of psychometric grounds (for a review, see Christie, 1991). In recent years, however, Altemeyer (1988) has proposed a balanced 30-item measure that appears to have corrected many of the problems characteristic of the original scale and is regarded as " the best current measure of the essence of what the authors of the *Authoritarian Personality* were attempting to measure " (Christe, 1991, p. 522). Moreover, there appears to be renewed interest in RWA as a way of predicting individual differences in people's behaviors across a variety of domains, including attitudes towards minority groups (e.g., Peterson, Doty, & Winter, 1993; Lambert & Chasteen, 1996) and the sorts of allocation decisions that people make about AIDS victims (Skitka & Tetlock, 1992).

At first blush, the construct of authoritarianism would seem to have little, if any, relation to perceived risk. Indeed, the construct has been used primarily to predict the kinds of reactions that people have towards others (especially members of racial and ethnic minority groups) and we are not aware of any published work that examines the role of RWA in moderating perceptions of risk. Nevertheless, careful scrutiny of the *theoretical* underpinnings of RWA suggests that this personality construct could, in fact, play this sort of moderating role. In his recent book *Enemies of Freedom*, Altemeyer (1988) has briefly discussed the possible role of RWA in this regard and briefly alludes to some (unpublished) findings that bear on these considerations:

Both authoritarian students and parents are...more afraid of becoming the victims of terrorist attacks, automobile accidents, and contracting AIDS through blood transfusions, food preparation, drinking fountains, and so on. The correlation between authoritarianism and any of these fears is usually low, about .20. *But overall, Highs perceive the world as a significantly more dangerous place than others do* (Altemeyer, 1988, p. 147; emphasis added).

Why might authoritarians tend to view the world as a risky, dangerous place? Although we are not aware of any developmental data that speak to this point directly, Altemeyer (1988) has speculated that authoritarianism may arise, in part, in response to parental warnings that the world is a dangerous place and that strict laws and codes of moral conduct are needed to impose order and keep these malevolent forces at bay. This defensive reaction to perceived threat is seen also in the earlier writings of Adorno et al. (1950), although their framing of threat and perceptions of danger were couched in more psychodynamic terms. In particular, authoritarianism was thought to serve an ego-defensive function wherein rules and moral guidelines (e.g., "nudist camps are wrong") develop in response to the emergence of unacceptable id impulses rather than through parental warnings per se. Setting aside these theoretical differences (which are not of central concern here), the general point being made by both Adorno et al. and Altemeyer is that authoritarians tend to view the world as a dangerous, threatening place and that their belief system represents an attempt to impose order on these threatening elements.

3. JUST WORLD BELIEFS AND RIGHT-WING AUTHORITARIANISM COMPARED

The reader may have already noted some interesting similarities among the two personality constructs reviewed above. For one thing, previous research has found that BJW and RWA tend to be positively correlated, although the magnitude of this relation is often quite modest (in the .10 to .30 range); we find correlations of similar magnitude in our own work. Thus, although there is a slight tendency for people who believe in a just world to also score high in authoritarianism, being high on one dimension does not preclude one from scoring low in the other and vice versa. In addition, the two constructs are both associated with a tendency to be punitive of others, although the reasons for this punitiveness (and the likely targets of this punishment) may actually be quite different. For example, persons high in RWA tend to be generally punitive toward stigmatized persons (e.g., gays), regardless of whether these persons have experienced any misfortune or not. On the other hand, the "blaming" effects characteristic of people scoring high in BJW appear to be a more general response to hearing about the misfortunes of others, independent of whether the person, or the cause of the misfortune itself, is stigmatized per se.

As for their effects on perceived risk, BJW and RWA could, in principle, have either independent or interactive effects. Evidence for an independent effect would manifest itself simply as strong correlations between BJW and/or RWA and perceived risk, in which the relation between BJW and risk does not depend on whether people were relatively high vs. low in RWA and vice versa. Interestingly enough, the considerations raised above suggest that although BJW and RWA are weakly positively related to each other, they ought to be related in *opposite* ways to perceived risk. In particular, although BJW should be negatively correlated with perceived risk, RWA should be positively correlated with such perceptions.

The other possibility is that BJW and RWA could have interactive, rather than independent, effects on perceived risk. This would imply that the effects of BJW on perceived risk would depend, in turn on whether people were relatively high or low in authoritarianism and vice versa. In considering this latter possibility, it is worth noting that one construct (RWA) is theoretically linked to *general* perceptions of whether the world is a threatening place or not (*external threat component*) and the other variable (BJW) is linked to whether the self feels *personally* at risk for these threats (*personal buffer component*). A moment's reflection suggests that BJW should play a greater role in mediating personal vulnerability precisely when these "worldly" risks are most acute, that is, for high authoritarians. On the other hand, if the world is viewed in relatively safe terms (a state of affairs which should be true for low authoritarians), it could be the case that the presence or absence of a personal buffer—and, hence, one's level of BJW—would not play such a critical role in this case. Our research was designed, in part, to explore the viability of these different predictions.

4. TWO EMPIRICAL INVESTIGATIONS

Given the paucity of empirical work in this area, one of our main goals—at least in the beginning stages of our work—was to make the obviously important leap from theory to data and explore the empirical relation between the three main theoretical constructs at hand here, namely, BJW, RWA, and perceived risk. In our initial efforts, therefore, we (Lambert, Burroughs, & Ngyuen, 1996; Experiment 1) relied on a relatively simple methodological paradigm. Specifically, we first brought participants into our laboratory (N = 40) and measured individual differences in both RWA and BJW. The former construct was measured using Altemeyer's balanced RWA scale, which asks participants' personal agreement with a series of 30 statements (e.g., *It is always better to trust the judgment of proper authorities in government and religion than to listen to noisy rabbble-rousers in our society who are trying to create doubt in people's mind.*) Consistent with previous work by Altemeyer (1988), we find the RWA to have an excellent internal reliability, typically in the low .90s. For BJW, we used an 18-item measure of BJW derived from recent work by Dalbert and Yamauchi (1994) which presents participants with a series of statements (e.g., *I usually get what I deserve*) and asks them to indicate their relative agreement or disagreement with it. As in the case of RWA, we find this scale to have excellent levels of reliability (above .90).[1]

Two months later, participants were asked to participate in an ostensibly unrelated study. (In all cases, both the experimenter as well as the physical location of this latter experimental session was different from that of the earlier session.) In this latter session, participants were asked to complete a "Perception of Risk Scale," in which they provided probability estimates that 34 different types of negative events might happen to the self along a scale from 0% (no chance this would ever happen to me) to 100% (certain to happen to me). These events varied from life-threatening calamities (*get hit by lightning, contract AIDS*) to relatively mundane events (*lose one's wallet, catch cold*). In our research, we find that BJW and RWA reliably moderate only life-threatening, but not mundane, levels of risk. In the present chapter, therefore, we concentrate only on the former type of risk estimate.

A few observations on these sorts of severe risks are necessary before proceeding further. First, we have found that these perceived risks tend to be highly correlated with one another. Thus, the same people who feel relatively at risk for one event (e.g., getting hit by lightning) are the same people who feel at risk for another (e.g., dying of leukemia). Indeed, in our research we repeatedly find one primary "severe risk" factor to emerge out of principal component analyses on which the following specific estimates of risk load highly on the same factor: (*getting hit by lightning, dying in a flood, getting hit by a tornado, dying in a plane crash, getting hijacked, dying of hepatitis, dying of leukemia, contracting AIDS.*) (In the present study we report analyses for all of these risks separately as well as on an average across all 8 risks; alpha = .92). Although we of course do not claim that these represent an exhaustive list of all possible life-threatening events facing students, these appear to be a reasonable assortment of such risks. Finally, as one might expect, the distribution of probabilities for these events tend to be highly positively skewed, indicating that most, although not all, students view these events as relatively unlikely. Hence, we always

[1] The 18-item measure described here consists of items referring to beliefs about justice as they apply both to the self as well as to others in general. In our research we find very similar findings regardless of whether we focus on either the self or other-related beliefs about justice and thus our measure of BJW is based on the average across all 18 items.)

subject these estimates to log transformations and then convert these values to z-scores before analyzing further.

The question of primary theoretical interest concerned the relation between these perceptions of risk and individual differences in BJW and RWA. As we had noted earlier, BJW and RWA could, in principle, have either independent or interactive effects on perceived risk. Preliminary analyses revealed that neither variable was, in itself, a particularly good predictor of perceived risk. On the one hand, it was true that BJW and RWA were indeed related in opposite ways to perceived risk. However, the magnitude of these effects was not very impressive. Averaging across all 8 types of risk, BJW was correlated −.25 (p > .10) with perceived risk, indicating a modest tendency for people high in BJW to perceive that life-threatening events are less likely to happen to them compared to people low in BJW. In contrast, there was a slight tendency for RWA to be positively correlated with perceived risk, although the magnitude of this effect (r = .13) was trivial.

Although these data give some hint that BJW, at least, was related to perceived risk, further analyses showed that the strength of this relationship was strongly contingent on whether people were relatively high or low in RWA. The simplest way of showing this effect is to examine the relation between BJW and perceived risk separately for participants who were high vs. low in RWA (as discerned on the basis of a median split of this latter variable). The pattern of correlations corresponding to this analysis is shown in Table 1. Here we show perceptions of risk for the overall composite as well as the 8 specific risks to show the generalizability of our effects.

TABLE 1. Experiment One

Risk	Correlation between BJW and RWA with perceived risk (all participants)		Correlation between BJW and perceived risk (authoritarians only)	
	BJW	RWA	High[a]	Low[a]
Average of all risks	−.26	.10	−.57***	.06
Lightning	−.10	.10	−.26	.04
Floods	−.19	.17	−.34	−.02
Tornadoes	−.25	.18	−.54***	.15
Plane crash	.25	.18	−.54***	.12
Hijacking	−.17	−.03	−.41***	.08
Hepatitis	−.23	−.01	−.59***	.20
AIDS	−.29	.06	.43*	−.12
Leukemia	−.19	.09	−.35	−.04

Note: Correlations represent relation between individual differences in just world beliefs (BJW) and authoritarianism RWA with risk.
[a]"High" and "Low" refer to high authoritarians and low authoritarians, respectively.
*p < .10; **p < .05; ***p < .01

This table shows that, overall, BJW was strongly and negatively correlated with perceived risk among high authoritarians but BJW and perceived risk were literally uncorrelated when participants were low in RWA. (Supplemental analyses showed that this asymmetry was not due to differences in either the mean or standard deviation of BJW across these two conditions.) Furthermore, regression analyses revealed that these two corelations were significantly different from one another (p < .05), although the BJW × RWA interaction term in the relevant regression did not quite reach conventional levels of significance (p = .09). This shows, therefore, that people high in BJW view the world as a much less risky place than people who are low, but this was true only among high authoritarans. When people are low in authoritarianism, BJW showed no relation to perceived risk at all. Another way of looking at these findings is shown in Figure 1, which shows the regression of BJW on perceived risk for high vs. low authortarians.

4.1. A Working Theoretical Framework

How can these provocative results be explained? At this point, we present the outline of a working model that provides a possible conceptualization of these results. Following this, we present some findings that replicate and extend the implications of the first preliminary investigation.

As we had noted earlier, one way of conceptualizing perceived risk is in terms of two components, namely, (a) the extent to which one gener-

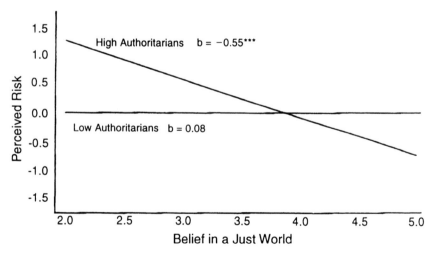

FIGURE 1.   Regression of belief in a just world on perceived risk for high vs. low authoritarians.

ally views the environment in relatively safe vs. threatening terms (*external threat component*), and (b) the extent to which one does, or does not, feel personally buffered from these potential threats (*personal buffer* component). Theoretically, RWA is primarily associated with the first "safety vs. threat" component, such that authoritarians generally tend to see the world in more threatening terms than non-authoritarians. Theoretically, BJW is primarily associated with the second, personal buffer component, such that people high in BJW feel less personally vulnerable to threat than people who are low.

If these assumptions have merit, then one may posit a straightforward model (depicted in Figure 2) which shows how these components are likely to act in combination with each other. We should mention at the outset that this model provides a highly schematic, simplified account of perceived risk and in no way is meant to capture all of the complexities of the processes underlying perceptions of risk. Nevertheless, we believe that it presents a heuristically useful summary of how BJW and RWA might act together to moderate perceived risk. As one can see in Figure 2, the first consideration is whether the perceiver feels relatively safe or threatened at the time of judgment. If one feels relatively safe, then perceived risk should naturally be low. Although this is not surprising in itself, it points out that the presence or absence of a personal buffer should not make a difference under this condition. On the other hand, if there is a high "baseline" level of potential threat (i.e., the perceiver generally views the world as threatening) then the extent to which the perceiver *does* feel personally threatened should indeed depend on the presence or absence of a personal buffer (i.e., a sense that the self is personally protected from the threatening elements of the environment).

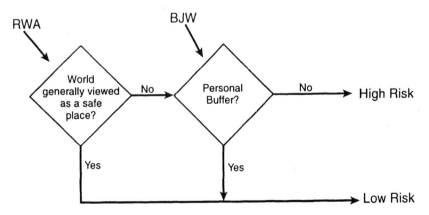

FIGURE 2. Theoretical roles of RWA (right wing authoritarianism) and BJW (belief in a just world) on perceived risk.

According to our model, the extent to which people view the world in threatening terms is determined, in part, by one's level of RWA and the extent to which one feels *personally* buffered by these threats is driven by BJW. We should note that we make no claims as to the exclusive role of either RWA or BJW in these considerations. That is, it seems reasonable to suppose that more than one kind of variable (other than RWA) could drive one's view of the world as a threatening place and, similarly, that BJW would not be the only variable that could act as a psychological buffer. (Toward the end of this chapter we discuss some likely candidates in this regard.) For present purposes, we assume only that RWA and BJW represent *two examples* of personality traits that could play the kind of interactive role depicted in Figure 2.

Readers familiar with the social support literature may have noted some overlap between the theoretical framework presented in Figure 2 and the assumptions underlying the "buffering hypothesis" postulated by Cohen and Wills (1985; see also Stroebe & Stroebe, 1995). Specifically, Cohen and Wills (1985) have argued that the presence or absence of a social support network should have an effect on well-being only under high levels of stress. In such cases, well-being should be greater among people who have high rather than low levels of social support. However, the presence or absence of a social support network should make less of a difference when stress is low. We are making an essentially similar argument in this domain. Specifically, the presence or absence of a psychological buffer (BJW) should make a difference in perceived risk only when stress is high (true of people high in RWA) than when it is low.

4.2. An Additional Test

Although we feel that the model presented in Figure 2 provides a reasonable account of our initial findings, one shortcoming of that earlier study is the failure to obtain a statistically significant RWA X BJW interaction, which is implied directly by this model. Thus, we (Lambert et al., 1996, Experiment 2) sought to gather additional support for our arguments by replicating and extending our earlier findings with a much larger sample size (N = 93). As before, we measured individual differences in BJW and RWA and, two months later, measured people's perceived risk to the same series of life-threatening events described earlier. In order to further understand the different roles of BJW and RWA in perceptions of risk, the risk estimate task was preceded by an ostensibly unrelated experiment in which participants either were, or were not, asked to read an newspaper article about the death of a fellow college student to AIDS. Importantly, the exact reason why the person contracted AIDS was deliberately left ambiguous, leaving it open (for example) as to whether he was heterosexual or homosexual.[2]

The primary reason for this manipulation was to explore the boundary conditions of the relation of BJW and RWA to perceived risk and, in particular, whether this relation would hold across conditions of high vs. low threat. On a priori grounds, two possibilities presented themselves. On the one hand, it could be that the dual effects of BJW and RWA had in moderating perceptions of risk (cf. Figure 2) represent a relatively stable, enduring process that holds regardless of whether the self had recently been primed with threatening information. On the other hand, it could be that the strength of the moderating effect of BJW and RWA would be augmented (or changed in some other way) through recent exposure to threatening stimuli in the environment. The analytic approach for this investigation was similar to the previous investigation, except that we explored the relation the role of BJW and RWA in moderating risk for (a) the combined sample of participants, collapsed over the type of prior article read, (b) those participants who had read the control passage and (c) those participants who had read the AIDS article.

The overall pattern of findings were similar to that of the first study. Collapsed over prime type, hierarchical regression analyses performed on the overall risk composite revealed the predicted BJW x RWA interaction ($p < .01$) with no significant main effect of either BJW or RWA. This interaction was due to the fact that a significant negative correlation emerged between BJW and perceived risk among high authoritarians ($r = -.36$, $p < .01$) but not among low authoritarians ($r = .18$, ns). Again, this shows that among high authoritarians, BJW moderated risk such that persons high in just world beliefs estimated that a number of life-threatening risks were less likely to occur to them compared to people low in just world beliefs. However, this relation disappeared (and, if anything, was slightly reversed) among low authoritarians.

Supplemental analyses revealed a similar contingency across the two levels of the priming manipulation. Among high authoritarians, BJW was negatively correlated with perceived risk, regardless of whether partici-

---

[2] We chose to present our participants with information about an AIDS-related death (as opposed to some other cause of death) for two reasons. First, we knew of few issues that can represent the level of threat posed by AIDS, especially for college-age students, many of whom are either sexually active or at least considering such activity in the near future. Second, Altemeyer's work on RWA led us to believe that the tendency for authoritarians to generally perceive higher levels of threat might be driven by a more specific fear of (what authoritarians perceive to be) immoral or deviant behavior on the part of others and the threat posed by AIDS victims in either a direct sense (e.g., through contamination of the blood supply or through the infection of others) or though the more "symbolic" threat to one's sense of old-fashioned values.

pants had earlier been exposed to the AIDS target or not (rs = −.35 vs. −.38). Among low authoritarians, this negative relation completely disappeared, and this was true in both the AIDS prime condition (r = −.02) as well as the control condition, in which the relation between BJW and risk was actually reversed (r = .31). Although it is not entirely clear why BJW would be *positively* correlated with perceived risk among low authoritarians (at least in the control condition), the most important implication of these findings is that they replicate the general picture emerging from the first investigation, which showed that BJW acts as a personal buffer with respect to perceived risk for high, but not low, authoritarians.

This is not to say, however, that the presentation of the AIDS article had no effects on perceived risk. Another way of analyzing perceived risk is in terms of the *mean* level of perceived risk across experimental conditions (which is not readily apparent from the regression analyses presented above). For all participants, presentation of the AIDS article produced a sort of "global defensiveness" effect such that overall perceived risk was lower (not only for AIDS, but for all risks) if participants had recently read about the death of a college student to AIDS than if they had not. This effect is generally consistent with the tendency for most people to respond with a certain degree of defensiveness and self-servingness in order to maintain their sense of well-being by (for example) dissociating themselves from the plight of others, especially stigmatized others (cf. Taylor & Brown, 1988). The observant reader may have already noted, however, that there ought to be one notable exception to this global defensiveness effect. Specifically, our working model (cf. Figure 2) suggests that one specific "type" of person—those high in RWA, but low in BJW—ought to show a pronounced *absence* of such defensiveness effects. This is because such individuals are especially fearful of such threats and, moreover, lack a personal buffer to protect the self. This is generally what we found. Specifically, unlike other individuals, such persons were the only group that showed a general *increase* (rather than decrease) in perceived risk in the AIDS condition compared to the control condition. This pattern is consistent with our general framework, which suggests that the combination of being high in RWA (high threat component) but low in BJW (low buffer) would leave one especially vulnerable to the impact of a potentially threatening information (such as hearing about the recent death of a college student) on general feelings of risk.

5. LOOKING AHEAD: THEORETICAL IMPLICATIONS AND ISSUES TO BE ADDRESSED IN FUTURE WORK

When we asked undergraduates about their perceived risk of life-threatening events happening to the self, the results of two experiments showed that these estimates depended on the joint influence of individual differences in both BJW and RWA. Although neither variable alone is particularly good at predicting estimates of risk, knowing information about the person's standing on both variables yielded considerably more leverage. In particular, when people were relatively high in authoritarianism, BJW strongly moderated risk such these perceptions were much lower if people believed in a just world than if they did not. In contrast, BJW was not reliably related to risk among low authoritarians. On a theoretical level, these findings are consistent with a model (Figure 2) in which perceived risk is conceptualized in terms of two components (underlying threat, personal buffer) wherein RWA is primarily associated with the first component and BJW is associated with the second.

It goes without saying, of course, that the present results hardly constitute a definitive statement on the role of BJW and RWA in perceived risk. Additional theoretical and empirical work is obviously needed to address some important questions left unanswered by the work presented above. In the space below, we consider some of the issues and questions that arise out of the present findings and offer some suggestions in terms of how these questions might be profitably addressed in future work.

5.1. Single versus Dual Influence Models of Perceived Risk

One of the more provocative aspect of our model is that it suggests that the processes underlying subjective risk can be decomposed in terms of two components, namely external threat and personal buffer. From the standpoint of parsimony, one might wonder if a single-influence "optimism" model would be preferable. For example, an alternate conceptualization of perceived risk is that people who score high in dispositional optimism (cf. Carver & Scheier, 1987) generally feel lower at risk. Such a model is obviously simpler in that it does not require one to make the distinction (central to the proposed model here) between "external threat" and personal buffer. Such an alternative model would, instead merely assume that certain people generally view all aspects of the environment (including the self) in more optimistic terms than others.

Although this alternative model is attractive in its simplicity, it would seem to have difficulty accounting for the findings we have reported in this chapter. For one thing, it suggests that measures that tap general optimism (as would presumably be the case for BJW) would predict perceived risk in its own right, but this clearly did not happen, at least for the kinds of life-threatening risks we focused on. We should also note that on a priori grounds, it seems useful to distinguish one's view of the external environment (and whether there are potential threats arising from it) and whether the self is ultimately protected from such threats. Relatedly, unlike a single influence model (which assumes that people generally view all elements of their environment in either optimistic or pessimistic terms) the kind of dual-influence model proposed in this chapter leaves room for a disparity between one's appraisal of one's surroundings (threatening or not) and one's appraisal of personal susceptibility to these dangers (buffered or not).

5.2. Aren't There Other Personality Variables (Aside from BJW and RWA) That Could Moderate Risk?

As we noted earlier, it would be foolish to assume that BJW and RWA are the only variables that would moderate perceptions of risk. Indeed, our model suggests that to the extent that other variables might drive one's underlying sense of safety vs. threat or, alternatively, a relatively strong vs. weak personal buffer, these other variables should moderate risk as well. For example, the observant reader may have already noted that RWA plays a role in this model only to the extent that this variable is indeed linked to the underlying threat of the environment. Our model suggests, therefore, that one should get similar findings with a more direct measure of perceived threat, such as might be obtained in a measure of chronic worry or anxiety.

Finally, there are at least two measures of "chronic optimism" that have been proposed in the literature, namely, the construct of hardiness (Kobasa, 1979) and a measure of dispositional optimism developed by Scheier and Carver (1987). Both constructs theoretically tap people's ability to withstand stress and cope with negative events in a more effective manner, although recent theorists (e.g., Watson & Pennebaker, 1989) have argued that the effects of both hardiness as well as dispositional optimism are actually due to the fact that both measures tap differences in negative affect (NA), and that the effects of both constructs disappear once NA is controlled for. Be that as it may, our current work is aimed at understanding the relation among BJW and RWA with hardiness, optimism, and NA in order to gain further insight into chronic differences in perceived risk.

5.3. Are There Any Conditions under Which BJW Moderates Perceived Risk Independent of Other Personality Variables?

Another provocative aspects of our findings is that BJW seems to reliably predict risk only under certain boundary conditions, namely, when people are high in authoritarianism. This naturally raises the question of whether the processes mediating other "types" of risk judgments might be somewhat different. In this regard, it is important to acknowledge that the research discussed in this chapter focused on a relatively narrow type of perceived risk, namely, probability estimates of severe or life-threatening events. Although we feel we have a reasonably good understanding of how BJW plays a role in this particular setting, it is equally important to understand how BJW might play different roles in other types of risk estimates.

In fact, some of our recent work (Chasteen, Smith, & Lambert, 1996) has looked at the role of BJW in a more circumscribed domain, namely, the role of this variable in moderating people's general level of optimism about their own aging process. In this research, we ask people to indicate their general level of optimism vs. pessimism regarding their own old age (e.g., "I feel optimistic about getting older" or "I have to admit that I dread getting older because my physical appearance will change"). We find that people are significantly more favorable in their appraisals of their aging process if they are high in BJW than if they are not. More importantly for present purposes, such effects are not contingent on RWA (nor does RWA moderate risk in it own right).

This obviously raises the question of why BJW would be contingent on RWA for one type of risk assessment (the probability of life-threatening risks happening to the self) but not another (general appraisals of the quality of life as a senior citizen). Although purely speculative, one possibility is that the component of external threat should tend to play a role only insofar as the type of risk under consideration is strongly tied to factors that are believed to be *outside* one's control, either because they are due to sheer chance (e.g., getting hit by lightning) or through the malevolence of others (e.g., getting hijacked). For these types of events, variables such as RWA play a role insofar as they can predict what sorts of people typically see the external world as threatening. On the other hand, people may view the quality of life in later years as more under their control and, hence, the question of whether the world is seen as a threatening place might play a somewhat more minor role. At this point, however, this line of reasoning remains highly speculative and one of our overriding goals in our future work is to gain a better understanding of the various processes underlying perceptions of self vulnerability and the possibly different role of BJW across these different substantive and methodological domains.

6. CONCLUDING COMMENTS

In a recent review of the literature on BJW, Furnham and Procter (1989) noted that research on BJW has gone through three distinct stages, including (a) initial recognition of the phenomenon and its test in laboratory settings, (b) development and validation of individual difference measures, and (c) examination of the multidimensionality of the individual difference measure and a more general examination of the original construct. Although current research has unquestionably entered the third stage (cf. Lipkus et al., 1996) we would modestly venture to suggest the possibility of an additional stage that we see being developed in the recent work on BJW. This would be the extension of research into conceptual/methodological domains that were not originally envisioned in the original formulation of the construct. We believe that such extensions often leads to a greater understanding of the construct and its implications for social thought and behavior. We see the recent work by Tomaka and Blascovich (1994) as a particularly provocative example of this movement, as they consider the role of BJW in moderating physiological reactions to stress. It is our hope that the present chapter adds something valuable to these sorts of recent extensions and will spark further investigation of the role of just world beliefs (either on its own, or in combination with other variables) in people's subjective understanding of their world and their reactions to it.

ACKNOWLEDGMENTS

We wish to thank Mike Strube, Scott Madey, and Bruce Friedman for their helpful comments on an earlier draft.

REFERENCES

Adorno, T.W., Frenkel-Brunswick, E., Levinson, D. J., & Sanford, R. N. (1950). The authoritarian personality. New York: Harper & Row.
Altemeyer, R. (1988). Enemies of Freedom: Understanding right-wing authoritarianism. San Francisco: Joessy-Bass
Chasteen, A. L. Smith, C., & Lambert, A. J. (1996). Attitudes towards the elderly and about getting old: The role of gender and belief in a just world. Unpublished manuscript.
Christie, R. (1991). Authoritarianism and related constructs. In J. P. Robinson, P. R. Shaver, & L. S. Wrightsman (Eds.), Measures of personality and social psychology attitudes (pp. 501–571). San Diego, CA: Academic Press.
Dalbert, C. (1993). Gefährdung des Wohlbefindens durch Arbeitsplatzunsicherheit: Eine Analyse der Einflußfaktoren Selbstwert und Gerechte-Welte-Glaube. Zeitschrift fur Gesundheitpsychologie 4, 294–310.
Dalbert, C. & Yamauchi, L. A. (1994). Belief in a just world and attitudes towards immigrants and foreign workers: A cultural comparison between Hawaii and Germany. Journal of Applies Social Psychology, 24, 1612–1626.
Furnham, A., & Procter, E. (1989). Belief in a just world: Review and critique of the individual difference literature. British Journal of Social Psychology, 28, 365–384.
Johnson, E., & Tversky, A. (1983). Affect, generalization, and the perception of risk. Journal of Personality and Social Psychology, 45, 20–31.
Kahneman, D., & Tversky, A. (1979). Prospect Theory. Econometrica, 47, 263–291.
Kahneman, D., & Tversky, A. (1984). Choices, values, and frames. American Psychologist, 39, 341–350.
Kobasa, S. C. (1979). Stressful life events, personality, and health: An inquiry into hardiness. Journal of Personality and Social Psychology, 37, 1–11.

Lambert, A. J., & Chasteen, A. L. (1996). Perceptions of deviance vs. disadvantage: political values and prejudice toward the elderly vs. Blacks. Manuscript submitted for publication.

Lambert, A. J., Burroughs, T., & Nguyen, T. Exploring the interface between perceptions of self vulnerability and prejudice: Belief in a just world and right-wing authoritarianism. Manuscript submitted for publication.

Lerner, M. J. (1965). Evaluation of performance as a function of performer's reward and attractiveness. Journal of Personality and Social Psychology, 1, 355–360.

Lerner, M. J., & Miller, D. T. (1978). Just world research and the attribution process: Looking back and ahead. Psychological Bulletin, 85, 1030–1050.

Lerner, M. J. (1980). The belief in a just world: A fundamental delusion. New York: Plenum.

Lerner, M. J., & Somers, D. G. (1992). Employees' reactions to an anticipated plant closure: The influence of positive illusions. In L. Montada, S. H. Filipp, & M. Lerner (Eds.) Critical life events and the experience of loss in adulthood. (pp. 229–253). Hillsdale, NJ: Erlbaum.

Lipkus, I. M. (1991). The construction and preliminary validation of a global belief in a just world scale and the exploratory analysis of the multidimensional belief in a just world scale. Personality and Individual Differences, 12, 1171–1178.

Lipkus, I. M., Dalbert, C., & Siegler, I. C. (1996) The importance of distinguishing the belief in a just world for self versus others: Implications for psychological well-being. Manuscript under review.

Lipkus, I. M., & Siegler, I. C. (1995). Do comparative self-appraisals during young adulthood predict adult personality? Psychology and Aging, 10, 229–237.

Peterson, B. E., Doty, R. M., & Winter, D. G. (1993). Authoritarianism and attitudes towards contemporary social issues. Personality and Social Psychology Bulletin, 19, 174–184.

Rosenberg, M. (1965). Society and the adolescent self-image. Princeton, NJ: Princeton University Press.

Rubin, Z., & Peplau, L.. A. (1975). Who believes in a just world? Journal of Social Issues, 31, 65–90.

Scheier, M. F., & Carver, C. S. (1987). Dispositional optimism and physical well-being: The influence of generalized outcome expectancies on health. Journal of Personality, 55, 169–210.

Skitka, L. J. & Tetlock, P. E. (1992). Allocating scarce resources: A contingency model of distributive justice. Journal of Experimental Social Psychology, 28, 33–37.

Slovic, P. (1987). Perceptions of risk. Science. 236, 280–285.

Slovic, P., Fischoff, B., & Lichtenstein, S. (1982) Response mode, framing, and information processing effects in risk assessment. In R. Hogarth (Ed.) New directions for methodology of social and behavioral science: Question framing and response consistency. (pp. 21–36). San Francisco: Jossey Bass.

Taylor, S. E., & Brown, J. D. (1988). Illusions and well-being: A social psychological perspective on mental health. Psychological Bulletin, 103, 193–210.

Tomaka, J. & Blascovich, J. (1994). Effects of justice beliefs on cognitive appraisal of subjective, physiological, and behavioral responses to potential stress. Journal of Personality and Social Psychology, 67, 732–740.

Watson, D. & Pennebaker J. W. (1989). Health complaints, stress, and distress: Exploring the central role of negative affectivity. Psychological Review, 6, 234–254.

Weinstein, N. D. (1980). Unrealistic optimism about future life events. Journal of Personality and Social Psychology, 39, 806–820.

Weinstein, N. D. (1982). Unrealistic optimism about susceptibility to health problems. Journal of Behavioral Medicine, 5, 441–460.

Chapter 8

The Belief in a Just World and Willingness to Accommodate among Married and Dating Couples

ISAAC M. LIPKUS[1] and VICTOR BISSONNETTE

Since the mid 1960s, the effects of individual differences in one's *Belief in a Just World* (BJW; Lerner, 1980; Lerner & Miller, 1978; Rubin & Peplau, 1975) has been applied to various domains. One area that seems particularly promising is the understanding of how the BJW might be related to a number of important indicators of relationship functioning and well-being. In this chapter, we will review some preliminary findings that have been obtained from samples of married and dating couples relating the BJW to one style of handling interpersonal conflict, willingness to accommodate.

---

[1] Data collected for the younger married and dating couples was collected while the first author was at the University of Wisconsin, Whitewater. All correspondence regarding this chapter should be addressed to Isaac Lipkus, Duke University Medical Center, Box 2949, Durham, NC 27705.

ISAAC M. LIPKUS • Duke University Medical Center, Box 2949, Durham, North Carolina 27710. VICTOR BISSONNETTE • Southeastern Louisiana University, Box 401, Hammond, Louisiana 70402.

Responses to Victimizations and Belief in a Just World, edited by Montada and Lerner. Plenum Press, New York, 1998.

1. THE BELIEF IN A JUST WORLD AND WILLINGNESS TO ACCOMMODATE

No matter how well relationship partners get along with each other, from time to time they manage to hurt each others' feelings by behaving in a way that is destructive to the relationship (e.g., by being selfish or rude, by ignoring the other partner, by raising one's voice, etc.). When one relationship partner behaves poorly, the second partner must decide how to behave *in response* to the first partner's negative behavior. We are interested in understanding how the BJW might influence this decision.

Rusbult and her colleagues (Rusbult, Zembrodt, & Gunn, 1982; Rusbult & Verette, 1991; Rusbult, Verette, Whitney, Slovik, & Lipkus, 1991) have suggested that one might respond to their partner's potentially destructive behavior in one of four ways:

1. *Exit:* Actively harming the relationship by leaving, by threatening to leave, or by being abusive toward one's partner (e.g., yelling or hitting).
2. *Voice:* Actively trying to improve the relationship by constructively discussing problems in the relationship and suggesting solutions to these problems, or finding other ways (e.g., therapy or discussion) to make positive changes in the relationship.
3. *Loyalty:* Patiently waiting for things to improve (e.g., praying for better moments).
4. *Neglect:* Ignoring or avoiding the partner, or any other behavior that prevents discussing problems and finding solutions (e.g., sulking).

Based on this scheme, *Exit* and *Neglect* represent relatively destructive reactions to a partner's negative behavior, whereas *Voice* and *Loyalty* represent relatively constructive reactions to a partner's poor behavior.

Research on married and dating couples have consistently demonstrated that the survival and welfare of intimate relationships depend on relationship partners' willingness to: a) respond to each others' negative behavior constructively, and b) not respond to each others' negative behavior destructively (e.g., Billings, 1979; Gottman, 1994; Gottman & Levenson, 1992; Gottman, Markman & Notarius, 1977; Margolin & Wampold, 1981; Rusbult, Bissonnette, Arriaga, & Cox, 1995; Rusbult, Johnson, & Morrow, 1986). Rusbult and her colleagues have used the term, *accommodation*, to describe this strategy of choosing a constructive rather than a destructive response to a partner's negative behavior (Rusbult et al., 1991).

Although engaging in accommodation is beneficial to the relationship, it is not always one's first choice when deciding how to respond to a partner's negative behavior (Rusbult et al., 1991; Rusbult et al., 1995;

Yovetich & Rusbult, 1994). Rather, when faced with a partner's negative behavior, one typically experiences an initial "gut level" desire to reciprocate the partners potentially destructive behavior with *Exit* or *Neglect*. However, in many cases, the individual decides not to act out their initial reaction, but rather, to respond with *Voice* or *Loyalty*. Therefore, a discrepancy often emerges between an individual's initial and actual reaction to their partner's potentially destructive action (Yovetich & Rusbult, 1994).

Several authors have suggested that this discrepancy is partially a function of a prosocial *transformation of motivation* (Kelly & Thibaut, 1978; Yovetich & Rusbult, 1994). When faced with a partner's negative behaviors, the individual will often "implicitly or explicitly take account of broader considerations such as the long-term goals for the relationship, social norms, or knowledge of and concern for a partner's outcomes" while deciding how to respond (Yovetich & Rusbult, 1994, p. 12). In other words, the more an individual takes into account the broader consequences of their reaction to their partner's negative behavior, the more he or she is likely to "tone down" his or her initial reaction to respond destructively and instead respond constructively. Thus, willingness to accommodate involves a willingness to sacrifice for the good of the relationship—to forsake one's immediate self-interests in order to satisfy other long-term relationship goals (e.g., to maintain the relationship and to maintain the satisfaction level of both partners).

As we have argued elsewhere (Lipkus & Bissonnette, 1996), other "broader considerations" that may contribute to this prosocial transformation of motivation would include factors that are related to one's sense of justice in their world. A partner's negative behavior, in the absence of any reasonable justification for this behavior, may be perceived by the nonoffending partner as unjust (e.g., "I did not deserve to be treated that way."). We argue that an individual's perception of the unfairness and the severity of their partner's negative behavior may be affected by the person's own BJW. People with a strong BJW may be disinclined to attribute negative qualities to their partner's behavior under all but the most severe transgressions (Lerner, 1980, Lerner & Miller, 1978). These more benevolent attributions are likely to facilitate one's willingness to accommodate. Thus, people with a strong BJW should be more willing to accommodate. Furthermore, we suggest that there exist several important mediating variables relating the BJW to greater willingness to accommodate. Our research has focused on three potential mediating variables: perspective-taking, trust, and reciprocity of accommodation (Lipkus & Bissonnette, 1996).

Rusbult and her colleagues have argued that one's willingness to accommodate is partially a function of one's willingness to consider the offending partner's situation or point of view. They have found that individuals who exhibit higher levels of perspective-taking are more willing to accommodate (Rusbult et al., 1991). There is indirect evidence showing that individuals who have a stronger BJW exhibit a more other- and less self-centered orientation. For example, people with a stronger than a weaker BJW have been found to be more responsive to the needs of others (Bierhoff, Klein, & Kramp, 1991; Miller, 1977, experiment 1; Zuckerman, 1975), and the BJW has been shown to be a component of the "altruistic personality" (Bierhoff, Klein, & Kramp, 1991). These results suggest that individuals with a strong BJW should exhibit relatively higher levels of perspective-taking than individuals with a weaker BJW. If strong believers in a just world are more likely to consider their partner's perspective, we should expect them to be more willing to accommodate than individuals with a weaker BJW.

The BJW also may be related to one's willingness to accommodate via the level of trust that one has in his/her partner. Accommodation inherently involves some degree of risk. The accommodating individual hopes that his/her self-sacrifice (e.g., forsaking immediate self-interests) will be perceived by the partner as a benevolent and constructive relational gesture that will eventually be reciprocated. Unfortunately, there is no guarantee that this will occur.

Perceived trust in one's partner is likely to strengthen one's resolve that the partner will make these attributions and ultimately reciprocate the accommodating person's needs and desire—thereby encouraging accommodation (Boon, 1994; Boon & Holmes, 1991; Holmes, 1991; Wieselquest, Rusbult, Agnew, & Foster, 1994). Importantly, individuals with a stronger BJW have been found to be more trusting of others (Lipkus, 1991; Zuckerman & Gerbasi, 1977) than individuals with a weaker BJW. Strong believers in a just world are likely to view accommodation as an investment in the relationship that will be repaid by the partner with positive relational rewards (cf. Lerner, Miller, & Holmes, 1976).

This latter view suggests that the BJW may be related to greater accommodation via the perception that the partner will also be accommodating. Accommodation is likely to be a reciprocal process that is consistent with the use of a tit-for-tat strategy (Pruit & Carnevale, 1994) and the norm of reciprocity (Gouldner, 1960). Furthermore, as a relationship progresses, the relationship partners probably develop "routinized" methods of resolving conflict, which if they are of a prosocial nature, are likely to lead to stable, benevolent attributions of the partner's motives; this may include viewing him/her as accommodating (Rusbult et al., 1991; Rusbult et al., 1995). Thus, a third reason to expect individuals with a strong BJW to be more accommodating is that we would expect them to perceive their partners as being more accommodating.

In sum, we would argue that the BJW is likely to play an important role in how people resolve conflicts in relationships. We expect individuals with a stronger BJW to be more willing to accommodate when faced with their partners' negative behavior. The relationship between the BJW and accommodation is hypothesized to be mediated by perspective-taking, trust, and the perception that the partner is and will be accommodating. We now present data from married and dating couples that lend support to some of these predictions.

2. RELATIONSHIP BETWEEN THE BELIEF IN A JUST WORLD AND ACCOMMODATION AMONG MARRIED COUPLES

We have investigated the relationship between one's BJW and willingness to accommodate in two samples of married couples. The first sample consisted of 55 younger married couples (average age = 35) recruited from Whitewater, Wisconsin and surrounding communities via newspaper advertisements; the second sample consisted of 60 older married couples (average age = 58) randomly selected from the Duke University Aging Registry. The average length of marriage was 8 and 30 years for the younger and older couples, respectively. These participants were mailed a questionnaire packet to their homes and asked to complete the measures (discussed below) in private without discussing them with their spouse.

The BJW was measured by a 9-item modified version of Lipkus' (1991) Global Belief in a Just World Scale. Participants were asked to rate on a seven-point scale ranging from strongly disagree (scored a 1) to strongly agree (scored a 7), how well the following statements applied to them only: (1) I feel I get what I am entitled to have in life; (2) I feel that my efforts are noticed and rewarded; (3) I feel that people treat me fairly in life; (4) I feel that I earn the rewards and punishments I get; (5) I feel that when I meet with misfortune, I have brought it upon myself; (6) I feel I get what I deserve; (7) I feel people treat me with the respect I deserve; (8) I feel that the world treats me fairly, and (9) I basically feel that the world is a fair place. This modified just world scale has been found to correlate highly with other global just world scales (Lipkus, Dalbert, & Siegler, 1996).

Accommodation was measured using a 16-item questionnaire that assessed separately *Exit*, *Voice*, *Loyalty*, and *Neglect* (Rusbult et al., 1991). Accommodation was operationalized as the sum of each subject's responses to the *Voice* and *Loyalty* items, minus the sum of their responses to the *Exit* and *Neglect* items. Each individual responded to two different versions of this scale: one asking them to report how they typically respond when their partner has behaved poorly (their own accommodation), and one asking them to report how their partner typically responds when they themselves have behaved poorly (spousal accommodation). Trust was measured using Rempel, Holmes, and Zanna's (1985) Trust Scale, and perspective-taking was measured using a slightly modified 7-item version of Davis' (1983) Perspective-Taking Scale. Perspective-taking and trust were collected only in the sample of younger married couples. All measures demonstrated good internal consistencies (alphas > .80).

We found among all our measures considerable interdependence between partners—husbands' and wives' scores across measures were correlated significantly. Consequently, we used *pooled regression* to analyze these nonindependent data (Kenny, 1996). Briefly, this technique partitions the covariance among variables into two mutually exclusive components: an actor and a partner effect. An *actor effect* represents the extent to which an individual's standing on a predictor variable affects his or her standing on a criterion variable (e.g., how a husbands BJW affects his willingness to accommodate). A *partner effect* represents the extent to which the *partner's* standing on a predictor variable affects one's standing on a criterion variable (e.g., how the wife's BJW affects the husband's willingness to accommodate). The obtained regression coefficient (beta) is divided by the standard error resulting in a t-test for statistical significance—specific details concerning the calculations of these effects can be found in Kenny (1996). We used this approach to test the following specific hypothesis: (1) in both samples, the BJW will be positively related to willingness to accommodate; (2) the relationship between the belief in a just world and accommodation will be mediated by trust, perspective-taking (younger couples only),and perceptions of spousal accommodation (both samples).

These data from both samples of married couples were submitted to a number of pooled multiple-regression analyses. All these analyses controlled for each individual's age, gender, and the length of their marriage. Furthermore, all analyses were one-tailed tests in the predicted direction. Effects were deemed significant a-prior at the $p < .01$ or smaller. The main results of the these analyses are presented in Table 1.

As predicted, in both samples we found a significant and positive actor effect between the BJW and one's own willingness to accommodate—refer to the top of Table 1. Individuals who more strongly believed in a just world were also more willing to accommodate when their partner had behaved negatively. We did not, however, find any significant partner effects. Thus, an individual's own willingness to accommodate was not affected by his/her spouse's BJW.

We then tested whether the relationship between accommodation and BJW was being mediated by trust, perspective-taking, and spousal accommodation. Before conducting these analyses, is was necessary to establish that these potential mediating variables were significantly related to both one's willingness to accommodate, and to the BJW (Baron &

TABLE 1. Pooled Regression Analyses Predicting Own Willingness to Accomodate among Married Couples

Model	Older married couples			Younger married couples		
	Actor effect	Partner effect	S.E.	Actor effect	Partner effect	S.E.
Main effects models						
Belief in a just world	.217*	.029	.086	.265**	−.084	.091
Perceptions of spousal accommodation	.457*	.302***	.087	.413**	.460***	.077
Trust	—	—	—	.438***	.306***	.082
Partner perspective-taking	—	—	—	.429***	.084⁺	.087
Mediational analyses						
Model 1						
Belief in a just world	.065	−.109	.071	.277**	−.100	.092
Perceptions of spousal accommodation	.444***	.330***	.088	−.039	.105	.087
Model 2						
Belief in a just world	—	—	—	.258**	−.079	.093
Trust	—	—	—	.039	−.045	.079
Model 3						
Belief in a just world	—	—	—	.256**	−.069	.091
Partner perspective-taking	—	—	—	.134+	−.103	.073

Note: Analyses control for age, gender, and length of marriage. Results at 12 < .01 or smaller were deemed significant. Degrees of freedom for the older married sample varied from 73 to 111. Degrees of freedom for the younger married sample varied from 78 to 100.
⁺one-tailed $p < .05$; *one-tailed $p < .01$; **one-tailed $p < .005$; ***one-tailed $p < .001$

Kenny, 1986). As reported in Table 1, our results revealed that the three potential mediating variables were indeed significantly and positively related to one's own willingness to accommodate. Individuals who were more trusting of, and took their partner's perspective, were more accommodating. Furthermore, in both samples, individuals who viewed their spouse as accommodating were more willing to accommodate. In addition, we found that individuals who more strongly believed in a just world were more likely to: (1) trust their partner, (2) take their partner's perspective, and (3) perceive their spouse as accommodating in both samples (Lipkus & Bissonnette, 1996). In sum, all the prerequisite relationships for conducting mediational analyses were obtained (Baron & Kenny, 1986).

Three pooled regression analyses were then performed including trust, perspective-taking, and perception of spousal accommodation in separate models. If any of these three were acting as mediating variables, then their inclusion in the model as covariates should render the BJW a nonsignificant predictor of one's own willingness to accommodate (Baron & Kenny, 1986). The results of these mediational analyses are depicted in Table 1—see under mediational analyses.

Overall, there was mixed support for our predictions. Perceptions of spousal accommodation proved to be a mediator for the older but not younger married couples. The BJW no longer predicted significantly accommodation in the older couples once perceptions of spousal accommodation had been added to the regression model. This suggests that among the older couples, spouses who more strongly believed in a just world were more willing to accommodate primarily because they viewed their spouse as more accommodating.

The results from the sample of younger married couples did not provide any evidence that trust, perspective-taking, and perceptions of spousal accommodation mediated the relationship between BJW and one's willingness to accommodate. Rather, the results suggested that the BJW mediated the relationships between trust, perspective-taking, perceptions of spousal accommodation and own willingness to accommodate. As revealed in Table 1, trust, perspective-taking, and perceptions of spousal accommodation became nonsignificant predictors of own accommodation with the inclusion of the BJW in the regression model. No other significant effects were found.

Overall, these findings provided strong support for our first hypothesis that the BJW would be a significant predictor of one's own willingness to accommodate. However, the results from these two studies did not support strongly our second hypothesis that trust, perspective-taking and perception of spousal accommodation would mediate the relationship between the BJW and one's own willingness to accommodate. Thus, while BJW was related to greater trust, perspective-taking, and a greater perception of spousal accommodation, the inclusion of these three constructs into the regression models did not render the BJW as a nonsignificant predictor of one's willingness to accommodate in most cases. Among the older married couples, perceptions of spousal accommodation appeared to serve as a mediating variable.

The pattern of results revealed by these studies indicate that the BJW contributes unique variance in predicting how individuals choose to respond to their partner's negative behavior. In an attempt to replicate and expand these findings, we conducted a similar set of analyses on a sample of dating undergraduate couples which we report here for the first time.

3. RELATIONSHIP BETWEEN THE BELIEF IN A JUST WORLD AND ACCOMMODATION AMONG DATING COUPLES

The third study consisted of 55 undergraduate dating couples enrolled at the University of Wisconsin-Whitewater who participated for extra credit applied towards their psychology courses. Participants' ages ranged from 17 to 26 years old (Mean = 19.25). Couples had been dating for an average of 19.77 months, and the majority were dating their partner exclusively. Participants completed the same questionnaires as used with the younger married couples to assess accommodation, perception of partner accommodation, trust, perspective-taking, and the BJW. Respondents completed these questionnaires in private and were informed that their partner would never see their responses.

These data were submitted to a series of pooled multiple regression analyses similar to those employed in the last two studies. The goal of these analyses was to test the relationship between the BJW and one's willingness to accommodate, and to examine if this relationship might be mediated by trust, perspective-taking, and one's perception of partner accommodation. All analyses covaried the individual's age, gender, and the length of the dating relationship. Furthermore, all analyses were one-tailed tests in the predicted direction. Effects were deemed significant a-priori at the $p < .01$ or smaller. The results from the analysis of this third sample of data are presented in Table 2.

The results of our pooled multiple regression analysis revealed no significant actor effect but rather a significant partner effect for the BJW. Thus, an individual's willingness to accommodate was predicted best by the partner's BJW rather than his or her own BJW. Furthermore, and as predicted, one's willingness to accommodate was strongly and positively predicted by trust, perspective-taking, and the perception that one has an accommodating partner—all actor but not partner effects (see Table 2).

Further analyses revealed that the BJW was sigificantly related to the trust and partner perspective-taking but not perceptions of partner accommodation. Individuals with a partner who had a stronger BJW were more willing themselves to take their partner's perspective (Beta$_{(partner)}$ = 2.14, S.E. = .095, two-tailed $p < .02$) and were more trusting of their partner

TABLE 2. Pooled Regression Analyses Prediting Own Willingness to Accommodate among Dating Couples

Model	Actor effect	Partner effect	S.E.
Main effects			
Belief in a just world	.14	.23*	.096
Perception of partner accommodation	.60**	.17	.078
Trust	.55**	.12	.096
Perspective-taking	.40**	.09	.095

Note: Analyses control for age, gender, and length of dating relationship. Results at 12 < .01 or smaller were deemed significant. Degrees of freedom varied from 69 to 90.
*one-tailed p < .01; **one-tailed p < .001

(Beta$_{(partner)}$ = 2.04, S.E. = .098, two-tailed $p < .05$). Moreover, an individual's own BJW predicted greater trust in one's partner (Beta$_{(actor)}$ = 1.75, S.E. = .098, two-tailed $p < .05$). No other significant effects emerged.

The overall analyses revealed that own accommodation was predicted differently by the BJW and the three proposed mediating variables. The BJW produced mainly partner but not actor effects, while trust, perspective-taking, and perceptions of partner accommodation all produced actor but not partner effects. Since the source of the effects differed, actor versus partner, it was not possible to engage in a systematic test of the potential mediating effects of these variables (e.g., assessing the impact of the *partner* effect of the BJW after covarying a *significant partner* effect for trust, perspective-taking, etc.). However, for exploratory purposes, we performed two pooled regression analyses predicting own accommodation including those variables that were related to the BJW: trust, and partner perspective-taking—thus approaching a true test of a mediational analyses. In both analyses, the BJW became a nonsignificant predictor of own accommodation although there remained a strong trend in the predicted direction (Beta$_{(partner)}$ = 1.37, S.E. = .077, one-tailed $p < .10$; Beta$_{(partner)}$ = 1.59, S.E. = .093, one-tailed $p < .06$; covarying trust and perspective-taking, respectively). Thus there was evidence to suggest that the inclusion of trust and perspective-taking did influence, albeit weakly, the effects of one's partner's BJW to predict own accommodation. However, these results should not be interpreted as strong mediational effects for trust and perspective-taking.

4. CONCLUSIONS AND FUTURE DIRECTIONS

In a series of three studies, we presented data using married and dating couples which suggested that the BJW may confer benefits to the maintenance of relationships by affecting one conflict resolution style, willingness to accommodate. Willingness to accommodate involves a prosocial transformation of motivation (Yovetich & Rusbult, 1994), that entails the consideration of several factors, of which we argue, themes related to justice is one. In this realm, individuals who more strongly believe in a just world are likely to perceive their partner as acting in a manner consistent with themes of deservingness, and hence expect that their own accommodation will ultimately be reciprocated for the well-being of the relationship. We suggested further that this willingness to accommodate is based, in part, on relying that the partner can be trusted, is likely to take one's perspective, and is perceived as an accommodating person—accommodation begets accommodation.

Although the BJW did predict accommodation across studies, the source of this effect, whether it was an actor and/or partner effect, differed among samples. A person's own BJW predicted own willingness to accommodate among married couples, while a partner's BJW predicted own accommodation among dating couples. It is unclear why this difference emerged across samples. One plausible explanation is that during the early establishment of relationships, individuals may focus and be more affected by characteristics of the partner (e.g., should I continue to date this person, is this person satisfying my needs in the relationship) than more established relationships. Similarly, and as mentioned previously, as relationships develop, individuals may develop "routinized" methods of handling conflict. It is plausible that as conflicts emerge, both individuals will attempt different strategies to handle these situations before establishing "routinized mechanisms" (Kelley & Thibaut, 1978). In the process, it is likely that individual differences, such as the partner's BJW, may play a larger role in shaping conflict resolution strategies. Both of these explanation should remain speculative especially in light of the fact that both suggest that more partner effects should have been observed among the dating couples. In any event, future researchers should attempt to replicate the findings obtained with these dating couples before rendering stronger conclusions concerning underlying processes.

These studies also examined whether three potential mediating variables could account for the relationship between the BJW and own accommodation. While the BJW was significantly and positively related to trust, partner perspective-taking, and the perceptions that the partner was accommodating among married couples, with similar trends observed among the dating couples, the BJW continued to predict own accommodation when these factors were covaried in the regression models—at least with the younger married couples. These results lend further support demonstrating the beneficial impact of the BJW on relational dynamics independent of other important relational constructs. Moreover, the relationship between the BJW and own accommodation cannot be explained as one positive variable (e.g., BJW) predicting another positive variable (e.g. accommodation) because the inclusion of similarly valenced constructs (e.g., trust, perspective-taking) did not appreciably change the results.

If trust, perspective-taking, and to a lesser degree perceptions of spousal accommodation do not mediate the relationship between the BJW and own accommodation, what other mechanisms may account for these findings? A case can be made that perhaps a stronger mediating variable explaining the relationship between the BJW and accommodation, is seeing the partner as being supportive overall. Greater perceived partner social support may more fully capture the combined themes related to partner perspective-taking, trust, and viewing the partner as more accommodating. We are currently collecting data using dating couples at Duke University to explore these issues. It is predicted that the BJW will correlate positively with greater partner social support—using the Quality of Relationships Inventory (Pierce, 1994)—and that perceived partner social support will most powerfully mediate the relationship between the BJW and own accommodation relative to trust, partner perspective-taking, and partner accommodation.

In addition, these couples are completing measures of depression, stress, and life satisfaction in order to further test whether the positive relationship between the BJW and psychological well-being (Dalbert, 1992; Lipkus, Dalbert, & Siegler, 1996; Ritter, Benson, & Snyder, 1990) is mediated by these interpersonal dynamics. Thus, an exciting and potentially fruitful new direction of research is to begin exploring the relationships among the BJW, interpersonal processes, and psychological well-being. It is hoped that the results presented in this chapter highlight the need to assess the impact of the BJW on interpersonal process and ultimately psychological well-being.

REFERENCES

Baron, R.M., & Kenny, D.A. (1986). The moderator-mediator variable distinction in social psychological research: Conceptual, strategic, and statistical considerations. Journal of Personality and Social Psychology, 51, 1173–1182.

Bierhoff, H.W., Klein, R., & Kramp, P. (1991). Evidence for the altruistic personality from data on accident research. Journal of Personality, 59, 263–280.

Billings, A. (1979). Conflict resolution in distressed and nondistressed married couples. Journal of Consulting and Clinical Psychology, 47, 368–376.

Boon, S.D. (1994). Dispelling doubt and uncertainty: Trust in Romantic relationships. In S. Duck (Ed). Dynamics of relationships, Vol. 4,.(pp. 86–111).

Boon, S.D., & Holmes, J.G. (1991). The dynamics of interpersonal trust: resolving uncertainty in the face of risk. In R.A. Hinde & J. Groebel (Eds.), Cooperation and prosocial behavior (pp. 190–211). Cambridge, United Kingdom: Cambridge University Press.

Dalbert, C. (1992, July). Belief in a just world as a source of subjective well-being. Paper presented at the 25th International Congress of Psychology, Brussels, Belgium.

Davis, M. (1983). Measuring individual differences in empathy: Evidence for a multidimensional approach. Journal of Personality and Social Psychology, 44, 113–126.

Gottman, J.M. (1994). What predicts divorce? The relationship between marital processes and marital outcomes. Hillsdale, New Jersey: Lawrence Erlbaum.

Gottman, J.M., & Levenson, R. (1992). Marital processes predictive of later dissolution: Behavior, physiology, and health. Journal of Personality and Social Psychology, 63, 221–233.

Gottman, J.M., Markman, H.J., & Notarius, C.I. (1977). The topography of marital conflict: A sequential analysis of verbal and nonverbal behavior. Journal of Marriage and the Family, 39, 461–478.

Gouldner, A. (1960). The norm of reciprocity: A preliminary statement. American Sociological Review, 25, 161–178.

Holmes, J.G. (1991). Trust and the appraisal process in close relationships. In W.G. Holmes, & D. Perlman (Eds.), Advances in personal relationships, Vol. 2, (pp. 57–104). London: Jessica Kingsley.

Kelley, H., & Thibaut, J., (1978). Interpersonal relations: A theory of interdependence, New York: Wiley.

Kenny, D.A. (1996). Models of interdependence in dyadic research. Journal of Social and Personal Relationships, 13, 279–294.

Lerner, M.J. (1980). The belief in a just world: A fundamental delusion. New York: Plenum Press.

Lerner, M.J., & Miller, D.T. (1978). Just world research and the attribution process: Looking back and looking ahead. Psychological Bulletin, 85, 1030–1051

Lerner, M.J., Miller, D.T., & Holmes, J.G. (1976). Deservingness and the emergence of norms of justice. In L. Berkowitz & E. Walster (Eds.), Advances in experimental social psychology, Vol. 9, (pp. 134–162). New York: Academic Press.

Lipkus, I.M. (1991). The construction and preliminary validation of a global belief in a just world scale and the exploratory analysis of the multidimensional belief in a just world scale. Personality and Individual Differences, 12, 1171–1178.

Lipkus, I.M. & Bissonnette (1996). Relationships among the belief in a just world, willingness to accommodate, and marital well-being. Personality and Social Psychology Bulletin 22, 1943–1956.

Lipkus, I.M., Dalbert, C., & Siegler, I.C. (1996). The importance of distinguishing the belief in a just world for self versus for others: Implications for psychological well-being. Personality and Social Psychology Bulletin, 22, 666–677.

Margolin, G., & Wampold, B. (1981). Sequential analyses of conflict and accored in distressed and nondistressed marital partners. Journal of Counseling and Clinical Psychology, 49, 554–567.

Miller, D.T. (1977). Altruism and threat to the belief in a just world. Journal of Experimental Social Psychology, 13, 113–126.

Pruit, D.G., & Carnevale, P.J. (1994). Negotiation in social conflict. Pacific Grove, Calif: Brooks Cole.

Rempel, J.K., Holmes, J.G., & Zanna, M.P. (1985). Trust in close relationships. Journal of Personality and Social Psychology, 49, 95–112.

Ritter, C. Benson, D.E., & Snyder, C. (1990). Belief in a just world and depression. Sociological Perspectives, 33, 235–252.

Rubin, Z., & Peplau, A. (1975). Who believes in a just world? Journal of Social Issues, 13, 65–89.

Rusbult, C.E., Bissonnette, V.L., Arriaga, X.B., & Cox, C.L. (1995). Accommodation processes during the early years of marriage. Manuscript in preparation.

Rusbult, C.E., Johnson, D., & Morrow, G. (1986). Impact of couple patterns of problem-solving on distress in dating relationships. Journal of Personality and Social Psychology, 50, 744–753.

Rusbult, C.E., & Verette, J. (1991). An interdependence analysis of accommodation processes in close relationships. Representative Research in Social Psychology, 19, 3–33.

Rusbult, C.E., Verette, J., Whitney, G.A., Slovik, L.F., & Lipkus, I. (1991). Accommodation processes in close relationships: Theory and preliminary empirical evidence. Journal of Personality and Social Psychology, 60, 53–78.

Rusbult, C.E., Zembrodt, I., & Gunn, L. (1982). Exit, Voice, Loyalty, and Neglect: Responses to dissatisfaction in romantic involvements. Journal of Personality and Social Psychology, 43, 1230–1242.

Wieselquist, J., Rusbult, C.E., Agnew, C.R., & Foster, C. (1994). Trust and commitment in marital relationships. Unpublished manuscript, University of North Carolina at Chapel Hill.

Yovetich, N.A., & Rusbult, C.E., (1994). Accommodative behavior on close relationships: Exploring transformation of motivation: Journal of Experimental Social Psychology, 30, 138–164.

Zuckerman, M. (1975). Belief in a just world and altruistic behavior. Journal of Personality
    and Social Psychology, 31, 972–976.
Zuckerman, M., & Gerbasi, K.C. (1977). Belief in a just world and trust. Journal of Research
    in Personality, 11, 306–317.

Chapter 9

Measuring the Beliefs in a Just World

ADRIAN FURNHAM

1. INTRODUCTION

Whilst it *may not* be totally clear who first used the term Belief in a Just World (BJW) it is certain that the ideas behind the concept can be found in the work of early attribution theorists (Heider, 1958) and indeed in the ideas of the great Greek Philosophers. People prefer to live in stable, orderly, predictable world where just works are rewarded and evil punished.

The term BJW has, however, come to be associated with Melvin Lerner whose pioneering studies over the past 30 years were elegantly summarized in his 1980 book entitled "The Belief in a Just World: A Fundamental Delusion." Since that time a considerable body of research has accrued that has attempted to understand the aetiology, structure and function of these beliefs. A "first time" reader of the research in this field will, no doubt, be frustrated by the multiple terms used by researchers all interested in the same concept. Hence terms like the "justice motive," "victim derogation," and "defensive attribution" are all used synonymously to discuss and describe the cognitive processes involved in the BJW.

This chapter, however, concerns how BJW beliefs are measured. It will focus specifically on the self-report psychometric tests that supposedly measure the BJW, their correlates and validities.

ADRIAN FURNHAM • Department of Psychology, University College London, 26 Bedford Way, London, WC1, Great Britain.

Responses to Victimizations and Belief in a Just World, edited by Montada and Lerner. Plenum Press, New York, 1998.

2. TWO MEASUREMENT APPROACHES

The two disciplines of scientific psychology, as Cronbach (1957) called them in his celebrated presidential address to the American Psychological Association, are the *experimental,* concerned with general laws, and the *correlation,* concerned with individual differences. He argued that they are both indispensable to a proper understanding of behaviour. More than that, one cannot properly exist without the other. Individual differences interact in almost every case with experimental and situational paradigms to produce results differing for individuals with different personalities, capacities, and motivations. Consequently, studies in experimental, social, educational, clinical or industrial psychology which do not take into account personality factors and individual differences in temperament, intelligence, character, attitudes an aptitudes inevitably throw away a great deal of potential information, and enlarge the error term in their analysis. Main effects are frequently swamped by interaction effects, and these are lost when personality variables are ignored in the research design. Conversely, the concepts and laws of experimental psychology are vital to any scientific understanding or interpretation of the results of work in understanding personality; if we are to explain the major factors of personality in scientific terms, we must make appear to the concepts used in experimental and physiological psychology.

The BJW literature is indeed nicely split between experimental social psychologists like Lerner (1965, 1977, 1978, 1981, 1980) himself and his colleagues (Miller, 1977; Miller & Smith, 1977; Miller & McCann, 1979; Miller et al., 1976) who have investigated the BJW experimentally, and the psychometricians like Lipkus (1991) and Schmitt (1993) who have been concerned with developing self-report measures of the BJW measures combined the correlational and the experimental research so providing validation for both approaches. However, recent reviews of the BJW literature would suggest that the psychometric approach is now more common (Furnham & Procter, 1989). There are long term consequences for the investigation of a concept like the BJW depending on whether one favours the experimental vs the correlational/psychometric paradigm. The experimental is more often about *process;* experiments are devised to test the tactics, strategies and motives of people confronted to threats in the BJW. It focuses on behaviour and infers cognitions and is self-evidently situation-specific.

The psychometric approach tends to focus on *content,* BJW scores are correlated with other attitude belief and personality measures to demonstrate concurrent validity. More importantly perhaps the assumption, though frequently unstated, of the psychometric researchers is that the BJW is trait-like in its stability. That is, the BJW is assumed to be stable over time and consistent across situations. Though there is little longitudinal evidence of this the internal and test-retest reliabilities that have been calculated are cited in evidence of this position (Furnham & Procter, 1989). In short, experimental social psychologists construct *situations* and psychometricians attitudinal *items* to "test" their hypotheses about the BJW.

3. THE DEVELOPMENT OF TRAIT MEASURES

The number of single-trait studies are legion and include such dimensions as authoritarianism, achievement motivation, A/B Type behaviour, field dependence-independence, conservatism, locus of control, assertiveness, Protestant Work Ethic beliefs, self-monitoring, etc. Three points need to be made about this list which may extend to nearly 80 traits or more. Firstly, although described as traits or dimensions, some researchers resist the term trait and prefer the terms type, style or need, because while they believe the dimension that they have isolated is stable over time and across situations, and highly predictive of certain types of behaviour, the term trait can have certain implications which are not necessarily inherent to their approach. For instance, in some contexts, the term trait suggests a biological, rather than a learned aetiology, or may imply a continuous variable where in fact the dimension is discontinuous and categorical. The BJW is conceived of as a bi-dimensional *belief system* and the word trait is seldom, if ever, used.

Secondly, the origin of these many trait measures is highly varied. Some have arisen from cognitive, social and clinical psychology, and some even from research on perception. Some, such as the trait of authoritarianism, might have first been articulated within a psychoanalytic framework, while others such as locus of control originated firmly within a behaviourist tradition. Hence there are very wide differences in how these traits are measured and the terminology employed in their use. The BJW appears to have arisen from the work of Rubin and Peplau (1973, 1975).

Thirdly, it is rare that any single-trait measure is entirely unique, in terms of the way it is conceived, described or measured. Although there are exceptions, it is frequently the case that researchers, after extensive reading, notice a consistence pattern in previous studies which makes sense of their results and which could be explained in terms of a "new" trait. Frequently then, the origin of a trait term can be ascribed to a particular source or research team, but the ideas that are articulated can be traced back to many other authors including those who were not psychologists or who never actively conducted research.

Despite the enormous number of "single trait" theories in psychology with variously different origins, terminologies and measurement techniques, they frequently shared similar histories. That is, the developmental history from the first published study on a new trait to world-wide research efforts often follows a standard pattern.

The development of single traits theories appears to go through most of the following stages sequentially (Furnham, 1990). There are, of course, many problems associated with any stage-wise theory—how long each stage lasts; what determines movement from the one stage to the next; whether one can skip a stage or not; whether one might return to an earlier stage; and whether all phenomena pass through all stages (Furnham & Bochner, 1986). Despite these obvious and important shortcomings, eight stages of development seem most common. The question is what stage have psychometric measures of the BJW reached.

3.1. Identification of the Phenomena

This may occur as a result of laboratory experimentation or observation in a clinic, at work or through critical reading. It may occur when a researcher operationalizes that which is well-known in literature into a psychological measure such as was the case with the Protestant Work Ethic (Furnham, 1990). But what is more normally the case is that a researcher observes a psychological phenomenon which he or she gives a name. Examples are legion; Seligman (1975) noticed learned helplessness, the behaviour in dogs which later become translated into an attribution-style questionnaire to identify the same behaviour in humans. Lerner (1980) reported on a extensive laboratory-based programme of research with many published studies before Rubin and Peplau (1973) developed the first instrument in the area. A number of points need to be made about this first stage. Firstly, the person or persons who originally make the observations need not necessarily be the ones who develop the single-trait theory or the self-report measure. Secondly, the phenomenon is often only new in the sense that it has not been recorded or reported before in quite the same way or received a particular label. Thirdly, this stage often occurs in the laboratory as a by-product of observational studies, or occasionally from the systematic recordings of clinical who note consistent relationships in the behaviour of their patients. Very rarely, if ever, are the researchers intentionally engage in developing a trait measure of theory.

3.2. Replication of the Effect

The second stage is characterized by replications and considerably more experimental work on the nature of the effect observed. An excellent illustration of this can be found in Lerner's (1980) book on Just World

Beliefs which reports on numerous experiments using the concept. The idea of this phase is to test the robustness of the findings, often by subtle yet simple a case of data gathering in an attempt to find support for observations made, while in others a series of studies attempts to test the various hypotheses that make up the nascent theory. These studies are usually reported in the first paper or book to describe the behaviour pattern/phenomenon.

3.3. The Development of a Self-Report Measure

Despite the fact that the original researchers may not be personality, clinical or social psychologists, and may in fact have little faith in self-report measures, the next stage does involve the development of a self-report measure. The questionnaires used may be of highly variable psychometric quality and the research that goes into establishing them somewhat inadequate. Reliability, validity and normative statistics may be fairly minimal to begin with, and it is unlikely that the first versions to be published are validated in a manner acceptable to psychometricans. Indeed, it is precisely because the originators of the concept are not psychometricians (being clinicians or experimentalists) that they do not always know the minimum criteria required of a good self-report measure. Frequently the self-report measure is developed some years after the concept/behaviour pattern has been described in the literature. In this case, which might occur is that over the space of a few years a number of similar (but not highly correlated) measures will be developed. In the first report using the BJW scale Rubin & Peplau (1972) reported

> As presented on the questionnaire, the Just World Scale consisted of 19 statements (plus two filler items) to which the subject indicated his agreement or disagreement on a six-point scale. The items were selected from a larger initial pool on the basis of a factor analysis of the responses of 66 Boston University undergraduates. Three of the 19 items were later eliminated from the scale on the basis of a further factor analysis of the responses of the draft lottery subjects. Of the remaining 16 items, nine are worded in the positive direction, with agreement reflecting the belief or perception that the world is just. The other seven items are worded in the negative direction. Coefficient alpha for the scale, based on the response of the 58 initial lottery subjects, was .79. The distribution of scores was skewed toward the low end of the scale, with a large majority of the subjects indicating more disagreement than agreement with statements that the world is just. There was nevertheless a wide range of scores of the scale, from total rejection to qualified acceptance of the "just world" ideology.

On the basis of this rather flimsy evidence, with no construct, concurrent of predictive validity many researchers have happily adopted the scale.

3.4. Validation of the Measure

The fourth phase may continue for some time and involves numerous experimental and correlational studies of various sorts, all aiming to
validate the measure and its underlying concepts. Studies are often of the
kind that make up a PhD and include a programmatic series aimed to test
corollaries of the theory. What links the studies is the uni-dimensional trait
measure used to assess the independent variable. A large number of these
studies are essentially attempts to establish the concurrent, construct and
predictive validity of the self-report scale by correlating it with other
well-known measures or behaviours. The danger of this sort of approach,
as Kline (1985) has pointed out, is that correlating a new measure with an
established but itself poorly psychometrized measure does not provide
good evidence of the validity of the theory or research. Whilst some studies
provide nice evidence of the construct validity of the measure, possibly
because of the difficulty and expense associated with longitudinal work,
a glance at the citation index of any well-know self-report measure shows
the extent to which validation studies are done, some by the original
author and his/her acolytes but more commonly by researchers from
different laboratories. Paradoxically, it is not lack of validity that prevents
research into a measure or concept, but more likely the extent to which the
measure taps the Zeitgeist of (North American) psychology. Furnham &
Procter (1989) review evidence of over 30 concurrent and construct validity
studies of the BJW.

3.5. Factor Analysis Work and Multi-Dimensionality

Although researchers may identify what they believe to be a single,
albeit complex, dimension or phenomenon, and hence develop a uni-dimensional scale, subsequent multivariate statistics (cluster analysis, factor
analysis, multi-dimensional scaling) nearly always show the measure to
be multi-dimensional with specific interpretable primary factors which
may be orthogonal or oblique. Assertiveness questionnaires, for instance,
have been shown to tap four quite different types of assertiveness depending on whether the behaviour is positive or negative, initiating or responsive (Furnham & Henderson, 1984). Locus of control scales have also
proved to be multi-dimensional though there is predictably some debate
as to the number of dimensions, their relationship and how they should
be labelled (Collins, 1974).

Factor analytic work usually poses problems for the original author
because the theory upon which the measure is founded usually assumes
a uni-dimensional concept. At least three responses are common. One is to
maintain that the concept, measure and trait are unified at a higher order

(i.e. super factors) and that although it may have various components, these are second order (secondary) distinctions/factors which do not threaten the theory. A second approach is to revise the scale, either by attempting to eradicate items that load on irrelevant factors or by building a truly multi-dimensional instrument. A third approach is to do a meta-analysis of factor-analytic studies, decide on the factor structure and accept the original scale as multi-dimensional. This phase may last many years but may help resolve equivocal findings when they can be attributed to the multi-dimensional structure of the trait measure. Both first and second responses have been made to factor analytic studies of the BJW.

3.6. Multiple, Multi-Dimensional Measures

The malaise following repeated psychometric investigations into an established uni-trait measure often leads scholars to despair because, as has been noted, it is uncertain at which level analysis should proceed. A common response however is for a team of psychometrically-oriented researchers to develop a new, better scale or self-report device. These new "improved" measures often have various specific features. Firstly, they are nearly always multi-dimensional in the sense that they provide subscale scores which may or may not be combined into a single score depending on the needs of the researchers. Hence, Levensohn (1974) developed a three-dimensional locus of control scale (internal, chance and powerful others). Secondly, many researchers develop sphere-specific scales to measure the trait, belief or behaviour system within a very restricted range of behaviours, as this has been shown to improve the predictive validity. Furnham and Steele (1993) found evidence of over 50 specific locus of control scales. There are, of course, problems with this proliferation of measures because studies using different measures are not strictly comparable. Secondly, it is possible that a person may score highly on one measure (internal economic locus of control), but low on a related measure (external mental health locus of control). Some authors have attempted to produce, not so much a multi-dimensional measure but sphere-specific measures which set out to measure the same beliefs (i.e. locus of control or just world) in different contexts (intra-, interpersonal, sociopolitical) (Furnham & Procter, 1989).

3.7. Doubts about the Original Concept

It is not infrequent that after a decade or so of intensive psychometric work on a measure/concept, authors begin to cast doubts about its conceptual and psychometric status. Consider Researchers concerned with the measurement of assertion construct now believe it is outmoded and should be relinquished." The construction has proven to be vague, difficult to define, and to be laden with assumptions reflecting traditional rather than more contemporary views of personality and behaviour change. In the future, we need to concentrate more on response- and situation-specific behaviour falling under the rubric of social skills - social competence and retire the assertiveness (assertion) construct" (Galassi, Galassi & Vedder, 1981, p. 330).

In other words, the complexity of measurement and the equivocal nature of the findings leads reviewers to conclude that the original concept/phenomenon/behaviour pattern, and all questionnaires that attempt to measure it should be abandoned either in favour of a new concept, usually a subscale of the former, or else that the original behaviour pattern is too unstable to be considered as a trait. This stage is characterized, not like the last two by increased empirical work, but theoretical reconceptualization. Naturally the commitment of researchers to a particular concept or scale means that they are loath to relinquish it, but happy to make further attempts to refine it. To a large extent this has not happened by the BJW though some researchers have argued that the belief tapped by the BJW are extremely naive and hardly likely to be believed by anyone.

3.8. Acceptance and "Text-Bookization"

Having gone through the above 7 stages and having survived the last one, the concept and its measures are usually accepted into the canon of individual differences measures. A sure sign of this process is the inclusion into the numerous, benevolent, eclectic text books on personality, social psychology or measurement. By this stage, there is probably a sizable literature on the concept and the measure, as citation counts show. However, one should not assume that because a test and concept have won through the above baptismal and confirmatory process, that it is therefore necessarily a psychometrically valid, theoretically important or diagnostically useful measure. Small bands of zealots wedded to the original ideas in the scale can propel a measure of dubious theoretical and psychometrical validity into the text books and research consciousness. Equally, extremely good measures based on sound theory and careful psychometric work can get "lost" and never make it to the laboratories of the world. Furnham (1995) has argued that the current zeitgeist in psychology seems more likely to determine measure popularity. However, like all stage-wise theories the above sequence has its limitations and unanswered questions. Do theories measures have to go through all the stages sequentially? Can some stages be skipped? Does development having to be linear or can it be cyclical? What prompts movement from one stage to another? Despite these unresolved questions it may be useful to adapt the above stage-wise model to evaluate the progress of a trait-like measure, or indeed to predict further developments.

4. THE RUBIN AND PEPLAU BJW SCALE

The Just World Scale requires the respondent to indicate how much he or she agrees or disagrees with 20 items on six-point continuum (the original Rubin & Peplau, 1973, version contained only 16 items). Half of these items refer to a just world where good deeds are rewarded, i.e. (11) 'By and large people deserve what they get,' while the other half refer to an unjust world where good deeds are no more likely to be rewarded than bad deeds, e.g. (4) 'Careful drivers are just as likely to get hurt in traffic accidents as careless ones.'

They showed BJW to be a unitary dimension (as have Ahmed & Steward, 1985, by factor analysis). There is no doubt that the Rubin & Peplau (1973, 1975) BJW Scale has stimulated most of the recent work on the just world. Indeed, there are over 50 references to the scale in the Social Science Citation Index between 1975 and 1985. One emphasis seems to have been on testing the construct validity of the scale and on factor analysing it to explore some of its possible components. A great deal of the studies using the scale have attempted to examine the validity of the measure in relation to juror behaviour (Arbuthnot, 1983; Gerbasi, Zuckerman & Reis, 1977; Kassin & Wrightsman, 1983; Moran & Comfort, 1982) and general attitudes to justice (Karniol, 1980; Nelsen, Eisenberg & Carrol, 1982). A second topic that has been frequently used to validate self-report BJW measure is accidents, misfortunes and fate (Asch, 1984; Burke, 1985; Dodd & Mills, 1985; Karuza & Carey, 1984; Keicolt-Glaser & Williams, 1987; Langer, 1977; Miller, Smith, Ferree & Taylor, 1976; Parker, Brewer & Spencer, 1980).

BJW as measured by the scale has been correlated with authoritarianism, religiousness, belief in the Protestant work ethic, internal locus of control beliefs, tendency to admire political leaders / social institutions and tendency to have negative attitudes towards the underprivileged, as well as other psychological demographic factors.

In order to test the validity of the scale, Rubin & Peplau (1973, 1975) used real life subjects whose fate (whether or not they would be sent to fight in Vietnam) was to be decided by the national draft lottery, which was broadcast on radio. Prior to listening to the live broadcast, the subjects completed the Just World Scale. The self-esteem of those who were drafted was much lower than the lucky ones who were not, irrespective of BJW. Overall, the drafted men were treated with sympathy and were better liked. Looking specifically at the third who scored highest on the BJW Scale, it was found, as predicted, that they were more likely to condemn the innocent victims of the draft lottery, Zuckerman, Gerbasi, Kravitz & Wheeler (1975) in one of the earliest studies using the questionnaire replicated some of the earlier experiments which had explained observers' reactions to victimization in terms of just world theory (Alderman, Brehm & Katz, 1974; Godfrey & Lowe, 1975; Lerner & Simmons, 1966). Those observers who scored highly on the scale (above the median) were much more likely to derogate the victim that those who did not hold a strong BJW. This was true across all three experimental conditions.

The Rubin & Peplau BJW Scale thus opened up a whole new area of research for just world theory. It provided a measure which could be used to make more direct links between the way people react to events in their environment and their BJW. Initially, research was intent on validating the scale. Recently, the focus has been on finding the many correlates of BJW and attempting to refine the scale through factor analysis.

However, Lerner (1980) made extensive and important criticisms of the Just World Scale. He accused the scale of having unsuitable items and tapping a very naive view of social reality, while still feeling that the findings generated by the scale provide:

> A pattern of correlates [that] is impressive and extremely persuasive. There certainly does seem to be an important dimension that is tapped by that scale and it appears to reflect beliefs about the extent to which one lives in a just world. Although related to other dimensions in meaningful ways, it is psychologically distinct from the Authoritarian syndrome, the acceptance of Protestant Ethic related beliefs, or an Internal versus External locus of control (p. 155).

Yet central to Lerner's (1980) concern was how to conceptualize individual differences in connection with the BJW. He suggestion was that the scale might be better conceptualized as an index of different styles people use to *maintain the BJW* rather than as a measure of the degree to which people believe in a just world. Thus the BJW is seen as a type of attribution 'style' rather than a present personality 'dimension' (Ellard & Lerner, 1982). This distinction has important implications for the stability, consistency and coherence of BJW as well as correlations with other measures. For instance, it seem much easier to change or strengthen styles of thinking than stable dispositions. Secondly, if the scale measures beliefs which maintain the BJW, it does not necessarily follow that the scale taps beliefs that are important in a the aetiology of those beliefs. Thus, specific experiences and/or beliefs may lead a person to adhere to the beliefs that the world is basically just and the BJW is maintained by the sort of belief that the Just World Scale measures.

A great deal of the value of this later research must depend on the psychometric properties of this scale which are not particularly impressive. There is little evidence, for instance, of test-retest reliability and the validity studies have concentrated most on concurrent rather than construct or predictive validity. The coefficient alpha of the scale was reported at 0.79 (Rubin & Peplau, 1973), while Smith & Green (1984) reported on alpha of 0.67 for the 20-item scale and Ma & Smith (1985) an alpha of 0.78. Furnham (1993), who administered the 16-item scale to over 2000 subjects from a dozen cultures, found alphas between 0.53 and 0.81. One serendipitously discovered but replicated finding is that the just and unjust world items are not strictly comparable in th sense that they have similar correlates (Furnham, 1993; Heaven & Connors, 1988). This suggests that the BJW is not a unitary dimension which is a theme pursued by various other researchers. Furnham & Procter (1989) argued that one may believe in the existence of either two of diametrically opposed worlds; the just world where people get what they deserve in the sense that the good and virtuous are rewarded and the bad and wicked are punished, or an unjust world where precisely the opposite occurs and the good are unrewarded or punished. Similarly, bad or wicked deeds have equal chances of being caught and punished, ignored and unapprehended, or even praised. In a sense, believers in a random or just world are midpoint scorers on this scale. It could be argued that the face, concurrent and predictive validity of the scale is satisfactory because it has been shown to correlate significantly and predictably with many other self-report measures (see below) and furthermore, 'experimental' studies using BJW scores as an independent variable have usually found these scores predictably related to specific behaviour. The major problem, however, concerns whether the scale measures the same concept of BJW as set out by the theory (Lerner, 1980).

5. THE DEVELOPMENT OF OTHER MEASURES

For over 20 years the Rubin & Peplau (1973, 1975) scale has been used by Just World researchers to measure the BJW. However over the past five to ten years some researchers have attempted to devise, other concurrently valid but psychometrically improved measures.

All three research groups have appeared to be concerned with the multidimensional structure of BJW. However they have reacted very differently to this problem. Two research groups—the one in Germany and the other in America—have devised much shorter questionnaires with no reverse items (Dalbert et al., 1987; Lipkus, 1991) while a British group has devised on longer explicitly multi-dimensional questionnaire with reverse items on all three subscales.

Table 1 gives details of five BJW scales. Dalbert et al. (1987) devised a German language scale which was validated in Spain and has recently proved to be psychometrically sound in Great Britain (Furnham, 1995). This measure has gone through extensive validation by the Trier group

TABLE 1. Five Different Beliefs in a Just World Scales

Author	Scale name	No. of items	Response scale	Reliability	Validity	Comments
Rubin & Peplau (1973)	Just World Scale	16	6 point agree-disagree	Alpha .79	Construct	Relatively little pilot work before scale was used
Rubin & Peplau (1975)	Just World Scale (revised)	20	6 point agree-disagree	Alpha .80 Alpha .81	Concurrent	13 of 16 items from above plus 7 more
Dalbert, Montada & Schmitt (1987)	Glaube an eine gerechte Welt als Motiv	6	6 point agree-disagree	Alpha .82 German .82 English .81	Concurrent Construct Predictive	Extensively tested by the University of Trier group but not without its problems
Lipkus (1991)	Global Belief in a Just World Scale	7	6 point agree-disagree	Alpha .79 to .82	Concurrent	An interesting "one-off"
Furnham & Procter (1992)	Multidimensional Just World Scale	30	7 point agree-disagree	Alpha .63 scales from .58 to .63	Construct	Compared to the above scale by Lipkus (1991)

and some 20 papers have resulted through there remains serious doubt concerning the construct validity of the measure.

Lipkus (1991) on the other hand seems to have done a "one-off" study. In his concurrent validity study he compared it to the Furnham and Procter (1989) measure and found though his simple 7 item measure showed considerably better internal reliability the latter measure showed better concurrent validity.

Furnham (1985) has argued that it is quite different believing that the world is not just as opposed to being unjust An examination of the items in the JWB Scale (Rubin & Peplau, 1975) show that approximately half intimate that the world is just and half unjust (to reduce response bias), but none that it is random. It could be argued that a midpoint response, i.e. neither just nor unjust, indicates the belief in a random world, but there are numerous problems associated with midpoint responses which suggest that there could be more than one reason for this particular response. Further recent evidence analyzing just and unjust world scores separately, suggest that they are indeed tapping into rather different belief systems (Connors & Heaven, 1987; Heaven & Connors, 1988).

More recently, Paulus (1983) has suggested that individual differences in perceived control could be apportioned into components associated with three different spheres of behaviour. These are personal (control over nonsocial environment such as in person achievement), interpersonal (control over other people in small or large groups), and socio-political (control over social, economic and political events and institutions). Sufficient robust empirical evidence was supplied to confirm this three factor structure in the development of a sphere-specific measure.

Furnham & Procter (1992) argue that it is possible that JWB-like locus of control beliefs are multi-dimensional in the sense that the beliefs circumscribe demonstrably different domains, hence it is possible to have just world beliefs about one domain but not about others. It is not necessarily inconsistent for people to believe in a just world in the personal domain but an unjust world in the political domain, or vice versa. For instance, one may believe that in one's interpersonal relationship the world is essentially just, but in the socio-political world, it is unjust.

In a study on attitudes to AIDS Furnham & Procter (1992) provide some construct validity for the scale though there remains serious doubt about its internal reliability.

Psychometric development are to be welcomed in this area. But they do have limitations and psychological consequences. Lerner (1980) has called these self-report measures "peek-a-scopes" that do little to understand the victimization process or explain the aetiology, development or change in these beliefs. Psychometric measures tend to turn the BJW into an individual difference variable that ends up being treated as a stable trait. Being seen as stable few studies in the psychometric tradition thus attempt to investigate how, when and why it changes. It has always been argued that the BJW is motivational in its origins yet traditionally psychometric tests have been poor at exploring motivation issues.

6. BJW BELIEFS: FUNDAMENTAL AND UNIVERSAL

Lerner (1980) has always argued that BJW are fundamental in the same way that the fundamental attribution error is fundamental. That is to follow the dictionary definition the just world process that leads to rationalization and victimization is essential, primary and original. Lerner (1980) and subsequently argues that there is now sufficient evidence that BJW and the motivational basis underlying it is fundamental in the sense that the process is powerful and widespread. But is it universal in the sense that it is pancultural?

One way of answering this is to examine the distribution of BJW in other countries and whether they have similar or different correlates.

When Furnham and Procter (1989) reviewed studies correlating just world beliefs with other variables, they found that subjects for seven countries (America, British, Canada, India, Japan, South Africa and Taiwan) had been administered Rubin and Peplau's (1973) Just World Beliefs Scale. Only three of these studies concerned societal differences; two examined national differences and one examined Black-White differences in America. Furnham (1985) found the White South African school children and undergraduates believed more strongly in a just world than did their matched British counterparts. Mahler, Greenberg & Hayaski (1981) compared the just world beliefs of Japanese and American undergraduates and found the former scored significantly lower than the latter. Smith and Green (1984) related sex, race, educational attainment, occupational prestige, personal income and age to belief in a just world and found that Blacks scored significantly lower than did Whites, that low income groups scored lower than high income groups did, and that for women, only age was positively correlated with belief in a just world. These results do provide some evidence of the cross-cultural equivalence of the meaning of the scale, though, admittedly, no other evidence exists.

Furnham (1985) has argued that beliefs in a just world may exist in an unjust society like than in South Africa because such a belief helps explain and justify numerous and obvious injustices in South African society.

However, this review ignored the very significant research effort of Montada, Dalbert, Schmidt and others in Germany. Work has also taken place in Poland (Dolinski, 1991). But Furnham reported on a study of 1,659 subjects from 12 countries (see Table 2).

TABLE 2. Details on the Twelve Populations and Their Mean Scores on the Two Measures

Country	n	Alpha			Just world			Unjust world		
		Total scale	Just world	Unjust world	M	SD	Rank	M	SD	Rank
America	172	.71	.77	.77	37.83[c]	7.25	3	22.95[d]	5.11	11
Australia	93	.62	.68	.60	36.11[c]	7.25	6	23.55[c]	5.51	8
Britain	189	.55	.59	.59	32.73[d]	7.74	11	24.24[d]	4.99	7
Germany	97	.62	.63	.68	34.41[c]	7.18	9	23.23[d]	3.90	9
Greece	123	.59	.59	.58	36.81[c]	10.82	5	27.61[c]	6.49	4
Hong Kong	117	.48	.54	.57	34.87[c]	5.83	7	25.34[d]	4.38	6
India	144	.58	.59	.62	44.20[a]	7.94	1	31.27[a]	4.69	1
Israel	224	.61	.66	.68	32.65[d]	9.28	12	22.56[c]	6.57	12
New Zealand	180	.46	.53	.50	34.62[c]	6.91	8	23.17[d]	4.66	10
South Africa	122	.68	.71	.70	41.19[b]	7.91	2	27.80[c]	4.79	3
West Indies	125	.63	.64	.61	34.04[c]	7.61	10	29.48[b]	5.27	2
Zimbabwe	103	.69	.68	.70	37.50[d]	8.13	4	25.79[d]	6.19	5

Note: scores with the same superscripts are not significantly different.

The just world and unjust world scores for the various groups are contained in Table 2. An analysis of variance (ANOVA), followed by paired comparisons, was calculated across the various samples. Both demonstrated striking significant differences in just world beliefs. Notably, the Spearman rank correlation for just and unjust world beliefs across the different countries was small, non significant and positive (vs. large, significant and negative), suggesting, as others have hypothesized, that just and unjust world beliefs are not opposites and may even be complementary. However, this finding could also indicate a response bias or specific acquiescent response bias on the subjects part.

The rank ordering of the just and unjust world scores (by country) and the rank ordering of the countries on the four orthogonal dimensions isolated by Hofstede (1984) in his analysis of cross-cultural differences is shown in Table 3.

Based on a survey of the literature, theoretical reasoning and a statistical analysis of all his data, Hofstede concluded that cultures differ along four orthogonal dimensions that indicate significant correlations with demographic, economic, geographic, historical and political indicators. The first dimension, *power-distance,* refers to the extent to which various societies weigh inequalities in areas such as prestige, wealth and power. The second dimension. labelled *uncertainty avoidance*, refers to the extent to which cultures cope with uncertainty through technology, law and religion. The third dimension, labelled *individualism,* refers to the way people live together in a society and to the relationship between the individual and the collective society. The fourth and final dimension, labelled *masculinity,* refers to the sex roles that are seen in families, schools, peer groups and the media.

Two countries, the West Indies and Zimbabwe, could not be ranked and compared because their data did not appear in Hofstede's work. Rank order correlations were then computed between the just and unjust world belief scores and the four dimensions. Three of the correlations were significant: Just world scores correlated, $r = .75$, $p < .05$, with power distance scores, whereas unjust world scores correlated $r = .92, p < .01$ with power distance and $r = .51, p < .05$, with individualism. Both correlations of the just and unjust world scores with uncertainty avoidance were negative, but neither reached significance. Just and unjust world rank order scores were also correlated with rank ordered gross domestic product scores (for 1985) derived from Lynn (1991). Whereas the just world scores did not reach significance, the unjust world scores did, $r = .84, p < .01$, indicating that the higher a country's gross domestic product, the lower its citizens' unjust world scores.

As predicted in the first hypothesis, the dimension that was most salient to just world beliefs is power distance, which correlated

TABLE 3. Rank Ordering of Ten Countries on Just and Unjust
World Beliefs and on Hofstede's (1984) Dimensions

	Type of belief		Hofstede's dimensions			
Country	Just world	Unjust world	Power distance	Uncertainty avoidance	Individualism	Masculinity
America	3	9	5	7	1	4
Australia	5	6	6	4	2	5
Britain	9	5	7.5	9	3	1.5
Germany	8	7	7.5	3	5	1.5
Greece	4	3	3	1	9	7.5
Hong Kong	6	4	2	10	10	7.5
India	1	1	1	8	8	9
Israel	10	10	10	2	7	10
New Zealand	7	8	9	5.5	4	6
South Africa	2	2	4	5.5	6	3

significantly and positively both with just world beliefs an with unjust world beliefs. Clearly those who have more property, wealth and power would have strong just world beliefs, whereas those who have little or no power and wealth would have unjust world beliefs. Furnham's study demonstrated that just world beliefs were negatively but not significantly correlated with uncertainty avoidance and individualism, and positively correlated with masculinity. One of the most robust findings in the literature is the fact that just world beliefs help people cope with disturbing or threatening events (rape, poverty, racism) an that the shared experience of these events causes people to develop a consensual view of reality. Because just world beliefs reduce or prevent feelings of guilt, they are retained and passed on to succeeding generations. In Third World countries, just world beliefs held by the rich and powerful condemn or devalue the poor. Some people believe in a just world because of their personal pathology and experiences (individual functionalism), but there is evidence that just world beliefs are a function not only of personal experience, but also of societal functionalism, (i.e. a country's structural and societal factors). In this sense just world beliefs are variables of both personality and social psychology.

7. FUTURE DEVELOPMENTS

The development of a robust, reliable and valid measure takes time. Over half of the published studies on the BJW (in English) have used the Rubin and Peplau (1975) scale uncritically (Furnham & Procter, 1989). Although the results from some studies are equivocal it is probably true to say that most studies were successful in confirming their hypotheses regarding the relationship of BJW scores and some dependent variable. Two major questions remain: the psychometric validity of the now various scales used to measure the BJW and the epistemic and theoretical yield from all this research. There has been concern about the dimensionality and indeed the validity of all the current measures of the BJW. More than that the items of many of the scales seem too unsubtle and therefore possible vulnerable to dissimulation or other forms of faking. Studies that have investigated the psychometric properties of these scales have been some what perfunctory. The exception is the admirable and extensive work of Schmitt (1994) and his colleagues whose studies have, however, led them to be non commital about the validity of their measure. Too many studies simply do not yield the predictive and construct validity data that one might hope for.

A second criticism is more important. After twenty years of BJW research using self report measures the question remains as to how much the research has advanced our understanding of the BJW. It is probably true to say that we know now that there is some evidence of the cross-cultural validity of the measures and that BJW beliefs relate to a very wide range of attitudes, beliefs and behaviours. But has it helped us understand the processes and mechanisms that lead to and maintain the justice motive? Critics of the psychometric tradition might argue that more indepth studies of individual actions backed up by social psychological experiments ultimately yield more insightful results. Yet one must agree with Cronbach that both research traditions have their place and together yield a better understanding of the BJW.

REFERENCES

Ahmed, S.M. & Stewart, R.A. (1985). Factor analytical and correlational study of just world scale. Perceptual and Motor Skills, 60, 135–140.

Alderrman, O., Brehm, S., & Katz, L. (1974). Empathetic observation of an innocent victim; The just world revisited. Iournal of Personality and Social Psychology, 29, 342–347.

Arbuthnot, J. (1983). Attribution by simulated jurors. Psychological Reports, 52, 287–298.

Asch, A. (1984). The experience of disability. American Psvchologist, 39, 529–536.

Braband, J. & Lerner, M.J. (1975). A little time and effort: Who deserves what from whom? Personality and Psychological Bulletin, 1, 177–181.

Burke, R. (1985). Beliefs and fears underlying Type A behaviour. Journal of General Psychology, 12, 133–145.

Collins, B.E. (1974). Four separate components of the Rotter I-E Scale: Beliefs in a difficult world, a just world, a predictable world and a politically responsive world. Journal of Personality and Social Psychology, 29, 381–391.

Connors, J. & Heaven, P. (1987). Authoritarianism and just world beliefs. Journal of Social Psychology, 127, 345–346.

Cronbach, L. (1957). The two disciplines of scientific psychology. American Psycholoist, 12, 671–689.

Dalbert, C., Montada, L. & Schmitt, M. (1987). Glaube an eine gerecht Welt als Motiv. Psychologische Beiträge, 29, 596–615.

Deutsch, M. (1985). Distributive Justice. New Haven: Yale University Press.

Dodd, D.K. & Mills, L.C. (1985). Fadis: A measure of the fear of accidental death and injury. The Psychological Record, 35, 269–275.

Dolinski, D. (1991). What is the source of the belief in an unjust Polish world. Polish Psychological Bulletin, 22, 43–51.

Ellard, J., & Lerner, M..J. (1982). The belief in a just world: Dimension or style. Paper presented at the annual meeting of the American Psychological Association, Washington DC.

Feinberg, R.A., Powell, A., & Miller, F.G. (1982). Control and belief in the just world: what's good can also be bad. Social Behaviour and Personality, 10, 57–61.

Finamore, F. & Carlson, J. (1987). Religiosity, belief in a just world and crime control attitudes. Psychological Reports, 61, 135–138.

Furnham, A. (1985). Just world beliefs in an unjust society: A cross-cultural comparison. European Journal of Social Psychology, 15, 363–366.

Furnham, A. (1990) The Protestant Work Ethic: The psychology of work-related beliefs and behaviours. London: Routledge.

Furnham, A. (1992). The Just World Belief in Twelve Cultures. Journal of Social Psychology, 133, 317–329.

Furnham, A. (1995). The just world, charitable giving and attitudes to disability. Personality and Individual Differences, 19, 577–583.

Furnham, A. & Bochner, S. (1986). Culture Shock: Psychological Consequence of Geographic Movement. London: Methuen. Pp. 298. (Translated into Japanese). Reprinted 1989, 1990, 1992.

Furnham, A., & Gunter, B. (1984). Just world beliefs and attitudes to the poor. British Journal of Social Psychology, 23, 265–269.

Furnham, A.& Henderson, M. (1984). A content and correlational analysis of five assertiveness inventories. Behavioural Assessment, 6, 79–88.

Furnham, A. & Procter, E. (1989). Just world beliefs and AIDS: A validational study of new multidimensional Just World Belief Scale. Unpublished paper.

Furnham, A. & Procter, E. (1992). Sphere-specific just world beliefs and attitudes to Aids. Human Relations, 45, 265–280.

Furnham, A. & Steele, H. (1993). Measuring locus of control: A critique of general, children's, health, and work-related locus of control questionnaires. British Journal of Psychology, 84, 443–479.

Galassi, J., Galassi, J. & Vedder, M. (1981). Perspectives on assertion as a social skills model. In J. Wane & H. Smye (Eds.) Social Competence. New York: Guildford Press.

Gerbasi, K., Zuckerman, M. & Reis, H. (1977). Justice needs a new blindfold: A review of mock jury research. Psychological Bulletin, 84, 323–345.

Godfrey, B.W., & Lowe, C.A. (1975). Devaluation of innocent victims: An attribution analysis within the world paradigm. Journal of Personality and Social Psychology, 31, 944–951.

Gruman, J.C., & Sloan, R.P. (1983). Disease as justice: perceptions of victims of physical illness. Basic and Applied Social Psychology, 4, 39–46.

Heaven, P. (1987). Belief about the spread of the acquired immune deficiency syndrome. The Medical Journal of Australia, 147, 272–274.

Heaven, P., & Connors, J. (1988). Personality, gender, and 'Just World' Beliefs. Australian Journal of Psychology, 40, 261–266.

Heider, F. (1958). The Psychology of Interpersonal Relations. New York: Wiley.

Hofstede, G. (1981). Cultures Consequences. London: Sage.

Hyland, M.E., & Dann, P.C. (1987). Exploratory factor analysis of the just world scale using British undergraduates. British Journal of Social Psychology, 26, 73–77.

Karniol, R. (1980). A conceptual analysis of immanent justice responses in children. Child Development, 51, 118–130.

Karuza, J. & Cary, T.O. (1984). Relevance preference and adaptiveness of behavioural blame for observers of rape victims. Journal of Personality, 52, 249–262.

Kassin, S. & Wrightsman, L. (1983). The construction and validation of a juror-bias scale. Journal of Research in Personality, 17, 423–442.

Kerr, K.L., & Kurtz, S.T. (1977). Effects of a victim's suffering and respectability on mock juror judgements: Further evidence on the just world theory. Representative Research in Social Psychology, 8, 42–56.

Kiecolt-Glaser, J. & Williams, D. (1987). Self-blame, compliance and distress among burn patients. Journal of Personality and Social Psychology, 53, 187–193.

Kline, P. (1985). Personality. London: Hutchinson.

Langer, E.J. (1977). The psychology of chance. Journal for the Theory of Social Behaviour, 1, 184–195.

Lerner, M.J. (1965). Evaluation of performance as a function of performer's reward and attractiveness. Journal of Personality and Social Psychology, 1, 355–360.

Lerner, M.J. (1977). The justice motive in social behaviour: Some hypotheses as to its origins and forms. Journal of Personality, 45, 1–52.

Lerner, M.J. (1978). Belief in a 'just world' versus the 'authoritarianism' syndrome.. by nobody liked the Indians. Ethnicity, 5, 229–237.

Lerner, M.J. (1980). The Belief in a Just World: A fundamental delusion. New York: Plenum Press.

Lerner, M.J. (1981). The justice motive in human behaviour: Some thoughts on what we know and need to know about justice. In M.J. Lerner & S.C. Lerner (Eds.), The justice motive in social behavior: Adapting to times of scarcity and change (pp. 11–35). New York: Plenum.

Lerner, M., & Miller, D. (1978). Just world research and the attribution process: Looking back and ahead. Psychological Bulletin, 85, 1030–1050.

Lerner, M.J., & Simmons, C.H. (1966). The observer's reaction to the "innocent victim": Compassion or rejection? Journal of Personality and Social Psychology, 4, 203–210.

Levenson, H. (1974). Activism and powerful others: Distinctions within the concept of internal-external control. Journal of Personality Assessment. 38, 377–383.

Lipkus, I. (1991). The construction and preliminary validation of a global belief in a just world and the exploratory analysis of the multi-dimensional belief in a just-world scale. Personality and Individual Differences, 12, 1171–1178

Long, E.T. & Lerner, M.J. (1974). Deserving the 'personal contract' and altruistic behaviour by children. Journal of Personality and Social Psychology. 29, 551–556.

Lynn, R. (1991). The Secret of the Miracle Economy. London: SAU.

Ma, L., & Smith, K. (1986). Individual and social correlates of the just world belief: A study of Taiwan college students. Psychological Reports, 57, 35–38.

Mahler, I., Greenberg, L. & Hayashi, H. (1981). A comparative study of rules of justice: Japanese versus American. Psychologia, 24, 1–8.

McFatter, R.M. (1978). Sentencing strategies and Justice: Effects of punishment philosophy on sentencing decisions. Journal of Personality and Social Psychology, 36, 1490–1500.

Miller, F.D., Smith, E.R., Ferree, M.M. & Taylor, S.E. (1976). Predicting perceptions of victimization. Journal of Applied Social Psychology, 6, 352–359.

Miller, D.T. & McCann, C.D. (1979). Children's reactions to the perpetrators and victims of injustices. Child Development, 50, 861–868.

Miller, D.T. & Smith, J. (1977). The effect of own deservingness and deservingness of others on children's helping behaviour. Child Development, 48, 617–620

Montada, L. (1991). Life stress, injustice and the question "Who is responsible?" In H. Steensma & R. Vermunt (Eds.) Social Justice in Human Relations (pp. 9–30). New York: Plenum.

Moran, G. & Comfort, J.C. (1982). Scientific juror selection. Journal of Personality and Social Psychology, 42, 1052–1063.

Moroi, K. (1983). An experimental study of causal attributions for an unjust outcome. Japanese Journal of Psychology, 23, 61–73.

Nelsen, E.A., Eisenberg, N. & Carroll, J.L. (1982). The structure of adolescents' attitudes towards law and crime. Journal of Genetic Psychology, 140, 47–58.

Paulus, D. (1983). Sphere-specific measures of perceived control. Journal of Personality and Social Psychology, 44, 1253–1265.

Rubin, Z., & Peplau, L. (1973). Belief in a just world and reactions to another lot: A study of participants in the national draft lottery. Journal of Social Issues, 31, 65–90.

Rubin, Z., & Peplau, L. (1975). Who believes in a just world. Journal of Social Issues, 31, 65–90.

Schmitt, M. (1994). Multiple Ambiguities of Belief in a Just World Measures. University of Trier. Unpublished Paper.

Seligmann, M. (1975). Helplessness: On Depression, Development and Death. San Francisco: Freeman.

Shorkey, C. (1980). Relationship between rational thinking and belief in a just world. Psychological Reports, 1, 161–162.

Simmonds, C.H. (1981). Theoretical issues in the development of social justice. In M.J. Lerner & S.C. Lerner (Eds.) The Justice Motive in Social Behaviour: Adapt to times of scarcitv and chance. New York: Plenum.

Sloan, R.P. & Gruman, J.C. (1983). Beliefs about cancer, heart disease and their victims. Psychological Reports, 52, 415–424.

Smith, K.B & Green, D.N. (1984). Individual correlates of the belief in a just world. Psychological Reports, 54, 435–438.

Spence, J. & Helmreich, R. (1972). The attitude toward women scale. JSAS Catalogue of Selected Documents in Psvchology, 2, 667–668.

Stewart, R.A.C. (1976). An experimental form of the Stewart Personality Inventory, a simplified format measure of major personality dimension. Perceptual and Motor Skills, 43, 813–814.

Thornton, B., Rykeman, R.M., & Robins, M.A. (1982). The relationships of observer characteristics to beliefs in the causal responsibility of victims of sexual assault. Human Relations, 35, 321–330.

Wagstaff, G. (1984). Correlates of the j ust world in Britain. Journal of Social Psychology, 121, 145–146.

Wagstaff, G., & Quirk, M. (1983). Attitudes to sex roles, political conservatism, and belief in a just world. Psychological Reports, 2, 813–814.

Wagstaff, G.F. (1982). Attitudes to rape: the "just world' strikes again? Bulletin of the British Psychological Society, 35, 277–279.

Wyer, R.S., Bodenhausen, G.V., & Gorman, T.F. (1985). Cognitive mediators of reactions to rape. Journal of Personality and Social Psychology, 48, 324–338.

Zuckerman, M. & Gerbasi, K.C. (1977b). Belief in a just world and trust Journal of Research in Personality, II, 306–317.

Zuckerman, M., Gerbasi, K.C., Kravitz, R.I. & Wheeler, L. (1975). The belief in a just world and reactions to innocent victims. JSAS Catalog of Selected Documents in Psychology, 326.

Zuckerman, M. & Gerbasi, K.C. (1977a). Dimension of the I-E Scale and their relationship to other personality measures. Educational and Psychological Measurement, 37, 159–175.

Zuckerman, M. & Gerbasi, K.C. (1977b). Belief in internal control or belief in a just world. Journal of Personality, 45, 356–378.

Chapter 10

Eight Stages in the Development of Research on the Construct of Belief in a Just World?

JÜRGEN MAES

Thirty years ago, Melvin Lerner published his first article on the construct of Belief in a Just World. He had conducted an experiment on subjects' evaluations of two men being rewarded by chance for working on a task. Regardless of the stimulus persons' performance, and regardless of the subjects' sympathy for one of the two stimulus persons, their evaluations were more positive for the one who had been accidentally rewarded. They seemed to convince themselves that he had deserved the chance outcome. Lerner therefore suggested a basic need to believe that the world is just. In the following years, he conducted additional experiments to clarify and elucidate this phenomenon (cf. Lerner & Simmons, 1966; Lerner, 1971). Since then, in more than two hundred published studies Lerner's assumptions on people's need to believe in a just world have been tested. The present article is a historical one, resuming thirty years of just world research (1965–1995). In the same moment it is examined whether the history of research on the construct can be adequately described by a typical developmental pattern proposed by Furnham (1990, see also Furnham's chapter in this volume).

JÜRGEN MAES • Department of Psychology, University of Trier, D-54286 Trier, Germany.

Responses to Victimizations and Belief in a Just World, edited by Montada and Lerner. Plenum Press, New York, 1998.

1. A STAGE SEQUENCE PROPOSED BY FURNHAM (1990)

According to this developmental pattern, a so-called "single trait personality theory" runs a typical sequence of eight stages from the identification of a phenomenon to its general acceptance in the scientific community. The first stage is the identification of a phenomenon. A phenomenon is discovered by laboratory research, by observation in a clinic or through critical reading. Typical for the second stage are replications and additional experimental efforts to elaborate the nature of the observed effect. The robustness and generalizability of the findings are examined by subtle variations in the dependent and independent variables. Regardless of whether the original researchers are clinical, personality or social psychologists, a self-report measure is developed in the third stage, normally some years after the concept or behavior pattern has been described for the first time. This stage is associated with a shift from experimental to correlational research on the same concept. The fourth stage involves attempts to test the concurrent, construct and (less often) predictive validity of the self-report measure. Some of the studies are done by the original author, but more commonly by researchers from different laboratories. Although the self-report measure is regarded as unidimensional in the beginning, subsequent multivariate statistics—which characterize the 5th stage—often show the measure to be multidimensional. In some, but not in all cases, the identified subdimensions help to resolve equivocal findings of previous research. But that is not the only possible effect. On the sixth stage, repeated psychometric investigations "often lead scholars to despair" (Furnham, 1990, p. 926). Frequently, researchers tend to develop a new better scale, and these better scales often are multi-dimensionaland/or sphere-specific in order to measure the trait in a restricted range of behavior like politics or mental health. Finally, this leads to the seventh stage which is characterized by doubts about the original concept, especially doubts about its conceptual or psychometric status. In contrast to the other stages, this stadium is not characterized by increased empirical research but by theoretical reconceptualization. When a concept survives this critical stadium it reaches the eighth stage which is called acceptance and "text-bookization" by Furnham (1990): the concept then is "accepted into the canon of individual difference measures" (p. 927), which becomes visible through its inclusion in numerous text-books on personality. According to Furnham this developmental pattern can be observed in nearly all "single trait theories" regardless of whether the traits have their origins in cognitive, social or clinical psychology, and regardless of whether their authors like to call their concepts trait, type, style, behavior pattern, cognitive belief system or whatsoever. "Single trait personality theory" is only separated with Hampson (1982) from multi-trait theories which aim to describe the entire personality.

2. DEVELOPMENT OF JUST WORLD RESEARCH

Just World Theory has been continuously developed and supported from 1965 up to now. It is documented and summarized in great detail in one monograph (Lerner, 1980), two reviews (Lerner & Miller, 1978; Furnham & Procter, 1989), and several theoretical surveys (Lerner, 1976; Lerner, 1977; Lerner, Miller & Holmes, 1976). Since the beginning 1970s different research groups picked up Melvin Lerner's original conception, and since the beginning 1980s this conception is applied to larger social problems (cf. Lerner & Lerner, 1981; Albee, 1986). In order to establish the number and temporal distribution of studies on belief in a just world the APA database PsycLit and the German database PSYNDEX (drawn up by the ZPID at the university of Trier) were searched through. Studies older than 1974 were searched for in the Psychological Abstracts. Figure 1 shows the number of studies from 1965 up to 1994. Younger studies were not considered because experience teaches that it lasts up to two years until all the studies are included in the database.

Figure 1 shows that there is a rather continuous increase in studies since 1965 with peaks in the second half of the seventies, in the beginning of the eighties and even more in the beginning of the nineties. One might speculate that the first peak is due to the creation of a self-report measure, the second peak to the publication of Lerner's monograph "Belief in a just world—a fundamental delusion," and the last peak to grown popularity and world-wide research efforts. In the following, it is examined whether all the stages named by Furnham (1990) can be observed in the history of just world research as well.

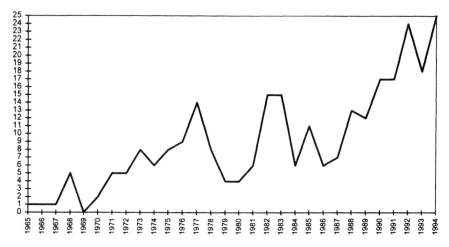

FIGURE 1.   Number of studies on just world theory.

2.1. Stage 1: Identification of a Phenomenon

According to Furnham (1990) a phenomenon is discovered more or less accidentally as a result of laboratory research, clinical observations or critical reading. It is given a name and it is worked out to describe and explain behavior. The discovery of belief in a just world cannot be reconstructed on the basis of Lerner's early publications which have been on topics like the organization of values (Lerner, 1960), working behavior of chronic schizophrenics (Lerner & Fairweather, 1963; Lerner, 1963a, 1963b), conformity and sibling position (Becker, Lerner & Carroll, 1966), psychoanalytic terms like identification with the aggressor (Baxter, Lerner & Miller, 1965), or convictions concerning a possible nuclear war (Lerner, 1965c; Novak & Lerner, 1966). The ideas for most of the early experimental studies were derived from popular social psychological conceptions of that time, like cognitive dissonance theory or cognitive balance. Failing attempts to explain experimental data with these conceptions drove the search for alternative explanations. The following quotation is typical for that period: "These data overall have negative implications for both conventional balance theory and the theory of cognitive generalization of similarities. . . . Taken together, however, these results create a rather consistent and somewhat surprising pattern. . . . It is clear that although the findings with both stimulus subjects appear to fit together, they do not support any available theoretical positions" (Lerner, Dillehay & Sherer, 1967, p. 484). Lerner and Becker (1962) had already demonstrated that the connection between similarity, liking and approaching only persists when no other motives become dominant on the part of the person. The term "belief in a just world" emerges as a explanatory construct for the first time in the experiment mentioned in the beginning (Lerner, 1965a). Another experiment—published by Lerner and Simmons (1966)—is regarded as the classical paradigm in just world research. Their subjects derogated a victim that got electric shocks in a pretended learning experiment. If the subjects could decide that the victim would receive reward instead of shock in the next round they did so and restored justice this way. But choice was not enough to prevent derogation, the subjects had to be sure that their decision would be successful in reducing the victim's suffering. Worst evaluations of the victim could be observed in the so-called "martyr" condition in which the victim only took part in the experiment for the subjects' benefit. The results of the first experiments can be summarized as follows: belief in a just world influences social judgments and evaluations of other people. Regardless of whether the stimulus persons' fate is portrayed as positive or negative, subjects seem to convince themselves that they deserve their fate. Thus, belief in a just world leads to derogation of losers, victims and underprivileged people (cf. Lerner & Simmons, 1966; Lerner, 1978) and to admiration of winners and privileged people (Lerner, 1965a; Lerner, 1978).

However, the first stage in just world research is not restricted to the discovering of a single phenomenon and its experimental demonstration, but includes theoretical formulations as well in order to describe different functions of the justice motive and to explain how it (the stage) comes about. These theoretical considerations cannot all be reported here, they are presented in detail by Lerner (1975, 1977, 1980) and by Lerner and Whitehead (1980). Moreover, additional questions and additional experimental designs were invented in order to demonstrate the complex functioning of people's justice motive. With these designs it could be shown how belief in a just world triggers and hinders not only social evaluations but a large set of behaviors like seeking and avoiding social contact (Novak & Lerner, 1968; Lerner & Agar, 1972), altruism (Miller, 1977a, 1977b), justification of one's own behavior (Lerner & Matthews, 1967; Lerner & Lichtman, 1968; Lerner, 1971; Chaikin & Darley, 1973), how it supports or impairs coping with life crises, and how experienced justice or injustice shapes behavior towards other people (Simmons & Lerner, 1968). Finally, it could be shown, that subjects even tend to portray their own fate as deserved (Comer & Laird, 1975; Bulman & Wortman, 1977). The theoretical formulations, the additional questions and experimental designs make the justice motive theory a rather complex theory which relates a large set of behaviors and convictions about the world and other people, and not just a "single trait personality theory."

2.2. Stage 2: Replication of the Effect

According to Furnham (1990) the second stage is characterized by numerous attempts to replicate the original findings. Many studies aim to test the robustness of the phenomenon by subtle changes in the dependent or independent variables. This stage is clearly demonstrable in the development of just world research. Most stimulating for replications was the Lerner-and-Simmons-paradigm. Similar patterns were found by Piliavin, Hardyck and Vadim (1968), Simons and Piliavin (1972), Johnson and Dickinson (1971). Lerner (1968), McDonald (1977) as well as Latta, Bernhardt, Hildebrand and Kahn (1974) could replicate the paradox of the "martyr" condition. Lerner, Miller and Holmes (1976, p. 139) summarize the results of several studies:

1. Most observers, if given the opportunity, would vote to end the victim's suffering and see to it that she received compensation for his/her suffering.

2. If they believed they were successful in rescuing and compensating the victim or that the victim would be compensated by a researcher in the end, they viewed him/her in a rather "neutral" objective light.
3. If they believed they both (the observer and the victim) had been vulnerable and the victim drew a critical ballot which decided their respective fates, she/he was not derogated, and in fact was often seen in a very positive light.
4. On the other hand, the observer's evaluation of the victim became increasingly negative, the greater her undeserved suffering.
5. The most derogation occurred when the victim was portrayed as a "martyr"—someone whose altruistic motives made him/her vulnerable for exploitation.
6. Observers who were either informed that the purpose of the research was to study the way people react to victims in society and/or made aware that the victim was merely acting and not actually being shocked did not portray the "victim" in negative manner or were they able to predict the derogation of the "innocent victim" or the "martyr."

Many replication studies have not merely confirmed or rejected the hypothesized effect but have drawn the attention to a large set of moderating or mediating variables. For example, a victim is not devalued

- if the subjects observe empathically (Aderman, Brehm & Katz, 1974),
- if the subjects expect interaction with the victim (Stokols & Schopler, 1973),
- if small group size is given (Brehm, Costanzo & Speck, 1972),
- if justified self interest is salient as a norm (Lerner & Lichtman, 1968),
- if the victim had the same chance to escape as the observer (Lerner & Matthews, 1967),
- if the subjects adhere to religion (Sorrentino & Hardy, 1974),
- if a dissimilar co-observer expresses sympathy for the victim (McKay & Lerner, 1977),
- if the victim can be hold "responsible" (Jones & Aronson, 1973),
- if it is socially desirable to feel sympathy with the victim (Lerner & Miller, 1978).

Zuckerman, Gerbasi, Kravitz and Wheeler (1975) have supposed that people use a "multiple response approach" (p. 326) to maintain belief in a just world. Their subjects did not only derogate the victim but evaluated the experiment as more important, more positive and less cruel.

2.3. Stage 3: The Development of a Self-Report Measure

The third stage involves the development of a self-report measure which is usually developed some years after the concept or behavior pattern has been described in the literature. In the case of just world theory it lasted eight years until Rubin and Peplau (1973) from UCLA presented a one-dimensional questionnaire to measure individual degrees of belief in a just world. This questionnaire contains 20 rather global items about the world in general, justice and injustice in several domains of life like traffic, law, education, sports, history and health. The questionnaire was applied for the first time in a field study during the "National Draft Lottery" (1973); with the data of that study they computed an alpha coefficient for internal consistency of $\alpha = .79$. Rubin and Peplau (1975) report two studies where they found alphas of .80 and .81. Later on, other authors found less sufficient alphas: Ambrosio and Sheehan (1989): .64, Feather (1991): .54 (high school) and .69 (university), Kristiansen and Giulietti (1991): .75, O'Quin and Vogler (1990): .70 (sample of sociology students) and .38 for prison inmates, Smith and Green (1984): .67 (large town in Texas), Whatley (1993): .56. Furnham (1993), using samples of psychology students in twelve different countries, found internal consistencies between $\alpha = .48$ and $\alpha = .71$.

2.4. Stage 4: Validation of the Measure

Experimental and correlational studies are used to validate the scale in the, sometimes long-lasting, fourth stage. In the case of just world theory, this stage lasted from 1973 to the end of the 1980s. Both sorts of studies are sifted through in the following. The first chance for Rubin and Peplau (1973) to validate their scale came with the National Draft Lottery in 1972. A good or bad fate (to have to go to Vietnam) was allocated by accident to a group of 20-year-old students. If the scale is a valid device—Rubin and Peplau concluded—then high scorers should evaluate co-students with a good fate positively and co-students with a bad fate negatively; the opposite pattern was expected for low scorers. In Rubin and Peplau's field study, 50 students not known to each other, listened to the live broadcast of the lottery per radio. There was an overall tendency for pity and compassion with the drafted ones in the whole group, but nevertheless the expected pattern was found for high scorers. The validity of the scale was confirmed by other experiments as well, as for example by a replication of the Lerner-and-Simmons findings by Zuckerman, Gerbasi, Kravitz and Wheeler (1975): high scorers were more prone to devalue the innocent victim than low scorers ($p < .03$). Zuckerman and Gerbasi (1977a) conducted three experiments and showed that high scorers were (1) less suspicious with regard to faking in social psychological experiments, (2) less suspicious when they were promised a gratis book, (3) less suspicious with regard to the government's position in a number of public affairs. Kleinke and Meyer (1990) found that high scoring men evaluated a videotaped rape victim less positive than low scoring men (but the opposite was true for women). Dion and Dion (1987) demonstrated that belief in a just world is an important cue in moderating evaluations of attractive stimulus persons. High scorers that were unfairly treated in an experiment convinced themselves that the procedure was not unfair and expressed less anger than low scorers (Hafer & Olson, 1989). Similarly, high scorers showed more conformity with their tormentor who had exposed them to unbearable noise in an experiment by Kerr and Gross (1978). Most studies using the Rubin-and-Peplau scale were correlational studies. These studies illustrate the construct validity of the scale. Some of the correlational patterns that are typically found are presented in the following:

2.4.1. Trust

The scale was found to correlate with Rotter's Interpersonal Trust Scale (r = .55) and with the subscales "institutional trust" (r = .42), "trust in other people's sincerity" (r = .34) and "trust that one will not be taken advantage of by others" (r = .32) (see Rubin & Peplau, 1975). Using a representative sample of London television viewers, Wober and Gunter (1985) found low scores on the just world items having more confidence in medical treatment for physical problems (but less confidence with respect to treatment of psychological problems and major surgical problems).

2.4.2. Religiousness

Because notions of a just world are implied in Western religions, correlations of just world scores with religious affiliations could be expected. Rubin and Peplau reported a correlation of r = .42 with self-reported church attendance and a correlation of r = .31 with belief in an active God. Furnham and Reilly (1991) found highly religious persons uttering higher just world beliefs in an British and in a Japanese sample. Similarly, Szmajke (1991) found a slightly higher belief in a just world in very religious Polish adults. Zweigenhaft, Phillips, Adams, Morse and Horan (1985) supposed that the association between BJW and religiousness found by Rubin and Peplau (1975) and by Sorrentino and Hardy (1974) is not true for all kinds of religious groups. They could show that the opposite pattern was true for Quakers The decisive variable was the manner in which people were religious, not simply whether or how much people were religious.

2.4.3. Protestant Work Ethic

Because McDonald (1972) had found that persons with high scores on the Protestant ethic scale developed by Mirels and Garrett (1971) were more prone to derogate victims, Rubin and Peplau (1975) supposed connections between both belief systems. Lerner (1978) found a correlation of $r = .35$. Furnham and Rajamanickam (1992) found rather high correlations between BJW and Protestant ethic: $r = .52$ in Great Britain ($r = .52$), $r = .49$ in India. Similar correlations were established by Wagstaff (1983) using Scottish adults ($r = .51$) and by Ma and Smith (1985; $r = .33$).

2.4.4. Authoritarianism

Rubin and Peplau (1975) supposed a connection because authoritarian people admire the powerful in society and just world believers devalue the weak. They obtained a correlation of $r = .56$ with Adorno, Frenkel-Brunswick, Levinson and Sanfords (1950) F-scale. Whereas Ma and Smith (1985) could only find a correlation of BJW and F-scale of $r = .06$ in a sample of students from Taiwan, Connors and Heaven (1987) calculated a correlation of $r = .33$ in a sample of students from Australia. Comparably, Finamore and Carlson (1987) found BJW to be associated with punitive criminal justice attitudes (but only for Protestant, not for Catholic students). Using the German just world scale (Dalbert, Montada & Schmitt, 1987), Dalbert (1992) found correlations between just world belief and authoritarianism of $r = .41$ (German students) and $r = .30$ (Spanish teachers). In spite of the partly considerable correlations between BJW and authoritarianism, factor analytic work done by Lerner (1978) showed that they can be and should be differentiated. Whereas authoritarianism was associated with a factor that reflected rejection of Indians, Metis, Americans, the poor and Jews, BJW was associated with another factor that reflected rejection of Indians and Metis, but admiration of Americans.

2.4.5. Locus of Control

Another pattern that is currently found is an association of BJW with internal locus of control sensu Rotter (1966). Rubin and Peplau (1975) report six studies that yielded correlations between .32 and .58. Similar correlations were found by Zuckerman and Gerbasi (1977c), Rim (1981), Lipkus (1991), Witt (1989), Hafer and Olson (1989), Bierhoff, Klein and Kramp (1991), and Clayton (1992).

2.4.6. Adaptability

Belief in a just world was often supposed to make adaptation to difficult situations easier, to let find meaning in life crises, and to contribute to better coping. In four different samples Feather (1991) found positive correlations between BJW and global self esteem sensu Rosenberg (1965), with correlations varying between .10 and .23. Ritter, Benson and Synder (1990) found a negative correlation between BJW and depression (scale by Radloff, 1977) in a study of coping with a difficult economical situation in Northern Ireland. Ma and Smith (1985) found BJW negatively related to alienation scales.

2.4.7. Political Attitudes and Voting Preferences

Rubin and Peplau (1975) reported positive correlations between BJW and positive attitudes towards political organizations (.37) and a positive attitude towards the government. High scorers uttered more conservative attitudes and had a more positive attitude towards President Nixon in the time when his impeachment was discussed. Additionally, they found a negative correlation (−.29) with political activism. Connors and Heaven (1987) found BJW to be correlated with a preference of right wing political parties (.30) and with a position on the right of the left-right-continuum (.16). Similarly, Wagstaff (1983) and Wagstaff and Quirk (1983) found that voters of the conservative party in England and Scotland had higher BJW scores. Comparable results were obtained by Furnham and Gunter (1984) for British voters and by Smith and Green (1984) for American voters. Dalbert, Montada and Schmitt (1987) and Montada and Schneider (1989) found a similar pattern in Germany with a German just world scale.

2.5. Stage 5: Factor Analytic Work and Multi-Dimensionality

The fifth stage is described as follows by Furnham (1990): although the self-report measure is regarded as unidimensional in the beginning, subsequent multivariate statistics often show the measure to be multidimensional. Different results of different studies lead to discussions about the number of dimensions, their relationship and their labeling. Can this stage be found for the development of just world research? In most of the studies attempting to validate the Rubin-and-Peplau scale the item sum was used as a measure for BJW. Thus, implicitly unidimensionality was presumed. Rubin and Peplau themselves conducted no factor analysis of the items. Nevertheless, there are a number of studies that show the scale to be multidimensional. The first factor analytic investigation was conducted by Fink and Wilkins (1976) with the data of 291 students. Principal component analyses with varimax rotation yielded three factors that were interpreted as: (1) Deserving (relationship between "inputs" and "outcomes"), (2) Denial of injustice, and (3) Judgment of a just world.

Only one of the numerous factor analytic studies shows the scale to be one-dimensional. Ahmed and Stewart (1985) administered the scale to 196 full-time and part-time students: The extraction of three factors would be statistically justifiable, but the first factor explains 65 percent of the variance. Except for one item, all items had substantial loadings on the first factor. This leads the authors to argue that the elimination of one item leads to a homogenous and reliable scale. Most of the other studies doubt the one-dimensionality. The most prominent investigation was done by Hyland and Dann (1987) who administered the Rubin-and-Peplau-scale to 226 psychology undergraduates and conducted a principal component analysis with varimax rotation. They obtained seven eigenvalues greater than 1, and according to the "scree" criterion they interpreted a four-factor solution explaining 38.7 percent of the variance. Factors were labeled as follows: (1) Justness of authority (the items refer to courts, parents, trial and referee), (2) The just world (items stress very generally that there is justice in the world), (3) The deserving person (items state that the person deserves something), (4) Consequences of prudence (items state that prudent actions lead to just outcomes).

In a sample of 283 adults from Northern Ireland, Ritter, Benson and Synder (1990) used only ten items which in their opinion correspond to the second factor interpreted by Hyland and Dann (1987). A principal component analysis over these ten items once again led to four factors that are not reported in detail. Their recommendation is to use only three items as a measure of BJW. These items state the prevalence of justice in the world in a very general way.

In a heterogeneous sample of 138 British residents, Harper, Wagstaff, Newton and Harrison (1990) interpreted three factors explaining 34.8 percent of the variance: (1) Pro Just World, (2) Anti Just World, (3) Cynical or Reserved Just World. Only the Pro Just World factor significantly correlated with blaming the poor for Third World poverty (r = .31).

O'Quin and Vogler (1990) administered the Rubin-and-Peplau scale to a sample of sociology students and to a sample of prison inmates. They did not only obtain strongly varying reliabilities (α = .70 for the students; α = .38 for prison inmates), but also different factorial structures. In both samples, there were eight eigenvalues above 1, according to the "scree" criterion two five-factor solutions were interpreted explaining 48 respectively 49 percent of the variance. Only the first two factors were comparable in both samples; the items stressed the triumph of the good and deserving persons—the other factors were totally different. Similarly, Whatley (1993) conducted factor analyses for different samples and obtained highly different factor structures. Examining the just world scores of an American undergraduate sample, Ambrosio and Sheehan (1990) found seven eigenvalues greater than 1 and interpreted a four-factor solution accounting for 19.4 percent of the total variance. They label the factors as: (1) Escape Justice, (2) Deserve what one gets, (3) Teach Justice, and (4) Prudence.

Unfortunately, the authors do not describe these factors in more detail. Moreover, separate analyses for the sexes led to different results, and reliabilities for the subscales were poor. Ambrosio and Sheehan (1991) conclude that the BJW scale should be revised basically. Equally, Ritter, Benson and Synder (1990) plead for more efforts to refine the concept's measurement.

2.6. Stage 6: Multiple Multi-Dimensional Measures

According to Furnham (1990), the sixth stage often leads researchers to despair: Repeated psychometric investigations lead to the development of new and better self-report measures; often these scales are multi-dimensionaland/or sphere-specific. This stage, also, can be observed in the development of just world research. Up to now, several questionnaires to measure belief in a just world exist, unidimensional as well as multi-dimensional, domain specific as well as general. These scales have different sources: partly they result from psychometric investigations of earlier scales, partly they were extracted more or less accidentally from attitude research in other domains, partly they were created as analogies to other instruments. An example for a scale that resulted more or less accidentally from attitude research is a study done by Hui, Chan and Chan (1989). These authors studied beliefs about the consequences of death and obtained five factors which they called Buddhist and Taoist belief (1), Naturalistic belief (3), Immortal Soul Belief (4), Protestant Belief (5) and Just World Belief (2). The items loading on that factor stress the conviction that good people ascend to heaven and evil people will descend to hell to suffer there. In contrast to this scale, other self-report measures were developed explicitly in order to get better or refined measures of BJW. Two examples for this are the one-dimensional just world scale developed by Lipkus (1991, 1992) and the German just world questionnaire developed by Dalbert, Montada and Schmitt (1987). Because a precise translation of the Rubin-and-Peplau scale didn't function in Germany (Dalbert, 1982), the latter authors strived for a refined German self-report device. They presented two homogeneous and reliable scales: one to measure general belief in a just world (GWAL), one to measure domain specific just world beliefs (GWBS). More recently, Dalbert and Yamauchi (1994) could show that an English version of the GWAL works as a homogeneous and reliable scale as well. Several studies confirm the usefulness of distinguishing general and domain-specific beliefs in a just world (cf. Montada & Figura, 1988; Montada & Schneider, 1989; Montada, Schmitt & Dalbert, 1986; Maes & Montada, 1989; Dalbert, Fisch & Montada, 1992). Lipkus' (1991) scale construction was a similar reaction to the insufficient psychometric properties and varying factor structures of the Rubin-and-Peplau scale: Like Dalbert, Montada and Schmitt with the GWAL, he uses only seven items which state the general prevalence of justice in the world. This scale proved to be homogeneous and reliable (Lipkus, 1991; Glennon, Joseph & Hunter, 1993). In contrast to these scale developments Furnham and Procter's (1992) sphere-specific questionnaire is a metaphorical transference from a sphere-specific measure of perceived control (Paulhus, 1983). In analogy to Paulhus (1983) who differentiated personal, interpersonal and sociopolitical beliefs in control, Furnham and Procter (1992) proposed to measure personal, interpersonal and sociopolitical belief in a just world. However, the internal consistencies of these scales were not really sufficient: they vary between α = .58 and α = .63 (Furnham & Procter, 1992, for a priori scales) and between α = .32 and α = .43 (Lipkus, 1991, who factor-analyzed the questionnaire).

2.7. Stage 7: Doubts about the Original Concept

After a decade of intensive psychometric work, the complexity of measurement and equivocal findings often lead scientists to cast doubts about the concept and its measurement. Either it is recommended to give up the concept, or it is argued that the phenomenon is too unstable to be regarded as a trait. In contrast to the other stages, this stadium is characterized by theoretical reconceptualization rather than increased empirical work (Furnham, 1990). It cannot be decided whether the just world construct has already reached this stage of basic doubt nor whether it will or will have to reach it: doubts were uttered from time to time concerning the psychometric properties of just world scales (Ritter, Benson & Synder, 1990), concerning the "ambiguous" interpretability of some empirical results (Schmitt, 1997, this volume) or concerning the quality of conceptualization (Lerner, Miller & Holmes, 1976)—the conception in itself, however, is enjoying a great acceptance in the scientific community. Critics are restricted to detail problems but do not imply a general questioning of the concept. For example, Bierhoff (1978) criticized that it is not clear how deserving, just-world belief and the matrix of social interactions developed by Lerner and Whitehead (1980) refer to each other. Kayser (1980) found the fact questionable that justified self-interest is regarded as a form of justice. O'Connor (1991) censured that researchers concentrated on effects of BJW and not on its sources. The most comprehensive evaluation of just world theory was performed from a philosophical perspective by Solomon (1989). In his personal opinion the study of belief in a just world is an "important but ultimately depressing study" (p. 351). He comments Lerner not only on the meticulous manner in which he describes "in painful detail" the various forms of self-deception concerning the fundamental delusion of "belief in a just world" which is ironically creating more injustice but as well on his adamant insistence that the issues he examines cannot be construed simply in terms of belief and the self-deceptions cannot be understood simply as reducing cognitive dissonance. Instead belief in a just world is regarded as a "deeply emotional matter, a question of deep personal investment, heavily tied up with self-esteem and other questions of self-worth, rather than an abstract philosophical belief" (p. 352).

But nevertheless he is insisting that no empirical study of justice can be value free. Because such a study is already embedded in a philosophical framework he is missing footnotes or bibliographical references to philosophical investigations in Lerner's fundamental book from 1980. In his opinion, the neglecting of this philosophical framework lead to a conception of justice as an ideal state of the world which inevitably directed the scientific attention to a catalog of rationalizations and deceptions described in just world research: "Once the divorce between the state of the world (just or unjust) and our conceptualization of justice is established, it is hard to imagine any possible outcome other than bitter resignation, revolutionary rebellion, or that tapestry of deceit catalogued in The Belief in a Just World: A Fundamental Delusion." This reminds him to Camus (1961) and his book "Myth of Sisyphus." Camus as well as Lerner suggest that seeing through the delusions is a precondition of becoming a just person. Even though he is recognizing in Lerner's work the same good-heartedness that won Camus the Nobel Prize, his critique culminates in the opinion that there is too little accent on the positive and too little description of those emotions and attitudes that make justice possible. While philosophers were only regarding justice as an abstract ideal up to now, Lerner is paying disproportionate attention to the unjust nature of the world and the etiology of the delusions in Solomon's opinion: "Justice is neither in the heavens nor is it merely in the mud of self-deception" (p. 355). Instead, he regards justice as a set of personal feelings, a way of participating in the world. One may concede that Solomon's critique offers some hints for the further development and elaboration of just world theory, but in all his remarks imply a great appreciation of Lerner's work.

2.8. Stage 8: Acceptance and 'Text-Bookization'

On the eighth stage, the inclusion of a concept in numerous textbooks on personality is a sign that a concept has survived the other stages and is accepted into the canon of individual difference measures (Furnham, 1990). In order to establish whether text-bookization of just world theory is in progress or not, all German and English text-books on personality psychology and on social psychology available in the university Library at the University of Trier were sifted through. On the basis of this sample of text-books, it can be ascertained that the text-bookization of just world theory has reached a considerable extent in social psychology and has begun in personality psychology. There are dozens of text-books on social psychology including references to just world theory, with the earliest examples in Wrightsman (1972), Baron and Byrne (1974) and the broadest mentioning in Bierhoff (1984). The inclusion of just world theory in text-books on social psychology did not stop up to now so that three text-books from 1995 with reference to just world theory could be detected (McKnight & Sutton, 1995; Smith & Mackie, 1995; Tesser, 1995). The extent of just world references in text-books on personality psychology is smaller and began later. It began slowly in the 1980s, with the earliest example in Samuel (1981) and the broadest mentioning in Krampen (1987).

The increasing acceptance of just world theory becomes not only visible with regard to beginning "text-bookization," and not only with regard to the quantitative increase of studies (see Figure 1), but as well with regard to the increase of subjects and topics that are analyzed as applications of just world theory. These topics reach from victimization by cancer (Gruman & Sloan, 1983; Sloan & Gruman, 1983; Stahly, 1988) or rape (Best & Demmin, 1982; Wagstaff, 1982; Wyer, Bodenhausen & Gorman, 1985), attitudes towards dying (Sherman, Smith & Cooper, 1982), altruism (Pancer, 1988), media effects and TV consumption (Hormuth & Stephan, 1981; Gunter & Wober, 1983), reception of stories (Jose & Brewer, 1984), jury decisions (Kerr, Bull & MacCoun, 1985; Shaffer, Plummer & Hammock, 1986), status generalization (Ellard & Bates, 1990) up to culture-specific beliefs about economy (Rasinski & Scott, 1990) academic job search and the review process in academic psychology journals (Ross & Ellard, 1986).

Moreover, the increasing acceptance becomes visible by the growing preparedness of researchers from different research domains to reinterpret their results in consideration of just world theory and to apply just world theory to their own research domain. Such applications can be found for attributions in school and education (Richey & Richey, 1978), sex roles (Larwood & Moely, 1979), job satisfaction (Stephan & Holahan, 1982), or criminal law (McFatter, 1982). Eventually, some authors have recognized the potential of just world theory to contribute to public information and enlightenment and the chance to use the explication and demonstration of just world effects to make a plea for more humanity and to reduce obstacles and deceptions on the way to a just society

(McDonald, 1973; Wagstaff, 1982; Albee, 1986; Deutsch & Steil, 1988; Lane, 1988; Cohen, 1989).

3. CONCLUSIONS

In sum, the history of just world research can at least partly be described by the stage sequence Furnham (1990) observed in the history of many personality constructs: The identification of BJW (stage 1) was followed by attempts to replicate the effects (stage 2), the development of the unidimensional just world scale (stage 3) and attempts to validate this measure (stage 4). Then, factor analytic work revealed the multi-dimensionality of the concept (stage 5) and led to multiple multi-dimensional-measures (stage 6). The last two stages show a large acceptance of just world theory, a beginning text-bookization in personality psychology and an advanced text-bookization in social psychology. But, it is not appropriate to settle the just world studies only along this stage sequence. Particularly, the theoretical elaboration and the multitude of phenomena that can be analyzed within the just world framework cannot be described adequately along this sequence. Also, researchers did not stop to conduct experiments and field studies as soon as a self-report measure was available. In fact, there were experimental studies from the beginning (Lerner, 1965a) up to now (Steensma, den Hartigh & Lucardie, 1994). The history of just world research is not only characterized by an increase in the number of studies (Figure 1) but as well by dispersion and diversification. More and more research groups all over the world have turned to the phenomenon discovered by Lerner. Just world research today is done on four continents, mainly in America (USA and Canada) and Europe (especially Great Britain and Germany), but as well in Australia and in Asia; merely from Africa no studies are known up to now. Besides responsibility attribution and person perception additional dependent variables were investigated, like altruism (e.g. Miller 1977a, 1977b; Pancer, 1987) or adaptive processes (e.g. Bulman & Wortman, 1977; Tomaka & Blascovich, 1994). In all stages, new and imaginative paradigms were created to demonstrate intriguing just world effects. For example, Gollob and Rossman (1973) had 38 undergraduates read a number of simple sentences and then asked to what degree the sentence subjects were "powerful and able to influence others." They observed that their subjects were inclined to perceive the power and ability to influence others as residing in the hands of good people rather than bad people and interpreted this finding in the light of just world theory. In summary: The stage sequence observed by Furnham (1990) is very well suited to describe the history of the just world scale but is not completely doing justice to the diversity of experimental research and to the subtle and deep structure of just world theory.

REFERENCES

Aderman, D., Brehm, S. S., & Katz, L. B. (1974). Empathic observation of an innocent victim: The just world revisited. Journal of Personality and Social Psychology, 29, 342–347.

Adorno, T. W., Frenkel-Brunswick, E., Levinson, D. J., & Sanford, R. N. (1950). The authoritarian personality. New York: Harper.

Ahmed, S. M. S., & Stewart, R. A. C. (1985). Factor analytical and correlational study of Just World Scale. Perceptual and Motor Skills, 60, 135–140.

Albee, G. W. (1986). Toward a just society: Lessons from observations on the primary prevention of psychopathology. American Psychologist, 41, 891–898.

Ambrosio, A. L., & Sheehan, E. P. (1990). Factor analysis of the Just World Scale. Journal of Social Psychology, 130, 413–415.

Ambrosio, A. L., & Sheehan, E. P. (1991). The just world belief and the AIDS epidemic. Journal of Social Behavior and Personality, 6, 163–170.

Baron, R. A., & Byrne, D. (1974). Social Psychology. Understanding Human Interaction. Boston: Allyn and Bacon.

Baxter, J. C., Lerner, M. J., & Miller, J. S. (1965). Identification as a function of the reinforcing quality of the model and the socialization background of the subject. Journal of Personality, 2, 692–697.

Becker, S. W., Lerner, M. J., & Carroll, J. (1966). Conformity as a function of birth order and type of group pressure: A verification. Journal of Personality and Social Psychology, 3, 242–244.

Best, J. B., & Demmin, H. S. (1982). Victim's provocativeness and victim's attractiveness as determinants of blame in rape. Psychological Reports, 51, 255–258.

Bierhoff, H. W. (1978). Equity und andere Formen der Gerechtigkeit. Zeitschrift für Sozialpsychologie, 9, 89–94.

Bierhoff, H. W. (1984). Sozialpsychologie: Ein Lehrbuch. Stuttgart: Kohlhammer.

Bierhoff, H. W., Klein, R., & Kramp, P. (1991). Evidence for the altruistic personality from data on accident research. Journal of Personality, 59, 263–280.

Brehm, S., Constanzo, P., & Speck, B. (1972). Observer's reaction to the "innocent victim": An alternative explanation and attempted replication. Catalog of Selected Documents in Psychology, 122, 16–17.

Bulman, R. J., & Wortman, C. B. (1977). Attributions of blame and coping in the "real world": Severe accident victims react to their lot. Journal of Personality and Social Psychology, 35, 351–363.

Camus, A. (1961). The Myth of Sisyphus. New York: Vintage.

Chaikin, A. L., & Darley, J. M. (1973). Victim or perpetrator? Defensive attribution of responsibility and the need for order and justice. Journal of Personality and Social Psychology, 23, 268–275.

Clayton, S. D. (1992). The experience of injustice: Some characteristics and correlates. Social Justice Research, 5, 71–91.

Cohen, R. L. (1989). Fabrications of justice. Social Justice Research, 3, 21–46.

Comer, R., & Laird, J. D. (1975). Choosing to suffer as a consequence of expecting to suffer: Why do people do it? Journal of Personality and Social Psychology, 32, 92–101.

Connors, J., & Heaven, P. C. (1987). Authoritarianism and just world beliefs. Journal of Social Psychology, 127, 345–346.

Dalbert, C. (1982). Der Glaube an eine gerechte Welt: Zur Güte einer deutschen Version der Skala von Rubin & Peplau (P.I.V.-Bericht Nr .3 = Berichte aus der Arbeitsgruppe "Verantwortung, Gerechtigkeit, Moral" Nr .10). Trier: University of Trier, Fachbereich I: Psychologie.

Dalbert, C. (1992). Der Glaube an die gerechte Welt: Differenzierung und Validierung eines Konstrukts. Zeitschrift für Sozialpsychologie, 23, 268–276.

Dalbert, C., Fisch, U., & Montada, L. (1992). Is inequality unjust? Evaluating women's career chances. European Review of Applied Psychology, 42, 11–17.

Dalbert, C., Montada, L., & Schmitt, M. (1987). Glaube an eine gerechte Welt als Motiv: Validierungskorrelate zweier Skalen. Psychologische Beiträge, 29, 596–615.

Dalbert, C., & Yamauchi, L. A. (1994). Belief in a just world and attitudes toward immigrants and foreign workers: A cultural comparison between Hawai and Germany. Journal of Applied Social Psychology, 24, 1612–1626.

Deutsch, M., & Steil, J. M. (1988). Awakening the Sense of Injustice. Social Justice Research, 2, 3–23.

Dion, K. L., & Dion, K. K. (1987). Belief in a just world and physical attractiveness stereotyping. Journal of Personality and Social Psychology, 52, 775–780.

Ellard. J.H., & Bates, D. D. (1990). Evidence for the role of the justice motive in status generalization process. Social Justice Research, 4, 115–134.

Feather, N. T. (1991). Human values, global self-esteem, and belief in a just world. Journal of Personality, 59, 83–107.

Finamore, F., & Carlson, J. M. (1987). Religiosity, belief in a just world and crime control attitudes. Psychological Reports, 61, 135–138.

Furnham, A. (1990). The development of single trait personality theories. Personality and Individual Differences, 11, 923–929.

Furnham, A. (1993). Just world beliefs in twelve societies. Journal of Social Psychology, 133, 317–329.

Furnham, A., & Gunter, B. (1984). Just world beliefs and attitudes towards the poor. British Journal of Social Psychology, 23, 265–269.

Furnham, A., & Procter, E. (1989). Belief in a just world: Review and critique of the individual difference literature. British Journal of Social Psychology, 28, 365–384.

Furnham, A., & Procter, E. (1992). Sphere-specific just world beliefs and attitudes to AIDS. Human Relations, 45, 265–280.

Furnham, A., & Rajamanickam, R. (1992). The Protestant Work Ethic and Just World Beliefs in Great Britain and India. International Journal of Psychology, 27, 401–416.

Furnham, A., & Reilly, M. (1991). A cross-cultural comparison of British and Japanese Protestant work ethic and just world beliefs. Psychologia - An international Journal of Psychology in the Orient, 34, 1–14.

Glennon, F., Joseph, S., & Hunter, J. A. (1993). Just world beliefs in unjust societies: Northern Ireland. Journal of Social Psychology, 133, 591–592.

Gollob, H. F., & Rossman, B. B. (1973). Judgments of an actor's "power and ability to influence others." Journal of Experimental Social Psychology, 9, 391–406.

Gruman, J. C., & Sloan, R. P. (1983). Disease as justice: Perceptions of victims of physical illness. Basic and Applied Social Psychology, 4, 39–46.

Gunter, B., & Wober, M. (1983). Television viewing and public trust. British Journal of Social Psychology, 22, 174–176.

Hafer, C. L., & Olson, J. M. (1989). Beliefs in a just world and reactions to personal deprivation. Journal of Personality, 57, 799–823.

Hampson, S. (1982). The construction of personality. London: Routledge.

Harper, D. J., Wagstaff, G. F., Newton, J. T., & Harrison, K. R. (1990). Lay causal perceptions of Third World poverty and the Just World theory. Social Behavior and Personality, 18, 235–238.

Hormuth, S. E., & Stephan, W. G. (1981). Effects of viewing "Holocaust" on Germans and Americans: A just-world analysis. Journal of Applied Social Psychology, 11, 240–251.

Hui, C. H., Chan, I. S., & Chan, J. (1989). Death cognition among Chinese teenagers: Beliefs about consequences of death. Journal of Research in Personality, 23, 99–117.

Hyland, M. E., & Dann, P. L. (1987). Exploratory factor analysis of the Just World Scale using British undergraduates. British Journal of Social Psychology, 26, 73–77.

Johnson, C., & Dickinson, J. (1971). Class differences in derogation of an innocent victim. University of St. Xavier: Unpublished manuscript (quoted in: Lerner, Miller & Holmes, 1976).

Jones, C., & Aronson, E. (1973). Attribution of fault to a rape victim as a function of respectability of the victim. Journal of Personality and Social Psychology, 26, 415–419.

Jose, P. E., & Brewer, W. F. (1984). Development of story liking: Character identification, suspense, and outcome resolution. Developmental Psychology, 20, 911–924.

Kayser, E. (1980). Der Stellenwert von Gerechtigkeit, individueller und kollektiver Rationalität in hypothetischen und realen Entscheidungssituationen. Zeitschrift für Sozialpsychologie, 11, 112–124.

Kerr, N. L., Bull, R. H., MacCoun, R. J., & Rathborn, H. (1985). Effects of victim attractiveness, care and disfigurement on the judgements of American and British mock jurors. British Journal of Social Psychology, 24, 47–58.

Kerr, N. L., & Gross, A. C. (1978). Situational and personality determinants of a victim's identification with a tormentor. Journal of Research in Personality, 12, 450–468.

Kleinke, C. L., & Meyer, C. (1990). Evaluation of rape victim by men and women with high and low belief in a just world. Psychology of Women Quarterly, 14, 343–353.

Krampen, G. (1987). Handlungstheoretische Persönlichkeitspsychologie. Konzeptuelle und empirische Beiträge zur Konstrukterhellung. Göttingen: Hogrefe.

Kristiansen, C. M., & Giuletti, R. (1990). Perceptions of wife abuse: Effects of gender, attitudes toward women, and just-world beliefs among college students. Psychology of Women Quarterly, 14, 177–189.

Lane, R. E. (1988). Procedural Goods in a Democracy: How One Is Treated Versus What One Gets. Social Justice Research, 2, 177- 192.

Larwood, L., & Moely, B. E. (1979). Sex role and developmental evaluations in the Just World. Sex Roles, 5, 19–28.

Latta, R. M., Bernhardt, V. L., Hildebrand, P. K., & Kahn, A. S. (1974). Attraction to a beneficent victim: Balance theory or "the just world"? Personality and Social Psychology Bulletin, 1, 107–109.

Lerner, M. J. (1960). Some factors in the organization of values. Dissertation Abstracts, 20, 3418.

Lerner, M. J. (1963a). Responsiveness of chronic schizophrenics to the social behavior of others in a meaningful task situation. Journal of Abnormal Social Psychology, 67, 295–299.

Lerner, M. J. (1963b). Social behavior of chronic schizophrenics in supervised and unsupervised work groups. Journal of Abnormal and Social Psychology, 67, 219–225.

Lerner, M. J. (1965a). Evaluation of performance as a function of performer's reward and attractiveness. Journal of Personality and Social Psychology, 1, 355–360.

Lerner, M. J. (1965b). The effect of responsibility and choice on a partner's attractiveness following failure. Journal of Personality, 33, 178–187.

Lerner, M. J. (1965c). The effect of preparatory action on beliefs concerning nuclear war. Journal of Social Psychology, 65, 225–231.

Lerner, M. J. (1968). Conditions eliciting acceptance or rejections of a martyr. University of Kentucky: Unpublished manuscript (quoted in: Lerner, 1974).

Lerner, M. J. (1971). Observer's evaluation of a victim: Justice, guilt, and veridical perception. Journal of Personality and Social Psychology, 20, 127–135.

Lerner, M. J. (1974). Social psychology of justice and interpersonal attraction. In T. Huston (Ed.), Foundations of interpersonal attraction, (pp. 331–351). New York: Academic Press.

Lerner, M. J. (1975). The justice motive in social behavior: Introduction. Journal of Social Issues, 31(3), 1–19.

Lerner, M. J. (1977). The justice motive in social behavior. Some hypotheses as to its origins and forms. Journal of Personality, 45, 1–52.

Lerner, M. J. (1978). ... but nobody liked the Indians. "Belief in a just world" versus a "Authoritarism" syndrome. Ethnicity, 5, 229–237.

Lerner, M. J. (1980). The belief in a just world. A fundamental delusion. New York: Plenum Press.

Lerner, M. J., & Agar, E. (1972). The consequences of perceived similarity: Attraction and rejection, approach and avoidance. Journal of Experimental Research in Personality, 6, 69–75.

Lerner, M. J., & Becker, S. (1962). Interpersonal choice as a function of ascribed similarity and definition of the situation. Human Relations, 15, 27–34.

Lerner, M. J., & Fairweather, G. W. (1963). Social behavior of chronic schizophrenics in supervised and unsupervised work groups. Journal of Abnormal Social Psychology, 67, 219–225.

Lerner, M. J., & Lerner, S. C. (1981). The justice motive in social behavior: Adapting to times of scarcity and change. New York: Plenum Press.

Lerner, M. J., & Lichtman, R. R. (1968). Effects of perceived norms on attitudes and altruistic behavior toward a dependent other. Journal of Personality and Social Psychology, 9, 226–232.

Lerner, M. J., & Matthews, P. (1967). Reactions to suffering of others under conditions of indirect responsibility. Journal of Personality and Social Psychology, 5, 315–325.

Lerner, M. J., & Miller, D. T. (1978). Just world research and the attribution process: looking back and ahead. Psychological Bulletin, 85, 1030–1051.

Lerner, M. J., & Simmons, C. H. (1966). The observer's reaction to the "innocent victim": Compassion or rejection? Journal of Personality and Social Psychology, 4, 203–210.

Lerner, M. J., & Whitehead, L. (1980). Verfahrensgerechtigkeit aus der Sicht der Gerechtigkeitsmotivtheorie. In G. Mikula (Hrsg.), Gerechtigkeit und soziale Interaktion, (pp. 251–300). Bern: Huber.

Lerner, M. J., Dillehay, R. C., & Sherer, W. C. (1967). Similarity and attraction in social contexts. Journal of Personality and Social Psychology, 5, 481–486.

Lerner, M. J., Miller, D. T., & Holmes, J. G. (1976). Deserving and the emergence of forms of justice. In L. Berkowitz (Ed.), Advances in Experimental Social Psychology Vol. 9, (pp. 133–162). New York: Academic Press.

Lipkus, I. (1991). The construction and preliminary validation of a global belief in a just world scale and the exploratory analysis of the multidimensional belief in a just world scale. Personality and Individual Differences, 12, 1171–1178.

Lipkus, I. M. (1992). A heuristical model to explain perceptions of unjust events. Social Justice Research, 5, 359–384.

Ma, L. C., & Smith, K. B. (1985). Individual and social correlates of the Just World Belief: A study of Taiwanese college students. Psychological Reports, 57, 35–38.

Maes, J., & Montada, L. (1989). Verantwortlichkeit für "Schicksalsschläge": Eine Pilotstudie. Psychologische Beiträge, 31, 107–124.

McDonald, A. P. (1972). More on the protestant ethic. Journal of Consulting and Clinical Psychology, 39, 116–122.

McDonald, A. P. (1973). A time for introspection. Professional Psychology, 4, 35–42.

McDonald, G. W. (1977). Innocent victim, deserved victim and martyr: Observers' reaction. Psychological Reports, 41, 511–514.

McFatter, R. M. (1982). Purposes of punishment: Effects of utilities of criminal sanctions on perceived appropriateness. Journal of Applied Psychology, 67, 255–267.

McKay, H. B., & Lerner, M. J. (1977). Sympathy and suffering: Reactions to the plight of an innocent victim. Criminal Justice and Behavior, 4, 282–289.

McKnight, J., & Sutton, J. (1995). Social Psychology. New York: Prentice Hall.

Miller, D. T. (1977a). Personal deserving versus justice for others: An exploration of the justice motive. Journal of Experimental Social Psychology, 13, 1–13.

Miller, D. T. (1977b). Altruism and threat to a belief in a just world. Journal of Experimental Social Psychology, 13, 113–124.

Mirels, H., & Garrett, J. B. (1971). The protestant ethic as a personality variable. Journal of Consulting and Clinical Psychology, 36, 40–44.

Montada, L., & Figura, E. (1988). Some psychological factors underlying the request for social isolation of Aids victims (= Berichte aus der Arbeitsgruppe "Verantwortung, Gerechtigkeit, Moral" Nr. 50). Trier: Universität Trier, Fachbereich I: Psychologie.

Montada, L., Schmitt, M. & Dalbert, C. (1986). Thinking about Justice and Dealing with One's Own Privileges. In H. W. Bierhoff, R. L. Cohen & J. Greenberg (Eds.), Justice in Social Relations (pp. 125–143). New York: Plenum Press.

Montada, L., & Schneider, A. (1989). Justice and Emotional Reactions to the Disadvantaged. Social Justice Research, 3, 313–344.

Novak, D. W., & Lerner, M. J. (1966). The effect of preparatory action on beliefs concerning nuclear war: A test of some alternative explanations. Journal of Social Psychology, 70, 111–121.

Novak, D. W., & Lerner, M. J. (1968). Rejection as a consequence of perceived similarity. Journal of Personality and Social Psychology, 9, 147–152.

O'Connor, B. P. (1991). How a relationship between thinking and feeling may give rise to a variety of human behaviors. Genetic, Social, and General Psychology Monographs, 117, 29–48.

O'Quin, K., & Vogler, C. C. (1990). Use of the Just World Scale with prison inmates: A methodological note. Perceptual and Motor Skills, 70, 395–400.

Pancer, S. M. (1988). Salience of appeal and avoidance of helping situations. Canadian Journal of Behavioural Science, 20, 133–139.

Paulhus, D. (1983). Sphere-specific measures of perceived control. Journal of Personality and Social Psychology, 44, 1253–1265.

Piliavin, I., Hardyck, J., & Vadim, T. (1968). Reactions to a victim in a just or non-just world. Berkeley, University of California: Unpublished paper (quoted in: Lerner, 1980).

Radloff, L. S. (1977). The CES-D Scale: A self report depression scale for research in the general population. Applied Psychological Measurement, 1, 385–401.

Rasinski, K. A., & Scott, L. A. (1990). Culture, values, and beliefs about economics justice. Social Justice Research, 4, 307–323.

Richey, H. W., & Richey, M. H. (1978). Attribution in the classroom: How just is the just world? Psychology in the Schools, 15, 216–222.

Rim, Y. (1981). Who believes in graphology? Personality and Individual Differences, 2, 85–87.

Ritter, C., Benson, D. E., & Synder, C. (1990). Belief in a just world and depression. Sociological Perspectives, 33, 235–252.

Rosenberg, M. (1965). Society and the adolescent self-image. Princeton, NJ: Princeton University Press.

Ross, M., & Ellard, J. H. (1986). On winnowing: The impact of scarcity on allocators' evaluations of candidates for a resource. Journal of Experimental Social Psychology, 22, 374–388.

Rotter, J. B. (1966). Generalized expectancies for internal versus external control of reinforcement. Psychological Monographs, 80 (Whole No .608), 1–28.

Rubin, Z., & Peplau, L. A. (1973). Belief in a just world and reactions to another's lot: A study of participants in the National Draft Lottery. Journal of Social Issues, 29(4), 73–93.

Rubin, Z., & Peplau, L. A. (1975). Who believes in a just world? Journal of Social Issues, 31(3), 65–89.

Samuel, W. (1981). Personality. Searching for the Sources of Human Behavior. New York: McGraw-Hill.

Schmitt, M. (1994). Multiple ambiguities of Belief-in-a-just-world-Measures. (this volume)

Shaffer, D. R., Plummer, D., & Hammock, G. (1986). Hath he suffered enough? Effects of jury dogmatism, defendant similarity, and defendant's pretrial suffering on juridic decisions. Journal of Personality and Social Psychology, 50, 1059–1067.

Sherman, M. F., Smith, R., & Cooper, R. (1982). Reactions toward the dying: The effects of a patient's illness and respondents' belief in a just world. Omega Journal of Death and Dying, 13, 173–189.

Simmons, C. H., & Lerner, M. J. (1968). Altruism as a search for justice. Journal of Personality and Social Psychology, 9, 216–225.

Simons, C., & Piliavin, J. A. (1972). The effect of deception on reactions to a victim. Journal of Personality and Social Psychology, 21, 56–60.

Sloan, R. P., & Gruman, J. C. (1983). Beliefs about cancer, heart disease, and their victims. Psychological Reports, 52, 415–424.

Smith, E. R., & Mackie, D. M. (1995). Social Psychology. New York: Worth Publishers.

Smith, K. B., & Green, D. N. (1984). Individual correlates of the belief in a just world. Psychological Reports, 54, 435–438.

Solomon, R. C. (1989). The emotions of justice. Social Justice Research, 3, 345–374.

Sorrentino, R. M., & Hardy, J. E. (1974). Religiousness and derogation of an innocent victim. Journal of Personality, 42, 372–382.

Stahly, G. B. (1988). Psychosocial aspects of the stigma of cancer: An overview. Journal of Psychosocial Oncology (=Special Issue: Clinical research issues in psychosocial oncology), 6, 3–27.

Steensma, H., den Hartigh, E., & Lucardie, E. (1994). Social Categories, Just World Belief, Locus of Control, and Causal Attributions of Occupational Accidents. Social Justice Research, 7, 281–299.

Stephan, C. W., & Holahan, C. K. (1982). The influence of status and sex-typing on assessments of occupational outcome. Sex-Roles, 8, 823–833.

Stokols, D., & Schopler, J. (1973). Reactions to victims under conditions of situational detachment: The effects of responsibility, severity, and expected future interaction. Journal of Personality and Social Psychology, 14, 199–209.

Szmajke, A. (1991). Religiousness, belief in a just world, authoritarianism and subjective image of social life in Poland at the decline real socialism. Polish Psychological Bulletin, 22, 33–42.

Tesser, A. (1995). Advanced Social Psychology. New York: McGraw-Hill.

Tomaka, J., & Blascovich, J. (1994). Effects of justice beliefs on cognitive appraisal of and subjective physiological, and behavioral responses to potential stress. Journal of Personality and Social Psychology, 67, 732–740.

Wagstaff, G. F. (1982). Attitudes to rape: The "Just World" strikes again? Bulletin of the British Psychological Society, 35, 277–279.

Wagstaff, G. F. (1983). Correlates of the just world in Britain. Journal of Social Psychology, 121, 145–146.

Wagstaff, G. F., & Quirk, M. A. (1983). Attitudes to sex-roles, political conservatism and belief in a just world. Psychological Reports, 52, 813–814.

Whatley, M. A. (1993). Belief in a Just World Scale: Unidimensional or multidimensional. Journal of Social Psychology, 133, 547–551.

Witt, L. A. (1989). Urban-nonurban differences in social cognition: Locus of control and perceptions of a just world. Journal of Social Psychology, 129, 715–717.

Wober, M., & Gunter, B. (1985). Television and beliefs about health care and medical treatment. Current Psychological Research and Reviews, 4, 291–304.

Wrightsman, L. S. (1972). Social Psychology in the Seventies. Belmont: Wadsworth.

Wyer, R. S., Bodenhausen, G. V., & Gorman, T. F. (1985). Cognitive mediators of reactions to rape. Journal of Personality and Social Psychology, 48, 324–338.

Zuckerman, M., Gerbasi, K. C., Kravitz, R. I., & Wheeler, L. (1975). The belief in a just world and reactions to innocent victims. Catalog of Selected Documents in Psychology, 5, 326.

Zuckerman, M., & Gerbasi, K. C. (1977a). Belief in a just word and trust. Journal of Research in Personality, 11, 306–317.

Zuckerman, M., & Gerbasi, K. C. (1977b). Belief in internal control or belief in a just world: The use and misuse of the I-E- scale in prediction of attitudes and behavior. Journal of Personality, 45, 356–378.

Zuckerman, M., & Gerbasi, K. C. (1977c). Dimensions of the I-E- scale and their relationship to other personality measures. Educational and Psychological measurement, 37, 159–175.

Zweigenhaft, R. L., Phillips, B. K. G., Adams, K. A., Morse, C. K., & Horan, A. E. (1985). Religious preference and belief in a just world. Genetic, Social and General Psychology Monographs, 111, 331–348.

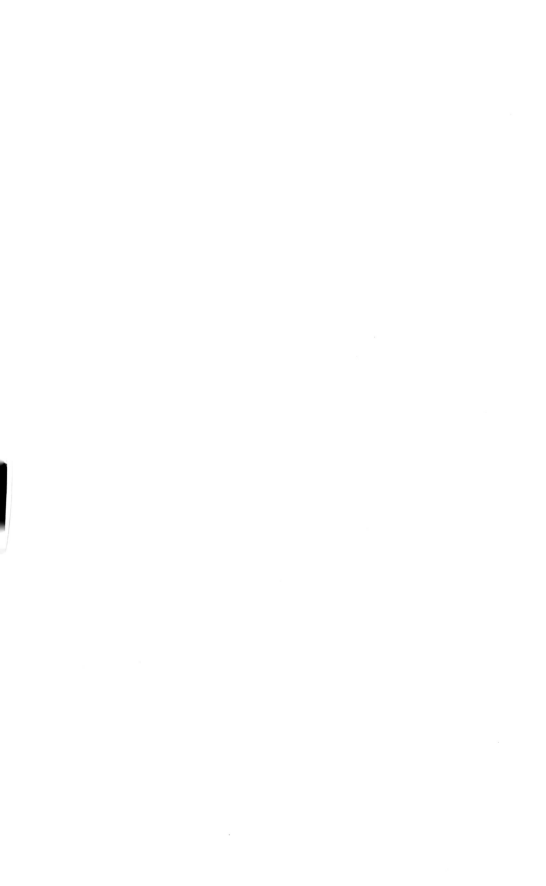

Chapter 11

Methodological Strategies in Research to Validate Measures of Belief in a Just World

MANFRED J. SCHMITT

1. HISTORY AND AIMS OF THIS CONTRIBUTION

When I first came across Justice Motive Theory (JMT) and related research (Lerner, 1970; Lerner & Simmons, 1966), I was initially confused, then puzzled, and eventually fascinated by the idea that certain social judgments and behaviors, such as blaming victims for their misfortune, might be motivated by the exact opposite of what these judgments and behaviors seemed to reflect on first sight: a need for justice. Given my interest in personality and individual differences, I was attracted to Rubin and Peplau's (1973, 1975) suggestion that the justice motive (JM) might differ between individuals just like other motives and needs do (power, achievement, approval, etc.).

In 1980, Leo Montada invited Claudia Dalbert and me to participate in his work on relative privilegation (Montada, Schmitt, & Dalbert, 1986). Our model for predicting reactions to underprivileged groups, such as reactions to citizens from the developing countries, included Lerner's

---

MANFRED J. SCHMITT • Department of Psychology, Universität Trier, D-54286 Trier, Germany.

Responses to Victimizations and Belief in a Just World, edited by Montada and Lerner. Plenum Press, New York, 1998.

(1980) Justice Motive Theorie (JMT). Based on the core premise of JMT, we predicted that Belief in a Just World (BJW) as an indicator of the JM would affect the way in which people perceive, explain, evaluate, and react emotionally and in action to the fate of disadvantaged groups and suffering victims. Accordingly, we assumed that BJW would influence the way in which privileged individuals deal with their own advantages, for example, whether they justify their privileges as deserved or feel guilty about them (cf. Montada, this volume).

Following Rubin & Peplau's (1973, 1975) reasoning, we chose BJW as the best available indicator of the JM. For several reasons, we decided to develop a new self-report questionnaire (Dalbert, Montada, & Schmitt, 1987). Our BJW inventory consists of two scales. The general BJW scale (GBJW) contains items whose content is most general. Our domain specific BJW scales (SPBJW) address justice regarding privileges which distinguish our subjects from disadvantaged comparison groups (cf. Montada, this volume). Our GBJW scale contains six items (e.g.: "Basically, the world is a just place.") which are very general in three regards: (1) Unlike our domain-specific scale, the Furnham & Procter (1992) questionnaire, and the Maes (1992) scales, they do not specify domains or spheres of justice. (2) Unlike some of the Rubin and Peplau items, the items of our scale refer neither to specific rules of distributive justice (such as equity, equality, or need) nor to specific criteria of procedural justice (such as process control, outcome control, consistency, nonpartiality, acuracy, lack of bias, correctability, representativeness). (3) Unlike some of the Rubin and Peplau items, no agents are mentioned who violate or protect justice. This general format was chosen to make it possible for subjects to select their own domains, justice criteria, agents, and means when expressing their BJW.

The general format we used seemed feasable because JMT does not imply *what* justice is and *how* it can be attained. More specifically, a general format does not confound belief in justice with domains, criteria, agents, and so forth. Statements in which justice is related specifically to domains, criteria, agents, means, etc., introduce additional sources of variance and may harm construct validity. For example, answers to items in which justice is linked to a certain criterion such as equality are ambiguous. Consider an item claiming that men and women have equal career chances. Agreeing to such an assertion indicates BJW only if equality of career chances is accepted as just. A second argument for the general format was that unspecific items allow individuals to associate their personal themes of justice, i.e., justice issues which are important for them. It can be assumed that the JM is most powerful in domains which people care about (cf. Montada, this volume). A third argument for the format was parsimony.

The estimated internal consistency reliability of our GBJW scale ranges from .70 to .80 depending on the sample. Dalbert & Schneider (1995) report a peer rating validity of .41 when correlating the scale with the average scale scores attributed to the target subject by three acquaintances. This validity coefficient is not high in absolute terms but substantial given that belief in a just world cannot be linked as directly with observable behavior as other personality variables (such as sociability, dominance, anxiety, intelligence, etc.). Montada & Schneider (1989) report a six-month retest correlation of .75. The pattern of correlations obtained in question-naire studies between our GBJW scale and measures for other constructs appears to be coherent, theoretically conclusive and thus affirming the scale's construct validity according to Lerner's conception of BJW (for reviews see Dalbert, 1996; Montada, this volume; Reichle, Schneider, & Montada, this volume).

Given the widespread scepticism of experimental social psychologists toward survey research, I decided to additionally investigate the construct validity of our scale *experimentally*, treating BJW as an independent organismic variable and moderator of experimental factors—as others have done before with the Rubin & Peplau scale (e.g., Miller, 1977). In one of these experiments, which will be described in more detail later, subjects witnessed another person winning or losing money *by chance* (Schmitt et al., 1991). Afterwards, they were asked to rate the stimulus person on a number of favorable and unfavorable traits. It was predicted that subjects would upgrade the winner and downgrade the loser, and that the extent of this motivated bias would be larger for subjects with a strong BJW than for subjects with a weak BJW. The obtained pattern of results ran directly counter to these expectations: Subjects scoring high on our scale tended to *upgrade the loser* and *downgrade the winner*. Although a reasonable psychological interpretation for this result is possible (see below), it insti-gated, together with results from three other experimental studies (Schmitt, 1991, 1992; Schmitt & Herbst, 1993, see below), a process of reflecting about the meaning of BJW and the construct validity of GBJW scales. In this chapter, I will address some of these issues which have, in part, been raised by other authors before (Lerner, 1980, Chapter 10; Furn-ham & Procter, 1992; Maes, 1994a, this volume). Furthermore, I will dem-onstrate some methodological strategies for clarifying these issues and present some data from studies in which these strategies were used.

2. SYNERGETIC INTERACTION OF THE JUSTICE MOTIVE AND BELIEF IN A JUST WORLD

Construct validity can only be defined and explored empirically on the basis of a theory (Cronbach & Meehl, 1955). If the theory has been successfully applied many times for predicting observations implied by the theory, we will tend to attribute a false prediction with a new methodology to that methodology. Conversely, we will more likely dismiss a theory or revise it if contradicting observations were made using a well-tested method. Both conclusions may be wrong, but they are reasonable and common in the social sciences (Cattell, 1966).

What is the validity status quo of the JMT and BJW scales? JMT has been confirmed in many experimental studies (for reviews see Lerner, 1980; Lerner & Miller, 1978; Lerner, Miller, & Holmes, 1976). We may therefore use the predictions of JMT for testing the construct validity of BJW-measures. However, this strategy is reasonable if and only if we consider BJW to be an expression of the JM (cf. Montada, this volume). If BJW were not considered theoretically to be a manifestation of the JM, but a phenomenon independent from the JM, it would not be able to derive criteria for testing the construct validity of BJW measures from JMT. In this chapter, I start from the assumption, as many others have done beginning with Rubin & Peplau (1973), that BJW is a manifestation of the JM. It follows from this presumption that the construct validity of any BJW measure must be judged with regard to the core premises of JMT. According to my understanding of Lerner's writing (e.g., Lerner, 1980), one core premise of JMT is that the desire for justice will motivate individuals to help innocent victims if that is a possibility, if help is not too costly, and if help does not endanger the person's entitlements. Another core assumption of JMT is that individuals will tend to blame victims for their misfortune if helping them is not possible or too costly.

How can these central postulates of JMT be transformed into validity criteria for an individual difference measure of the JM? My suggestion is that such a measure should *moderate* every general effect of the JM such as helping innocent victims or derogating them. Every general effect that follows from JMT should be *stronger* for subjects with a high need for justice and *weaker* for subjects with a low need for justice. In other words, valid measures of the JM should *interact in a synergetic fashion* with situational factors that generate a general JM effect.

Several empirical studies have implemented this general methodological strategy for the Rubin & Peplau scale. The moderator hypothesis was fully supported by Zuckerman, Gerbasi, Kravitz, & Wheeler (1975) and by Miller (1977). Furthermore, the moderator effect was found for 4 out of 7 dependent variables by Rubin & Peplau (1973) and in one out of four experimental groups by Dion & Dion (1987). Finally, results from two experiments by Hafer & Olson (1989) have been interpreted as supporting the moderator hypothesis. No interaction effect was found in a study by Miller, Smith, Ferree, & Taylor (1976). To summarize, the pattern of results of available studies in which the Rubin & Peplau scale was used as a moderator of general effects of the JM, such as blaming or helping innocent

victims, provide some, but not equivocal, evidence for the construct validity of the Rubin & Peplau scale.

3. BELIEF IN A JUST WORLD VERSUS CENTRALITY OF JUSTICE AS INDICATORS OF THE JUSTICE MOTIVE

Moderator effects of the Rubin & Peplau scale or other BJW scales
may be that BJW is a rather indirect indicator of the JM. No item appears
in available BJW questionnaires which addresses the person's desire for
justice directly (Dalbert et al., 1987; Lipkus, 1991; Furnham & Procter, 1992;
Maes, 1992; Rubin & Peplau, 1973, 1975; Schmitt, Maes, & Schmal, 1995).
According to my knowledge, the only available instrument which comes
close to a more direct measure of the JM is a questionnaire developed in
our group for measuring what we called *Centrality of Justice* (Dalbert et al.,
1987; cf. Montada, this volume). Our Justice Centrality scale consists of six
items which have only one factor in common and which have a sufficient
internal consistency (alpha = .73): (1) there is hardly anything which
infuriates me as much as the observation of injustice; (2) I could not be
friends with someone who is insensitive to justice issues; (3) I feel that
injustices in our society have to be pointed out again and again; (4) I believe
that the observation of injustice makes me more upset than most other
people; (5) I feel guilty for a long time after I have done something unjust
or not stopped an injustice; and (6) people who don't care for justice make
me furious.

This scale and our GBJW scale were administered together in several
studies, e.g., in our first Existential Guilt Study (Montada et al., 1986) and
in a study by Herbst, Montada, & Schmitt (Herbst, 1992; Schmitt & Herbst,
1993). The latter research will be described in more detail later. In both
studies, the items from the Justice Centrality scale and the Justice Belief
scale (GBJW) loaded on separate orthogonal factors in a simultaneous
principle axes analysis. Consistent with this result, a small correlation of
.20 between the scales was obtained in the Herbst study. These results leave
open the question, of course, which of the two scales is a more construct
valid measure of the JM. It only shows that our measure for justice
centrality does not correlate with our GBJW scale.

4. DELUSION, KNOWLEDGE, AND JUSTIFICATION COMPONENTS OF BELIEF IN A JUST WORLD

If BJW were not a pure manifestation of the JM, what other origins
besides the JM might it have? Let's consider the wording of typical items

from BJW scales. What does it mean if a person agrees to assertions like "Men who keep in shape have little chance of suffering a heart attack" (Rubin & Peplau, 1975) or "People try to be fair when making important decisions" (an item from our GBJW scale)? One possibility is that the person wants to believe what these statements express in order to satisfy his or her JM. A second possibility is that the person agrees to these items on the basis of experience or knowledge. A third possibility is that the person acknowledges injustice but in public appeals to BJW assertions in a strategic manner, for example, in order to justify own advantages.

How can we empirically explore the extent to which these interpretations are appropriate? This question is perhaps posed too simply because different answers may be true for different individuals and for different domains. Yet it may be useful to begin with the question in its general form. As I see it, at least two methodological strategies can be employed for investigating the question empirically.

4.1. Empirical Distribution of Belief in a Just World

According to JMT, the observation of injustice motivates people to restore justice either by actions or by distorting their observations. Consequently, one would expect a fair amount of subjects endorsing items which claim a just world. Less agreement to just world items can be expected if it is assumed that they measure an unbiased aggregation of the subjects' knowledge. The media report on cases of injustice all the time and every educated and informed adult knows that the world is full of injustices. Rubin & Peplau (1975) report an average item mean of 3.08 for college students when using a six-point rating scale ranging from 1/total rejection of the just world premise to 6/total acceptance of the just world premise. Hence, there was slight average tendency to reject the notion of a just world. Rubin & Peplau (1975) cite an unpublished study (by Merrifield & Timpe) in which an average item mean of 3.79 was found for a student sample. Both values are rather close to the midpoint of the scale (3.5), and they do not provide compelling evidence either for the delusion assumption or the knowledge assumption.

Our GBJW scale also uses six-point rating scales. If keyed in the same way as the Rubin & Peplau items, the average item mean of our GBJW scale amounted to 1.57 in a demographically heterogeneous sample of more than 2000 subjects. In student samples, the item distributions were skewed even more toward the no-BJW end of the rating scales. For example, in a study by Mohiyeddini (1995), the average item mean obtained in a sample of 281 students was only 1.29. These values show that most individuals tend to reject the notion of a just world. This result seems to be more in line with the knowledge hypothesis than with the delusion hypothesis.

4.2. Group Differences in Belief in a Just World

As a second strategy for exploring the meaning of self-reported BJW, one could compare groups for whom different scores on BJW scales are to be expected under the delusion and knowledge assumptions. More specifically, one would expect a lower BJW under the knowledge hypothesis, but not under the motivation hypothesis, for groups whose members have experienced many or severe instances of injustice (refugees, victims of torture, etc.) in comparison to groups who have experienced fewer or less severe instances of injustice. Supporting the knowledge hypothesis, several studies have found that objectively disadvantaged groups have lower BJW compared to more privileged groups. For example, Smith & Green (1984) found lower BJW for blacks than for whites living in the same society. Using the Rubin & Peplau scale, Furnham (1993) compared BJW in twelve countries. For the negatively keyed items from the scale, he found a significant correlation between BJW and gross domestic product with BJW being lower in poorer countries. There are other studies, however, which have not found a correlation between objective disadvantages and BJW. For example, Rubin & Peplau (1975) report a correlation of .03 between social class and BJW. Finally, there is at least one data set which supports the delusion hypothesis. Lerner (1980, pp. 165–171) describes results from an unpublished study by Lerner & Elkinton suggesting a negative correlation between social class and BJW.

After the German reunification, East and West Germans have been compared in several social science research projects aimed at finding out the effects of living in different political and economic environments for almost two generations. If BJW was knowledge based, two counteracting mechanisms may cause East-West differences in BJW: (1) East Germans may have a higher BJW than West Germans due to the revolution and the reunification as two recent and salient experiences of justice. This assumption implies that knowledge based BJW is short-lived and changes with changing experiences. (2) East Germans may have a lower BJW than West Germans due to living in a basically unjust society for 40 years. This assumption implies that BJW is a trait which develops in a long process of experiences and changes slowly. Given evidence on the high stability of BJW, the knowledge hypothesis would predict that East Germans have a lower BJW than West Germans. At least six studies are available in which BJW was measured with our GBJW scale or with similar scales in East and West Germany. In one project, our GBJW scale was administered to more than 2500 East and West Germans (Schmitt, Maes, & Schmal, 1997). The sample was not representative but demographically heterogeneous. Data were collected in January 1996. East Germans displayed a significantly ($p < .01$) lower BJW than West Germans. Mean item scores were 1.40 and

1.57, respectively. The same result was obtained in three other studies (Limbach, 1992; Braun, 1993; Wegener & Liebig, 1994). In one additional study, the East-West-difference was in the same direction but not significant (Schmitt & Janetzko, 1993). Only Dalbert (1993) found the opposite pattern. She argues that East Germans may have a higher BJW because they were told to live in a much juster society than West Germans. One might wonder, however, why they would have reasons for wanting to overthrow their regime and strive so urgently for the reunification if they believed this propaganda.

Although the empirical evidence is rather clear, it is not unambiguous regarding the delusion versus knowledge hypothesis. The pattern of results is more favorable toward the knowledge hypothesis than toward the wishful thinking hypothesis, but only under the assumption that individual differences in BJW are stable across long periods of time. Considerable stability has been found for BJW scales, but in a sample whose members have not, unlike East Germans, experienced severe socioeconomic or sociopolitical changes.

4.3. Separating Belief in Justice and Belief in Control

Discriminant validity is a crucial criterion for the construct validity of psychological measures (Campbell & Fiske, 1959). The issue of discriminant validity of BJW scales needs to be addressed for several related reasons. First, alternative interpretations have been advanced for some of the phenomena that JMT seeks to explain (e.g., Miller et al., 1976; Sauer, 1984). Some authors (e.g., Shaver, 1985; Walster, 1966) have argued that blaming victims may be caused by a need for control (Burger, 1992). In order to test both explanations against each other, need for justice and need for control have to be conceptually and empirically separated (cf. Kordmann, 1991; Maes, 1994a). Regarding discriminant construct validity of self-reported BJW, it has to be explored whether, and to what extent, BJW reflects a need for control in addition to reflecting a need for justice.

The second reason is simply that correlations between measures for BJW and measures for Internal Locus of Control have been repeatedly reported in the literature (e.g., Clayton, 1992; Collins, 1974; Hafer & Olson, 1989; Lerner, 1978; Maes, 1994a; Rubin & Peplau, 1973, 1975; Zuckermann & Gerbasi, 1977). Whether this correlation is a problem of insufficient discriminant validity depends on the true correlation between belief in justice/need for justice and belief in control/need for control. If the correlation between the measures would match the true correlation, there would be no validity problem. Rather, depending on how close the true correlation is, there might be a problem with scientific parsimony.

A substantial true correlation between need for justice and need for control is not surprising if we consider the possibility that justice and control are confounded due to bidirectional influences. Under certain conditions, justice may imply control and control may imply justice. A just world is a predictable world, and to the extent that the rules are known, individuals can control their outcomes by choosing appropriate actions. Conversely, those who have power are capable of setting up a just world. This intrinsic relation between justice and control can be transferred to the need for control and the need for justice. A need for justice may reflect a more fundamental need for control. In this case, justice may not be desirable per se but as a means for control. Conversely, a need for control may reflect a more fundamental need for justice. In this case, control may not be desirable per se but as a means to obtain justice. An additional reason for a true correlation between need for justice and need for control may be that both serve the same underlying basic need for security and well-being.

Two methodological strategies can be used to clarify the issue of discriminant construct validity. (1) The first strategy is to devise measures for both constructs with the highest possible discriminant *content* or face validity (Maes, 1992). This means using only the most prototypical items possible and avoiding items that may also measure the reference construct. The correlations among such pure and prototypical indicators provide less biased estimates of the true correlations between the constructs (Borkenau, 1986). (2) The second strategy is to design experimental studies for investigating the discriminant *construct* validity of measures for both constructs according to the general rationale outlined earlier. This strategy requires experimental situations which stimulate *only one* of both motives but not both simultaneously. Under this condition, only the measure for the motive that was aroused should act as a moderator while the measure for the other motive must not.

5. CORRELATIONS AMONG MEASURES WITH DISCRIMINANT CONTENT VALIDITY

In a study by Herbst, Montada, & Schmitt (Herbst, 1992; Schmitt & Herbst, 1993), our Justice Belief (GBJW) scale and our Justice Centrality scale (see above) were used together with two control scales, a General Belief in Internal or Personal Control scale (e.g., "I believe that I can determine most things in my life.") and a Centrality of Control scale (e.g., "I rather rely on myself than on others."). Both scales were designed as similar as possible in level and scope to the justice scales. Also, the items were selected to be most prototypical and to not overlap with the justice domain.

The Control Centrality scale and the Control Belief scale were submitted separately to principle axes analyses. The results show that both sets of items have only one factor in common. Internal consistency reliability estimates alpha for the Centrality scale and the Belief scale were .76 and .67, respectively. While the coefficient for the Centrality scale is acceptable, the coefficient for the Belief scale is insufficient. Therefore, correlations between the scales should be corrected for attenuation (alphas for the GBJW and Centrality of Justice scale were .80 and .75, respectively, in the present study).

All four scales contain items with high discriminant content validity on the level of explicit item wording. No justice item refers to control issues, no control item refers to justice, no belief item refers to centrality issues, and no centrality item refers to belief issues. It seems as safe as possible, therefore, that the correlations between the four scales are not biased by shared method variance. The manifest correlations which were obtained from a demographically heterogenous sample of 182 adults are given in Table 1 (first value in a cell). Table 1 also contains the corrected coefficients (second value in a cell) and the probability of type I errors for the manifest correlations (third value in a cell).

The correlation between *Justice Belief and Justice Centrality* was discussed earlier. The correlation between *Control Belief and Control Centrality* is not crucial in the present context except for showing that wanting to have control and believing to have control are more closely related than wanting justice and believing in justice. The correlation between *Justice Centrality and Control Centrality* is important in the present context. This correlation is substantial on the true score level (.57). If both scales were valid need measures, the correlation would show that need for justice and need for control are truely correlated. This would be in line with the foregoing reasoning (a) that justice can be a means for control, (b) that control can be a means for justice, and (c) that justice and control can both be means for security and well-being.

The correlation between *Justice Belief and Control Belief* is also important in the present context. This correlation is considerably lower, even

TABLE 1. Correlations among Centrality
and Belief Scales for Justice and Control

	Justice belief[a]			Justice centrality[a]			Control belief[a]		
Justice centrality	.20	.26	<.01						
Control belief	.18	.25	<.05	.15	.21	>.05			
Control centrality	.12	.15	>.05	.43	.57	<.01	.40	.56	<.01

[a]First value: manifest correlation; second value: corrected correlation; third value: significance level.

when corrected for attenuation, than the average correlation of .40 reported in the literature for BJW scales and Internal Locus of Control scales. This finding suggests that the correlations reported in the literature between BJW and Internal Locus of Control are partly due to shared method variance (same or similar items in both measures) while the correlation obtained here is not. Therefore, the coefficients in Table 1 fulfill the classic criterion of discriminant validity with regard to our GBJW scale. The correlations of this scale with the three remaining scales are small enough to maintain the assumption that BJW reflects something unique —whatever that may be.

5.1. Experimental Investigation of Discriminant Construct Validity

The second strategy mentioned earlier for exploring discriminant validity was also employed in the Herbst study. The study was a vignette study containing four scenarios in which an unfavorable outcome occurred to the protagonist:

1. A bystander (protagonist) was hit by a rock during a rightist riot.
2. A car accident occurred to someone (protagonist) due to faulty repairs performed by a car repair shop.
3. A car accident occurred to a person (protagonist) while trying to avoid running over a child.
4. A car accident occurred to someone (protagonist) who ignored another's right of way.

The type of Scenario was varied within subjects, i.e., all scenarios were presented to all subjects. Two factors were varied between subjects and were fully crossed: (1) Need for Justice (evoked, fulfilled) and (2) Need for Control (evoked, not evoked).

Need for Justice was evoked by leaving the victim without compensation and letting the victimizer get away without punishment. This should provide a threat to the subject's sense of justice. In the Need-for-Justice-Fulfilled condition, the victim received full compensation and the victimizer was punished. This should affirm the subject's sense of justice. To avoid confounding justice and control, compensation depended on factors that were out of the victim's control. In the riot scenario, for example, compensation was possible because another bystander photographed the event allowing the victimizer to be later identified.

Adopting Shaver's (1985) concepts of personal and situational relevance, Need for Control was varied by describing the protagonist as similar (Need for Control evoked) or dissimilar (Need for Control not evoked) to the subject. Objectively, control was impossible in all cases. The control motive was kept silent by portraying the victim as dissimilar to the subject suggesting that the same misfortune could hardly happen to the subject. Need for control was evoked by letting the victim appear similar to the subject. In the first scenario, dissimilarity was operationalized by ethnicity. The victim was an African foreigner at whom the rock might have been thrown by one of the rightist rioters on purpose. Although this was not stated explicitely, it was a likely inference from the story. In the Need-for-Control-Evoked condition, the victim was German. In the second scenario, the dissimilar protagonist was a physically handicapped person whose car had complicated special mechanics suggesting that the car repair shop would not make a similar mistake when working on a regular car. In the third scenario, dissimilarity was suggested by age. In the Need-for-Control-Not-Evoked condition, the driver was a very old man suggesting that he may have wrecked his car due to slow reactions. In the fourth scenario, the dissimilar protagonist was from Great Britain suggesting that the fault may be due to unfamiliarity with continental traffic rules. Table 2 summarizes the between subjects part of the design and the operationalizations of the two need factors.

Several dependent variables and control variables were assessed. In the present context, only the indicators for blaming the victim are of interest. Six-point rating scales were used for measuring (1) the amount of the victim's causal contribution to the damage, (2) the extent of the victim's responsibility for the damage, and (3) the extent of the victim's moral blameworthiness (guilt).

What experimental (situational) effects on these dependent variables can be expected from JMT and from Control Motive Theory? The former would predict main effects of the Need for Justice Factor on all dependent variables because the subject cannot, in his or her role, compensate the victim. In order to make the complete event appear just, they have to justify it. This can be achieved by attributing a causal contribution, responsibility, and/or guilt to the victim. Control Motive Theory would predict main effects of the Need for Control Factor on the same dependent variables because guilt conceptually implies responsibility and responsibility conceptually implies control (Montada, 1992; Reichle, 1994; Shaver, 1985).

TABLE 2. Between Subjects Part of the Experimental Design of the Herbst Study

Need for justice	Need for control	
	Evoked	Kept silent
Evoked	Victim similar to subject receives no compensation	Victim dissimilar to subject receives no compensation
Fulfilled	Victim similar to subject receives compensation by mere chance	Victim dissimilar to subject receives compensation by mere chance

What effects can be expected from the organismic factors, i.e., from dispositional need for justice and from dispositional need for control? According to the general validation criterion exposed earlier, the main effects of the experimental factors (situational need) should be *moderated* by the *corresponding* dispositional need factors. More specifically, the main effects of the Need for Control Factor should be stronger for subjects with a high dispositional need for control than for subjects with a low dispositional need for control. Correspondingly, the main effects of the Need for Justice Factor should be stronger for subjects with a high dispositional need for justice than for subjects with a low dispositional need for justice. As a consequence of such ordinal moderator or interactions effects, main effects of dispositional need for justice and dispositional need for control can also be expected.

Discriminant construct validity of the measures for both needs requires that the moderator effects are specific or *unique*: Dispositional need for justice should only moderate the effects of situational need for justice but not the effects of situational need for control. Correspondingly, dispositional need for control should only moderate the effects of situational need for control but not the effects of situational need for justice.

Using multiple regression analyses with dummy-coded experimental factors and product terms for moderator effects (cf., Aiken & West, 1991), these expectations were tested separately for each scenario. The dependent variables (attribution of cause, responsibility, and guilt) were summed because the correlations between them were high within situations. Correspondingly, when principle axes analyses with all dependent variables were performed, the three attributions always loaded highly on the same common factor. Note, however, that the attributions did not generalize across situations. Therefore, separate regression analyses had to be performed for each situation. The dependent variable may be considered the best available indicator for *blaming the victim*. All significant effects are summarized in Table 3.

Regarding the effects of situational need for justice and control, JMT was supported by the results for two of the four scenarios (2, 3). If justice was reestablished, the victim was blamed less than when the victim was not compensated. No defensive attributions according to Control Motive Theory were found. Two main effects of situational need for control were significant, but they were in the wrong direction. In other words, victims similar to the subject were blamed less than nonsimilar victims. According to Shaver (1985), this may indicate a strong identification with the victim and an attempt to avoid blame instead of harm.

In the first scenario, main effects were found for the two belief scales. Subjects with strong beliefs in justice tended to blame the victim more than subjects with low scores on our GBJW scale. Accordingly, subjects with a

TABLE 3. Significant Effects (p < .05) of Situational and
Dispositional Needs for Justice and Control on Blaming
the Victim in the Herbst Study

	Scenario			
Effect	1	2	3	4
Main and interaction effects of experimental factors				
Need for justice		+	+	
Need for control	−			−
Need for justice × need for control				
Main effects of organismic factors				
Justice belief	+			
Justice centrality			−	
Control belief	+			
Control centrality				
Moderator effects of organismic factors on experimental effects				
Need for justice × justice belief				
Need for justice × justice centrality			+	
Need for control × control belief				
Need for control × control centrality				
Need for justice × control belief				
Need for justice × control centrality				
Need for control × justice belief	−			
Need for control × justice centrality				

Note: "+" for main effects indicates a positive effect of situational or
dispositional need/belief on blaming; "−" for main effects indicates a
negative effect of situational or dispositional need/belief on blaming;
"+" for moderator effects means that dispositional need/belief
amplified a positive situation effect; "−" for moderator effects means
that dispositional need/belief amplified a negative situation effect.

strong belief in personal/internal control tended to blame the victim more
than subjects with low scores on the Control Belief scale. In Scenario 3, a
negative main effect of Justice Centrality on blaming the victim was found.
This effect contradicts theoretical expectations.

Taken together, the pattern of results is inconsistent, nonconclusive,
and does not assert discriminant construct validity for any of the scales
used. One might object that vignette studies of this type are inappropriate
for investigating JMT and Control Motive Theory or that the design and
the procedure of the present study were inappropriate for testing discriminant construct validity. Regarding the control part, this objection seems
justified because the main effects of situational need for control contradicted theoretical expectations. Regarding the justice part, however, such
objections seem less convincing since, at least for two scenarios, the general

blaming effect was found. At least these two scenarios seem internally valid from the perspective of JMT. Note that in one of these two situations, one of the general blaming effects was amplified by Justice Centrality. If we had realized only this scenario, it would be tempting to conclude that the study adds weight to the discriminant construct validity, yet of the Justice Centrality scale, not of the BJW scale.

6. POSSIBLE MEANINGS OF LOW BELIEF IN A JUST WORLD

Several authors have reported orthogonal or fairly independent factors for positively keyed BJW items and for negatively keyed items (e.g., Dalbert, 1982; Maes, 1992; Schmitt et al., 1997). Accordingly, lower internal consistency coefficients were found for the Rubin & Peplau scale, which contains positively and negativly keyed items, than for subscales containing only positively or only negatively keyed items (Furnham & Gunter, 1984; Furnham, 1993; Heaven & Connors, 1988). The most popular interpretation for this result is that BJW and Belief in an Unjust World (BUW) are separate dispositions. This interpretation creates an intriguing conceptual and psychological problem: What do low scores on BJW scales and on BUW scales express psychologically? In regard to our GBJW scale which does not contain negatively keyed items, this question came up a while ago when an initial experiment was conducted to explore the construct validity of our GBJW scale experimentally (Schmitt et al., 1991). The results of this experiment initiated the present reflections on the construct validity of BJW scales and advanced the assumption that low scores on our GBJW scale reflect BUW. The design of the study is depicted in Table 4.

One hundred and forty-five students were recruited as subjects for the experiment and assigned randomly to one of four treatments. Subjects were told that they would participate in a study on the facial expression of emotions. They would observe via live video transmission another subject taking part in a gamble. They should watch carefully how the person reacted emotionally. They would later be asked to give their impression of

TABLE 4. Experimental Design of the Schmitt et al. (1991) Study

Value of fate	Direction of fate	
	Good luck	Bad luck
Low	Target wins 2 German Marks in a gamble	Target loses 2 German Marks in a gamble
High	Target wins 20 German Marks in a gamble	Target loses 20 German Marks in a gamble

the person and his emotions. The stimulus person was always the same male student. Because the outcome of the gamble had to be faked, subjects did not observe a real situation but a video film. This was disguised by having the experimenter communicate via phone with the experimenter of the gamble, pretending that they talked about the timing of the gamble, the transmission and so forth. No subject suspected seeing a film.

Subjects participated in groups of five. After arriving, they were given a questionnaire containing our GBJW scale and a German version of the Crowne-Marlowe (1960) Social Desirability Scale (Lück & Timaeus, 1969). The GBJW items were mixed with the Social Desirability items to keep them as nonsalient as possible. In order to further reduce the salience of the GBJW items, a second questionnaire was handed out that dealt with human emotions in great detail. Emotions were chosen for distracting subjects' attention from the GBJW items and for increasing the credibility of the cover story.

In the two Bad Luck or Losing conditions, the target was told by the gamble experimenter on arrival in the gambling room that he had been assigned by lot to the losing condition and that he could now only lose money. The amount of money he lost would depend on how well he betted in a roulette game. The gamble experimenter then asked the target to put 20 German marks of his own on the table (20 German marks were the equivalent of about 13 US dollars at the time of the experiment). The target was told that he had to bet on red or black in ten roulette trials. Each wrong bet would cost him 2 German marks. If he betted correctly, he could keep his money. In the Low Value condition, the person betted correctly in 9 out of the 10 trials and lost only 2 German marks. In the High Value condition, the person betted falsely in every trial and lost all his money (20 German Marks). In the two Good Luck or Winning conditions, the target was told that he had been assigned randomly to the winning condition and that he could win money depending on how well he betted in a roulette gamble. The experimenter then put 20 German Marks on the table. In the Low Value condition, the person betted correctly in 1 out of 10 trials, thus winning only 2 German Marks. In the High Value condition, the person always betted correctly and won 20 German Marks.

After subjects had watched the video film, they were given a questionnaire containing items for rating the stimulus person's emotions and personality. The emotion items served to maintain the cover story. Personality was rated on a list of 15 bipolar six-point scales which were adopted partly from the Lerner & Simmons (1966) study. A principle axes analysis of the 15 personality items revealed two common factors. The first factor loaded substantially (> .50) seven socially desirable traits: interesting-boring, bright-dull, lively-lame, likable-unpleasant (highest loading: .77), attractive-unattractive, warm-unfriendly, open-closed. The second factor was emotional stability (e.g., calm-nervous). The items of the first factor were chosen for measuring *derogation* as the dependent variable.

Based on JMT, it was expected that the target would be evaluated less favorably in the Losing conditions than in the Winning condition and that this main effect would be stronger if the person lost/won a lot rather than if the person lost/won a little, respectively. Finally and more importantly in the present context, it was expected that these experimental effects would depend in strength on BJW. Subjects with a high BJW were expected to upgrade the winner more and to downgrade the loser more than subjects scoring low on our GBJW scale. The only significant effect that emerged from moderated regression analysis was this two-way interaction ($F_{1,137}$ = 4.58; $p < .05$), but as can be seen from the fitted regression lines in Figure 1, the effect ran exactly counter to predictions.

Contrary to expectations, subjects who scored high on our GBJW scale tended to upgrade the loser and to downgrade the winner, while subjects with low BJW scores tended to upgrade the winner and downgrade the loser. Schmitt et al. (1991) offered the following interpretation: Subjects with a high BJW construe justice by assuming that losers in a gamble were more fortunate in real life due to an attractive personality which provides them with all kinds of desirable social outcomes. This construal corresponds to a popular German saying: "Pech im Spiel, Glück in der Liebe" (Bad luck with gambling, good luck in love). Accordingly, high BJW subjects assume that those who were lucky in the gamble were less fortunate in real life. Subjects with a low BJW construe their observa-

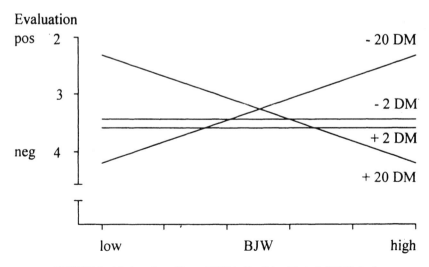

FIGURE 1. Moderating effect of BJW in the Schmitt et al. (1991) study.

tion as proof for their assumption that the world is an unjust place and that there are losers and winners.

Note that this interpretation does not start out from a deserving notion of justice but from a nonconditional equality principle. According to the Schmitt et al. (1991) reasoning, an attractive personality serves as a compensation for bad luck in a gamble, while winning in a gamble is a compensation for a less attractive personality. Accordingly, BJW means to believe in such an equality or compensation principle. Whether this belief is based on experience (knowledge) or wishful thinking is irrelevant for the explanation. Most importantly for the present discussion is that the interpretation implies that low scores on our GBJW scale reflect BUW. Only BUW, but not a low BJW or an indifferent belief can explain why an unfavorable personality is attributed to losers and a favorable personality to winners.

7. COMBINING BELIEF IN A JUST WORLD WITH PREFERENCES FOR DISTRIBUTIVE JUSTICE PRINCIPLES

The interpretation offered by Schmitt et al. (1991) for the results of their experiment is feasable under the assumption that the subjects' sense of justice did not accord to concepts of deserving but to concepts of equality and compensation. Indirect support for this assumption is provided by findings showing that German subjects in general and German students in particular consider the parity principle as more just than the equity, achievement, or deserving principle (Schmitt & Montada, 1982). Contrary to this pattern, North Americans prefer the equity principle over other principles, especially when material resources are to be distributed (Törnblom & Foa, 1983). This cultural difference may explain why the subjects in the Schmitt et al. (1991) experiment behaved other than subjects in some of the North American studies reviewed earlier.

In a follow-up study by Schmitt (1991), this speculation was tested directly. Subjects' attitudes toward equity and equality were measured in addition to BJW. Following the interpretation offered by Schmitt et al. (1991), it was assumed that subjects who favor the equality principle would behave like the subjects in the Schmitt et al. (1991) study, but in a more pronounced manner. Subjects who favor equity (as the principle which comes closest to the concept of deserving) were expected to show the opposite pattern of attributions. More specifically, it was assumed that subjects with a favorable attitude toward equity and high BJW would tend to upgrade winners and downgrade losers, while subjects with a favorable attitude toward equity *and* low BJW would downgrade winners and upgrade losers.

Subjects were shown a video film (presumably a live transmission) of an interview with a first-year psychology student. Questions were asked about five topics: Trier University, the housing situation for students in Trier, financial situation, most extraordinary events during the last year, activities during the semester break. A single experimental factor was varied between subjects: Good Luck vs. Bad Luck.

In the Good Luck condition, the student portrayed himself as a winner who had been exceptionally lucky and fortunate. (1) He had wanted to be a student at Trier University and he been admitted based on a lottery (a real possibility in Germany). (2) Given a lucky coincidence, he had found a very nice and cheap appartment. (3) He had just won money in a speculation that seemed hopeless. (4) Someone had ran into his old car and the insurance payed him more money than he had payed for the car. (5) He was lucky to have found a perfect job for the semester break. The target stressed that he owed these fortunate events to chance or factors that were outside his control. He mentioned several times that he didn't really deserve so much luck and that he thought he was a "Glückspilz" (lucky dog). These remarks were designed to create a need for justification by making it difficult to attribute the favorable events to willful actions on behalf of the target.

In the Bad Luck condition, the student portrayed himself as a loser who had been very unlucky. (1) He wanted to be a student in Hamburg but was assigned to Trier by the Central Agency for the Distribution of Students (a real institution in Germany). (2) Because of a broken public phone, he missed getting a nice and cheap appartment. (3) He had just lost money in a speculation that seemed safe. (4) Someone had ran into his special car, an oldtimer. The insurance would pay him much less than he had payed for the car. (5) Because a roommate told him too late to return a phone call, he missed the perfect job for the semester break. The target stressed that his misfortune was not his fault but due to unfortunate circumstances which were outside his control. He mentioned several times during the interview that he didn't deserve so much bad luck and that he thought he was a "Pechvogel" (unlucky fellow).

One hundred and twenty eight students participated in this experiment. BJW and attitudes toward equity and equality were measured independently. Subjects were assigned randomly to experimental conditions and watched the interview in groups of five or less. Subjects were told that the experiment was designed to find out how well the personality of a person could be judged from the person's description of current life. After subjects had watched the interview, they were distributed a questionnaire which contained a number of manipulation control items and the same personality ratings as in the Schmitt et al. (1991) study.

Two-way interactions between the experimental factor (Good Luck vs. Bad Luck), BJW, and attitude toward equity/equality were expected and

tested via moderated regression analyses. In addition, the three-way interaction (Experimental Factor x BJW x Attitude toward Equity x Attitude
toward Equality) was tested to explore the possibility that only subjects
with negative attitudes toward one principle *and* positive attitudes toward
the other principle would show the expected moderator effect of BJW. The
only significant effect from these analyses was a main effect for the experimental factor. In line with JMT and previous experimental findings (Lerner,
1980; Lerner & Miller, 1978; Lerner, Miller, & Holmes, 1976), the lucky target
was upgraded and the unlucky target was downgraded (mean item scores
amounting to 3.7 vs. 4.3, respectively, on six-point rating scales with 1/most
likable and 6/most unpleasant personality).

The failure to find the predicted interaction effects in the present
study must not be mistaken as a final answer to the question whether BJW
effects differ depending on the justice principle a person prefers in general
or in particular social context. Additional studies are needed to investigate
combined effects of BJW and attitudes towards justice principles in more
detail in different social settings and to explore the usefulness of the
general methodological strategy that was suggested here.

8. METHODS FOR CLARIFYING THE CORRELATIONS BETWEEN BELIEF IN A JUST WORLD AND POLITICAL CONSERVATISM

Several authors have reported positive correlations between BJW
and political conservatism (Dalbert et al., 1987; Dalbert, 1992; Furnham &
Gunter, 1984; Rubin & Peplau, 1973; Schneider, 1988; Wagstaff, 1983). The
causes for this correlation are not clear. At least three interpretations are
possible.

A *first* possibility is that conservatism and BJW are both manifestations of a need for law, order, continuity, stability, and predictability. This
interpretation is supported by the fact that political conservatism and BJW
both correlate with authoritarianism (Dalbert, 1992; Rubin & Peplau, 1973).

Consider a *second* interpretation: Conservatism means wanting to
preserve things as they are. If things are just, it is good to keep them.
According to this rationale, BJW is a causal explanation for conservatism.
Those who believe that the world is just want to keep the world as it is and
develop a conservative attitude towards societal issues.

A *third* causal interpretation suggests that BJW is a consequence of
preferring the current political system. Let's assume that a country is
governed by a certain political party. Citizens who favor this party and
voted for it will have an interest to preserve the status quo. At the same
time, citizens who favor opposed political parties will be dissatisfied with
the situation. Furthermore, it seems reasonable to assume that more politi-

TABLE 5. Order of Political Power and Order of BJW of Different
Political Parties during the Data Collection of Studies Reporting
a Positive Correlation between BJW and Conservatism

Study	Year of data collection	Order of political power, conservatism, and BJW
Dalbert et al. (1987)	1982	CDU/CSU > FDP > SPD > Grüne
Dalbert (1992)	1990	CDU/CSU > FDP > SPD > Grüne
Furnham & Gunter (1984)	≈ 1982	Tories > Labour
Rubin & Peplau (1973)	≈ 1971	Republicans > Democrats
Schneider (1988)	1984/1985	CDU/CSU > FDP > SPD > Grüne
Wagstaff (1983)	≈ 1981	Tories > Labour

cal decisions will be considered as fair by voters of the leading party than by voters of the opposed parties. This mechanism would lead to a positive correlation between a person's preference for the leading party and BJW.

At the same time, BJW should correlate negatively with the distance of the person's political attitude to the leading party (e.g., on a left-right or liberal-conservative continuum). In other words, BJW should be lowest among those whose political attitudes are most different from those of the leading party. This reasoning may sound like a bold speculation, but it is consistent with available data. As can be seen from Table 5, the order of conservatism, political power, and BJW were the same while the studies who reported a positive correlation between BJW and conservatism were conducted. Changes in the political power structure will provide opportunities to submit this hypothesis to further tests. More specifically, the hypothesis predicts that the correlation between BJW and conservatism should have turned negative in the US during the last years and will turn negative in Great Britain after the Labour Party has become the leading political force.

The correlation between BJW and political attitudes is only an example. Competing causal interpretations can easily be construed for the correlations between BJW and other variables such as well-being and emotions. It is not my intention to develop such causal interpretations here. Rather, I wanted to show that longitudinal research is needed to clarify the causal nature of the many correlations that have been reported between BJW and other variables. A great deal about the nature, origins, and functions of BJW could be learned from such research.

9. CONCLUDING CONSIDERATIONS AND SUGGESTIONS

Inconsistent and ambiguous data stimulate the refinement of theories and methods (Lakatos, 1978). This chapter was an attempt to contribute to such an advancement in the domain of BJW by presenting data and arguments which raise questions regarding the validity of BJW as an indicator of the JM. Certainly, only a few data have been presented. Nevertheless, I consider them sufficient for suggesting that it might be more difficult to measure individual differences in need for justice than has been acknowledged by researchers who have used BJW scales—including myself.

One possible reason for this has been discussed by Melvin Lerner on several occasions. Lerner assumes that people are mostly unaware of their need for justice. Accordingly, he has been sceptical about the use of BJW scales for measuring the JM (e.g., Lerner, 1980, Chapter 10). In his recent writings, Lerner (e.g., this volume) draws upon Epstein's level of processing model (Epstein, Lipson, Hostein, & Hub, 1992) to explain why blaming victims differs so greatly from our rational reactions to innocent suffering. Based on this model, Lerner suggests that basic beliefs and motives reside in the preconscious experiential system, they lead to quick and intuitive appraisals of situations, guide our behavior automatically, and cannot be accessed by introspection. The rational system operates logically, makes it possible to construe situations analytically, leads to conscious judgments based on knowledge, and provides a basis for planned behavior. Social norms as a domain of knowledge are part of the rational system. Both systems can operate independently from each other and often do so. The important consequence of this model for the validity of self-report measures for the JM is that the extent to which the JM and the need to believe in a just world are located in the experiential system, they cannot be accessed by introspection and cannot be transformed into answers to questionnaire items. Individuals may simply not know that they have a desire for justice and that they need to believe in a just world. To the extent that this is the case, self-report measures for JM will be difficult to obtain. Yet before giving up the use of BJW scales, it may be wise to continue exploring the psychological meaning of answers to BJW items.

Perhaps the first step toward a resolution is giving up the assumption or requirement that the construct validity of BJW scales is a *constant*. It may be more appropriate and more useful for the design of further research to consider construct validity as being a *variable* which might depend on third factors such as the research setting, the substantive context, and characteristics of the subjects. This way of thinking about the validity of tests and questionnaires is not very common in psychology. However, sufficient research evidence is available suggesting that it is feasible and useful to consider the validity of any measurement instrument as varying across various types of moderators (Schmitt & Borkenau, 1992). This general view calls for psychological reflections on situational and individual conditions on which correlations and effects of BJW may depend. Several lines of differentiation seem worth consideration.

A first line starts out from the fact that the individual difference perspective regarding the justice motive has been limited so far to its strength. It may be useful to additionally consider the possibility that individuals also differ in how the JM is transformed into specific emotions, cognitions, and actions. For example, individuals with an equally strong JM may differ in the means they prefer to use for defending or restoring their BJW. When observing a case of severe injustice, some individuals may choose to deny or to escape the situation while others may face the situation and try to do something to change it. These differences may be independent of the strength of the JM and exist in addition to situational factors suggesting one or another way of dealing with a threat to BJW. Given an equally strong JM, one person may tend to help an innocent victim while the other may prefer punishing the victimizer. It may be possible to resolve inconsistent findings partly by measuring individual differences in the means that are preferred for defending BJW. These preferences may be stable traits. For example, several studies have shown that individuals differ consistently and in a stable manner in altruism and helping behavior (e.g., Montada, Schmitt, & Dalbert, 1991; Silbereisen, Lamsfuss, Boehnke, & Eisenberg, 1991). If altruism as a trait is measured, it can be used as a moderator to allow tests for conditional effects of BJW. One would expect that for subjects scoring high on trait altruism, BJW has a stronger effect on helping innocent victims than for subjects scoring low on altruism. The opposite moderator effect can be expected for denial of responsibility as a trait (Schmitt, Montada, & Dalbert, 1991; Schwartz, 1977). To give a third example: Maes (1994b) has introduced the construct of draconity and proposed a self-report questionnaire for measuring individual differences in this trait. According to his data, individuals differ considerably in how harshly versus forgivingly they react to others who have made mistakes. It can be reasoned that for individuals with high draconity, BJW has a stronger effect on punishing victimizers than for individuals with low draconity.

A second line of differentiation seems necessary according to conceptual analyses (Lerner, 1980) and empirical evidence from research by Maes (1994a, this volume). According to these data, the observation of innocent victims has different impacts for individuals whose justice concept contains the notion of long-term compensation (ultimate justice) than for individuals who limit their justice analysis to a limited time frame. While for the latter, the observation of innocent victims is threatening and may lead to derogation, the latter group can more easily maintain their belief in justice by assuming that the victim will be eventually compensated. Consequently, there is no or less need to distort perceptions regarding the causes of the misfortune and no or less need for distorted evaluations of the victim.

A third line of differentiation deals with the justice standards or criteria that individuals prefer when judging distributions or decision-making processes. Independent of the inconsistent results obtained in the Schmitt et al. (1991) study and the Schmitt (1991) study, it seems necessary, on conceptual grounds alone, to control for the justice principles that can be applied in a particular situation. Depending on which justice principle a person prefers or has in mind when making a justice related observation, this observation may affirm or threaten the person's belief in justice. Accordingly, quite different behavioral consequences are likely in the same situation for individuals who compare the situation with different ideals. A similar problem is given when we compare answers from different individuals to BJW items. For example, belief in justice according to equity has a different meaning than belief in justice according to equality. Equal distributions challenge the first type of BJW while equitable distributions challenge the second type of BJW. One reason why we chose a very general format for our GBJW scale was that we wanted to avoid confounding belief in justice with attitudes toward justice principles. Yet without measuring theses attitudes or the person's specific justice concept in a particular situation, BJW remains ambiguous. Accordingly, it seems difficult to predict how the person will react in a particular situation. Simply asking subjects in the situation or shortly afterwards whether the situation was just or not ("manipulation control") can hardly provide the necessary information unless it were clear at what time defensive mechanisms began to operate. Whatever methodology may be more appropriate, well founded behavioral predictions from BJW according to JMT are only possible to the extent that we know the person's enduring justice concept and to the extent that the person refers to this concept when answering BJW items and when experiencing an experimental or real-life situation.

A fourth line of differentiation has been suggested by Montada & Mohiyeddini (this volume). These authors argue that the effects of BJW on prosocial reactions towards victims (sympathy, political activism directed toward reducing social inequality) and on antisocial reactions such as blaming victims depend on the person's justice self efficacy, i.e. their belief in having control regarding justice. Results reported by Montada & Mohiyeddini suggest that effects of BJW on pro- and antisocial behavior toward victims are stronger for individuals with low justice self efficacy.

Finally, it may be worth considering more direct indicators of the JM than BJW. A first possible candidate is *justice centrality*. Remember that justice centrality was the only organismic factor in the Herbst study which interacted synergetically with the equivalent situation factor. This is an isolated result, of course, which should not be given much weight before it has been replicated. But, there is research in the domain of attitudes showing that the consistency of attitudes and values with behavior is a function of attitude/value centrality (e.g., Krosnick, 1988). A second possible candidate may be *justice sensitivity*, a construct that was recently introduced to the social justice literature by Schmitt, Neumann, & Montada (1995). In several studies, we have been able to show that individuals differ consistently across situations and time in their perceptual threshold for observing cases of injustice, in the intensity of their emotional reactions to injustice, in the mental intrusiveness of such events, and in action tendencies aimed at restoring justice (Schmitt & Mohiyeddini, 1996; Mohiyeddini & Schmitt, 1997; Dörfel & Schmitt, 1997). This sensitivity is generalized across the different roles a person can play in any incidence of injustice (victim, observer, victimizer; Schmitt et al., 1997). In other words, a person who is more justice sensitive from the victim's perspective is also more sensitive from the remaining two perspectives. This generalized sensitivity and corresponding individual differences in the strength of action tendencies aimed at restoring justice may indicate a desire or need for justice according to JMT. Testing this possibility will require the adoption of the same kind of methodological rational used for exploring the construct validity of BJW scales.

REFERENCES

Aiken, L. S. & West, S. G. (1991). Multiple regression: Testing and interpreting interactions. Newbury Park: Sage.

Borkenau, P. (1986). Toward an understanding of trait interrelations: Acts as instances for several traits. Journal of Personality and Social Psychology, 51, 371–381.

Braun, M. (1993). Ideologie oder objektive Lage? Anmerkungen zur Interpretation von Unterschieden und Ähnlichkeiten in den Einstellungen von Ost- und Westdeutschen. ZUMA-Nachichten, 32, 7–21.

Burger, J.M. (1992). Desire for control. New York: Plenum.

Campbell, D.T. & Fiske, D.W. (1959). Convergent and discriminant validation by the multitrait-multimethod matrix. Psychological Bulletin, 56, 81–105.

Cattell, R.B. (1966). Psychological theory and scientific method. In R.B. Cattell (Ed.), Handbook of multivariate experimental psychology (pp. 1–18). Chicago: Rand McNally.

Clayton, S.D. (1992). The experience of injustice: Some characteristics and correlates. Social Justice Research, 5, 71–91.

Collins, B. (1974). Four components of the Rotter internal-external scale. Journal of Personality and Social Psychology, 29, 381–391.

Cronbach, L.J. & Meehl, P.E. (1955). Construct validity in psychological tests. Psychological Bulletin, 52, 281–302.

Crowne, D.P. & Marlowe, D. (1960). A new scale of social desirability independent of psychopathology. Journal of Consulting Psychology, 24, 349–354.

Dalbert, C. (1982). Der Glaube an eine gerechte Welt: Zur Güte einer deutschen Version der Skala von Rubin & Peplau (Berichte aus der Arbeitsgruppe "Verantwortung, Gerechtigkeit, Moral" Nr .10). Trier: Universität Trier, Fachbereich I: Psychologie.

Dalbert, C. (1992). Der Glaube an die gerechte Welt: Differenzierung und Validierung eines Konstrukts. Zeitschrift für Sozialpsychologie, 23, 268–276.

Dalbert, C. (1993). Psychisches Wohlbefinden und Persönlichkeit in Ost und West: Vergleich von Sozialisationseffekten in der früheren DDR und der alten BRD. Zeitschrift für Sozialisationsforschung und Erziehungssoziologie, 13, 82–94.

Dalbert, C. (1996). Über den Umgang mit Ungerechtigkeit. Bern: Huber.

Dalbert, C., Montada, L., & Schmitt, M. (1987). Glaube an eine gerechte Welt als Motiv: Validierungskorrelate zweier Skalen. Psychologische Beiträge, 29, 596–615.

Dalbert, C. & Schneider, A. (1995). Die Allgemeine Gerechte-Welt-Skala: Dimensionalität, Stabilität & Fremdurteiler-Validität (Berichte aus der Arbeitsgruppe "Verantwortung, Gerechtigkeit, Moral" Nr .86). Trier: Universität Trier, Fachbereich I - Psychologie.

Dion, K.L. & Dion, K.K. (1987). Belief in a just world and physical attractiveness stereotyping. Journal of Personality and Social Psychology, 52, 775–780.

Dörfel, M. & Schmitt, M. (1997). Procedural injustice in the workplace, sensitivity to befallen injustice, and job satisfaction (Berichte aus der Arbeitsgruppe "Verantwortung, Gerechtigkeit, Moral" Nr. 103). Trier: Universität Trier, Fachbereich I - Psychologie.

Epstein, S., Lipson, A., Holstein, C., & Hub, E. (1992). Irrational reactions to negative outcomes: Evidence for two conceptual systems. Journal of Personality and Social Psychology, 62, 328–339.

Furnham, A. (1993). Just world beliefs in twelve societies. Journal of Social Psychology, 133, 317–329.

Furnham, A. & Gunter, B. (1984). Just world beliefs and attitudes towards the poor. British Journal of Social Psychology, 23, 265–269.

Furnham, A. & Procter, E. (1992). Sphere-specific just world beliefs and attitudes to AIDS. Human Relations, 45, 265–280.

Hafer, C.L. & Olson, J.M. (1989). Beliefs in a just world and reactions to personal deprivation. Journal of Personality, 57, 799–823.

Heaven, P.C. & Connors, J. (1988). Personality, gender, and "just world" beliefs. Australian Journal of Psychology, 40, 261–266

Herbst, E. (1992). Zuschreibung von Verantwortlichkeit und Schuld gegenüber Opfern durch unbeteiligte Dritte in ihrer Abhängigkeit von Gerechtigkeits- und Kontrollierbarkeitsüberzeugungen sowie Gerechtigkeits- und Kontrollierbarkeitszentralität. Trier: Universität Trier, Fachbereich I - Psychologie (unpubl. diploma thesis).

Kordmann, P. (1991). Determinanten der Opferbeurteilung: Einflüsse von Gerechtigkeits- und Kontrollüberzeugungen auf den Attributionsprozeß. Trier: Universität Trier, Fachbereich I - Psychologie (unpubl. diploma thesis)

Krosnick, J.A. (1988). The role of attitude importance in social evaluations: A study of policy preferences, presidential candidate evaluations, and voting behavior. Journal of Personality and Social Psychology, 55, 196–210.

Lakatos, I. (1978). The methodology of scientific research programmes. Cambridge: Cambridge University Press.

Lerner, M.J. (1970). The desire for justice and reactions to victims. In J. Macaulay & L. Berkowitz (Eds.), Altruism and helping behavior (pp. 205–229). New York: Academic Press.

Lerner, M.J. (1978). ... but nobody liked the Indians. "Belief in a Just World" versus the "Authoritarianism" syndrome. Ethnicity, 5, 229–237.

Lerner, M.J. (1980). The belief in a just world: A fundamental delusion. New York: Plenum.

Lerner, M.J. & Miller, D.T. (1978). Just world research and the attribution process: looking back and ahead. Psychological Bulletin, 85, 1030–1051.

Lerner, M.J., Miller, D.T., & Holmes, J.G. (1976). Deserving and the emergence of forms of justice. In L. Berkowitz (Ed.), Advances in Experimental Social Psychology (Vol. 9, pp. 133- 162). New York: Academic Press.

Lerner, M.J. & Simmons, C.H. (1966). The observer's reaction to the "innocent victim": Compassion or rejection? Journal of Personality and Social Psychology, 4, 203–210.

Limbach, A.F. (1992). Die emotionale Verarbeitung von Arbeitslosigkeit. Trier: Universität Trier, Fachbereich I - Psychologie (unpubl. diploma thesis).

Lipkus, I.M. (1991). The construction and preliminary validation of a global belief in a just world scale and the exploratory analysis of the multidimensional belief in a just world scale. Personality and Individual Differences, 12, 1171–1178.

Lück, H.E. & Timaeus, E. (1969). Skalen zur Messung Manifester Angst (MAS) und sozialer Wünschbarkeit (SDS-E und SDS-CM). Diagnostica, 15, 134–141.

Maes, J. (1992). Konstruktion und Analyse eines mehrdimensionalen Gerechte-Welt-Fragebogens (Berichte aus der Arbeitsgruppe „Verantwortung, Gerechtigkeit, Moral" Nr .64). Trier: Universität Trier, Fachbereich I - Psychologie.

Maes, J. (1994a). Blaming the victim—belief in control or belief in justice? Social Justice Research, 7, 69–90.

Maes, J. (1994b). Drakonität als Personmerkmal: Entwicklung und erste Erprobung eines Fragebogems zur Erfassung von Urteilsstrenge (Drakonität) versus Milde (Berichte aus der Arbeitsgruppe "Verantwortung, Gerechtigkeit, Moral" Nr. 78). Trier: Universität Trier, Fachbereich I - Psychologie.

Miller, D.T. (1977). Altruism and threat to a belief in a just world. Journal of Experimental Social Psychology, 13, 113–124.

Miller, F.D., Smith, E.R., Ferree, M.M., & Taylor, S.E. (1976). Predicting perceptions of victimization. Journal of Applied Social Psychology, 6, 352–359.

Mohiyeddini, C. (1995). Sensibilität für widerfahrene Ungerechtigkeit als Disposition: kognitive, emotionale sowie behaviorale Reaktionen auf ungerechte Behandlung. Trier: Universität Trier (unpublished diploma thesis).

Mohiyeddini, C. & Schmitt, M. (1997). Sensitivity to befallen injusitce and reactions to unfair treatment in a laboratory situation. Social Justice Research, 10, 333–352.

Montada, L. (1992). Attribution of responsibility for losses and perceived injustice. In L. Montada, S.- H. Filipp, & M.J. Lerner (Eds.), Life crises and the experience of loss in adulthood (pp. 133–162). Hillsdale, NJ: Lawrence Erlbaum.

Montada, L. & Schneider, A. (1989). Justice and emotional reactions to the disadvantaged. Social Justice Research, 3, 313–344.

Montada, L., Schmitt, M., & Dalbert, C. (1986). Thinking about justice and dealing with one's own privileges: A study of existential guilt. In H.-W. Bierhoff, R.L. Cohen, & J. Greenberg (Eds.), Justice in Social Relations (pp. 125–143). New York: Plenum Press.

Montada, L., Schmitt, M., & Dalbert, C. (1991). Prosocial commitments in the family: Situational, personality, and systemic factors. In L. Montada & H.-W. Bierhoff (Eds.), Altruism in social systems (pp. 177–203). Toronto: Hogrefe & Huber Publishers.

Reichle, B. (1994). Die Zuschreibung von Verantwortlichkeit für negative Ereignisse in Partnerschaften: Ein Modell und erste empirische Befunde. Zeitschrift für Sozialpsychologie, 25, 227–237.

Rubin, Z. & Peplau, L.A. (1973). Belief in a just world and reactions to another's lot: A study of participants in the National Draft Lottery. Journal of Social Issues, 29(4), 73–93.

Rubin, Z. & Peplau, L. A. (1975). Who believes in a just world? Journal of Social Issues, 31(3), 65–89.

Sauer, C. (1984). Opfer und Beobachter: zwei experimentelle Untersuchungen von Reaktionen auf die Wahrnehmung von Ungerechtigkeit. Mannheim: Universität Mannheim - Fakultaet für Sozialwissenschaften (unpubl. dissert.)

Schmitt, M. (1991). Ungerechtes Schicksal und Personenbewertung. Zeitschrift für Sozialpsychologie, 22, 208–210.

Schmitt, M. (1992). Schönheit und Talent: Untersuchungen zum Verschwinden des Halo-Effekts. Zeitschrift für experimentelle und angewandte Psychologie, 39, 475–492.

Schmitt, M. & Borkenau, P. (1992). The consistency of personality. In G.-V. Caprara & G.L. Van Heck (Eds.), Modern personality psychology. Critical reviews and new directions (pp. 29–55). New York: Harvester-Wheatsheaf.

Schmitt, M. & Herbst, E. (1993). How to separate justice and control as motives for blaming the victims? Paper presented at the IV. International Conference on Social Justice Research in Trier.

Schmitt, M. & Janetzko, E. (1993). Verantwortlichkeitsüberzeugungen bei Ost- und Westdeutschen. In G. Trommsdorff (Hrsg.), Psychologische Aspekte des sozio-politischen Wandels in Ostdeutschland (S. 169–179). Berlin: Walter de Gruyter.

Schmitt, M., Kilders, M., Mösle, A., Müller, L., Pfrengle, A., Rabenberg, H., Schott, F., Stolz, J., Suda, U., Williams, M., & Zimmermann, G. (1991). Gerechte-Welt-Glaube, Gewinn und Verlust: Rechtfertigung oder ausgleichende Gerechtigkeit? Zeitschrift für Sozialpsychologie, 22, 37–45.

Schmitt, M., Maes, J., & Schmal, A. (1995). Gerechtigkeit als innerdeutsches Problem: Einstellungen zu Verteilungsprinzipien, Ungerechtigkeitssensibilität und Glaube an eine gerechte Welt als Kovariate (Berichte aus der Arbeitsgruppe "Verantwortung, Gerechtigkeit, Moral" Nr. 82). Trier: Universität Trier, Fachbereich I - Psychologie.

Schmitt, M., Maes, J., & Schmal, A. (1997). Gerechtigkeit als innerdeutsches Problem: Analyse der Meßeigenschaften von Meßinstrumenten für Einstellungen zu Verteilungsprinzipien, Ungerechtigkeitssensibilität und Glaube an eine gerechte Welt (Berichte aus der Arbeitsgruppe "Verantwortung, Gerechtigkeit, Moral" Nr. 105). Trier: Universität Trier, Fachbereich I - Psychologie.

Schmitt, M. & Mohiyeddini, C. (1996). Sensitivity to befallen injustice and reactions to a real life disadvantage. Social Justice Research, 9, 223–238.

Schmitt, M. & Montada, L. (1982). Determinanten erlebter Gerechtigkeit. Zeitschrift für Sozialpsychologie, 13, 32–44.

Schmitt, M., Neumann, R., & Montada, L. (1995). Dispositional sensitivity to befallen injustice. Social Justice Research, 8, 385–407.

Schneider, A. (1988). Glaube an die gerechte Welt: Replikation der Validierungskorrelate zweier Skalen (Berichte aus der Arbeitsgruppe "Verantwortung, Gerechtigkeit, Moral" Nr .40). Trier: Universität Trier, Fachbereich I: Psychologie.

Schwartz, S.H. (1977). Normative influences on altruism. In L. Berkowitz (Ed.), Advances in experimental social psychology (Vol. 10, pp. 221–279). New York: Academic Press.

Shaver, K.G. (1985). The attribution of blame: Causality, responsibility, and blame worthiness. New York: Springer.

Silbereisen, R.K., Lamsfuss, S., Boehnke, K., & Eisenberg, N. (1991). Developmental patterns and correlates of prosocial motives in adolescence. In L. Montada & H.-W. Bierhoff (Eds.), Altruism in social systems (pp. 177–203). Toronto: Hogrefe & Huber Publishers.

Smith, K. & Green, D. (1984). Individual correlates of the belief in a just world. Psychological Reports, 34, 435–438.

Törnblom, K.Y. & Foa, U.G. (1983). Choice of a distribution principle: crosscultural evidence on the effects of resources. Acta Sociologica, 26, 161–173.

Wagstaff, G.F. (1983). Correlates of the just world in Britain. Journal of Social Psychology, 121, 145–146.

Walster, E. (1966). Assignment of responsibility for an accident. Journal of Personality and Social Psychology, 3, 73–79.

Wegener, B. & Liebig, S. (1994). Hierarchical and social closure conceptions of distributive justice: A comparison of East and West Germans. In B. Wegener, A. Acisu, P. Davidson, S. Fischer, S. Kleebaur, R. Krämer, S. Liebig, & S. Steinmann (Eds.), Die Warhnehmung sozialer Gerechtigkeit in Deutschland im internationalen Vergleich (pp. 287–309). Berlin: Institut für Soziologie der Humboldt Universität.

Zuckerman, M. & Gerbasi, K. C. (1977). Belief in internal control or belief in a just world: The use and misuse of the I-E-scale in prediction of attitudes and behavior. Journal of Personality, 45, 356–378.

Zuckerman, M., Gerbasi, K. C., Kravitz, R. I., & Wheeler, L. (1975). The belief in a just world and reactions to innocent victims. Catalog of Selected Documents in Psychology, 5, 326.

Chapter 12

Belief in a Just World: A Hybrid of Justice Motive and Self-Interest?

LEO MONTADA

1. BJW: THE JUSTICE MOTIVE BLENDED WITH SELF-INTEREST

Ever since I read Melvin Lerner's article "The Justice Motive" (1977) I was fascinated by this construct, especially because it represented a contrast to "self-interest"—the basic motivation postulated in the *Economic Model of Man* and in *Rational Choice Theory*. I became convinced that it would be very worthwhile to contribute to the establishment of this construct as a basic human motivation in the Social Sciences.

Reading Lerner's work on "Belief in a Just World (BJW)" including his summarizing writings (1977, 1980) and further research literature on this concept, I was equally fascinated, not because BJW was a pure representation of the justice motive but because it seemed to be a powerful demonstration of human longing for justice even in cases of observed victimization and of the curious subjective constructions and fabrications of justice.

The construct BJW—this "fundamental delusion" as Lerner has characterized it—became prominent in social psychology as an explanation of the frequently observable phenomena of blaming innocent victims. Harm, losses, or disadvantages were undeserved if they resulted from bad luck;

LEO MONTADA • Department of Psychology, Universität Trier, D-54286 Trier, Germany.

Responses to Victimizations and Belief in a Just World, edited by Montada and Lerner. Plenum Press, New York, 1998.

they were unjust if they were afflicted or not prevented by agents or agencies unless a reasonable justification could be given. Every day we witness many cases of harm, hardship, and loss, and every day we are confronted with grossly disadvantaged people. Isn't this a challenge for our justice motive? How do these observations and encounters match or affect the way people view their world: Is it a just one or not? And how do prefabricated "dispositional" views of the world shape the understanding of observable facts? Lerner's hypothesis: Our understanding of and our responses to witnessed cases of harm, loss, and hardships are shaped in order to preserve a fundamental Belief in a Just World.

Principally, we have several options available to deal with facts challenging our intuitive conception of justice. We may try to remove the injustice by adequate intervention (e.g., by punishing the violators, political protest, individual help) or we may reappraise a case so that it appears less unjust to us. Blaming or derogating the victims are possibilities for this latter option. The question remains whether we can predict in what cases a particular option will most likely be chosen. Two of the hypotheses are that the choice of an option will depend on the subjective ability to remove the injustices and on the subjective costs such efforts would have (Miller, 1977).

The empirical evidence gathered in the 1970s was very convincing: Confronted with cases of bad treatment or poor living conditions, many subjects denied the existence of undeserved or unjust hardships and victimization. It was found that not everyone abstains from making attributional judgments when valid information about causation, responsibility, and deservingness is lacking. Apparently, people often interpret a case intuitively and in a biased manner (Lerner & Lerner, 1981).

It seems reasonable to expect that pre-existing subjective world views are a source of biased judgments and emotional appraisals. When they are traitlike stable and consistent conceptual and judgmental dispositions they may even trump contradicting information. The phenomena on blaming innocent victims becomes understandable when using the BJW hypothesis that people want to believe that the world is a just one where everyone gets what they deserve even if the immediately available observations and information challenge this view.

Some of the subjective views of incidents of hardship, loss, harm, or disadvantage motivated to preserve people's BJW may be objectively false, or at least one-sided, and to that extent unjust. This aspect was fascinating to me: the justice motive producing unjust evaluations of events and thus interfering with efforts to (re-)establish actual justice. How might this happen? Two hypotheses can be distinguished: (1) BJW may take on self-serving functions and will, therefore, be defended even at the cost of false evaluations of victims. (2) The justice motive is blended with self-interests. Self-interest may restrict the justice motive by limiting subjects' investments into reestablishing or maintaining justice "in the world" (Lerner &

Miller, 1978). This blending of justice motive and self-interests sometimes results in unjust blaming or derogating of victims. The conceptual question is the following: can BJW be conceived and operationalized as pure justice motive that occasionally competes with self-interests? Or is BJW the result of blending the justice motive with self-interest? In other words, is BJW (to be) conceived of as a hybrid of justice motive and self-interest?

What might be assumed to be the self-interest facet implied in BJW? At least those who do not feel burdened with inexpiated guilt should feel more safe by believing that they live in a just world where good people as they are will be rewarded. Besides this basic hypothesis, the defense of BJW by reappraising events that challenge BJW can be self-serving, for instance, in the following ways: (1) All those enjoying favorable living conditions would not feel obligated—for reasons of justice—to share with the less fortunate if they believe that the world in its current state is a just one. (2) All those who encounter or learn about other people's hardships wouldn't feel obliged to care about them if they believe the world is a just one. (3) All those who are confronted with cases of harmdoing would not have to intervene or to protest if they believe the world is a just one the way it is.

BJW may, however, also motivate people to correct observed cases of injustice or prevent injustices. Assuming that self-interest may come into play as a motivational factor limiting subjects' investments into reestablishing or maintaining justice requires thinking of a threshold for the interplay of justice motive and self-interest in the defense of BJW. The scientific problem is how to get knowledge ex ante of whether the justice motive will trump self-interests or not, or vice versa.

The blending of justice motive and self-interest in BJW is facilitated by the fact that views about deservingness and justice can be conceived of as social or personal constructions. Why? In principle, people always have options to apply with respect to rules or principles of justice as well as with respect to the attribution of responsibilities (cf. Montada, 1994). For instance, when appraising the case of a man who lost his job, several justice principles or justice criteria can be applied: the equality principle, the need principle, the equity principle, the seniority principle, the qualification principle, the principle of reciprocity, and so on. Besides the selection and weighting of a justice principle, the attribution of responsibility is crucial. Who is responsible for having caused or for not having prevented the dismissal: the dismissed employee, the employer, the workers' committee, the unions by their wage policy, the state by its economic or labor policies, or someone else? Or, is no one perceived as being responsible because the dismissal is attributed to more or less uncontrollable causes such as the constitutional poor health of the dismissed, the unfavorable overall economic situation, the globalization of markets, and so forth?

Given the spectrum of options that are principally available for appraisals of justice, the influence of self-interests on the social and personal constructions of justice becomes highly plausible, especially in cases where salient and valid information about causation of and responsibility for the injustice are lacking.

2. FACETS OF BJW

Belief in a Just World allows the assumption of interindividual and intraindividual variations along several facets. (1) BJW can be more or less strong meaning that subjects' views of the degree of justice realized in the world may vary. (2) The section of the world focused upon can vary, for instance, it can be "my personal world in the family and/or at the workplace," "my community," "my social class in society," "my society," or "all societies and human beings all over the world." (3) Different aspects of the world may be focused upon such as, for instance, close relationships, the market place, the political arena, the court systems, the social welfare system. (4) The conception of justice applied can vary: deserving with its different facets, need, parity, etc., or some mixtures. (5) The time period under consideration may vary. The world can be evaluated in its current state or over a prolonged period of time for the correction of currently observable injustices; current injustices can be believed to be corrected or compensated for in the future, even in a transcendental world, what Maes (1995, and in this volume) calls "Ultimate Belief in a Just World."

In all of our studies, we operationalized BJW as an individually varying disposition to perceive the world as just. In some studies, we used scales specifying some facets, e.g., the section of the world where BJW was assessed (specific BJW or SPBJW) or the time perspective. Most frequently we used a short general scale without any specification of facets (general BJW or GBJW, cf. Dalbert, Montada & Schmitt, 1987). One typical item in this scale is "In general, the world is a just one." This item allows for varying interpretations of the terms "world," "just," and "in general" and the scores assessed for such an item—scores on a rating scale from 1 (I agree perfectly) to 6 (I do not agree at all)—may have different meanings for different subjects and even for the same subjects on different occasions.

Nevertheless, we assumed that the responses to such an item represents a subject's BJW and thus, different scores represent interindividual differences in BJW. If such a belief could be considered a stable one that is not shaken by every contradictory event we might expect efforts to defend that view whenever it is challenged. And it is these efforts that are the motivational implications of BJW. Yet without knowing a subject's exact interpretation of such an item (and, consequently, of specific BJW facets rated by an individual subject), we do not know which cases are challenging the individual respondent's BJW. If, for example, the respondent answered the item with his or her workplace in mind, we could not predict whether the fate of children in a slum area somewhere in the world would challenge his/her BJW. This variation in the interpretation of items contributes to the error variance of the assessment scales and reduces their reliability as well as validity, and, consequently, the closeness of the theoretically expected relationships to other variables.

By assuming that the specified facets of BJW have varying impact on judgments, emotions, and behavior, many implications for research are given including the generation of experimental arrangements, the use of particular specified measurement devices (what, meanwhile, has been done, cf. Furnham, Maes, and Mohiyeddini & Montada in this volume), and the interpretation of data.

3. STUDIES ON BJW

I have conducted or supervised a series of studies that included BJW measures (GBJW, SPBJW). I will present an overview of some of the results generated in of 13 studies. The majority of these results are being published for the first time in this chapter. I will try to clarify the basic meanings of these scales and the various facets of the latent variable BJW which we tried to assess using these scales.

In experimental approaches to BJW assessment, the information that more or less threatens BJW is manipulated based on the assumption that in a randomized group design, interindividual differences are balanced out so that group differences can be interpreted as reflecting the impact of the manipulated variables (varying threat to BJW) on the dependent variable (e.g., derogation of victims). In questionnaire studies, individual differences in BJW are assessed and their impact on responses to selected cases that assumedly threaten BJW can be determined by correlational analyses. What both approaches have in common is that the investigators postulate hypotheses about the meaning of BJW as well as about cases which will probably challenge this presumed latent variable.

In the early 1980s we constructed the previously mentioned General BJW scale (GBJW) with six items stating that (1) in general, the world is a just one, (2) overall people get what they deserve, (3) justice generally wins, (4) everybody will be compensated for suffered injustice, (5) in all areas of life, injustices are the exception and not the rule, and (6) in important decisions, all those who are involved attempt to account for justice. The respondents rated their degree of agreement-disagreement on a 6-point scale from 1 (I perfectly agree) to 6 (I don't agree at all).

The available correlational patterns allow the identification of the construct validity or the meaning of the latent construct assessed with this scale. Before continuing, I should note, at the outset, that responses to this scale have consistently proven to be one-dimensional, with ade-

quate internal consistency coefficients and reliability."[1] The area-specific
scales—SPBJW—yield even better scale qualities.

3.1. GBJW and Phenomena of Blaming the Victim for Self-Infliction (BVSI)

In several studies we assessed tendencies to blame "victims" for
either having brought about their own hardships, losses, etc. or for having
failed to prevent them (BVSI), for instance, poor people in the Third World,
the handicapped, AIDS patients, accident victims, rape victims, cancer
patients, and some others."[2] BJW assessed by the GBJW scale turned out
to be significantly correlated with a tendency to blame victims (BVSI) in
all of these studies. A short overview is provided in Table 1.

3.1.1. Study 1

The question was: How do subjects having relatively favorable living
conditions respond to descriptions of misery, hardship, and problems of
relatively unfortunate people? The latter consisted of the poor in the Third
World, the handicapped, and Turkish foreign workers in Germany. For
each category of disadvantaged, three scenarios were designed which
contained vivid descriptions of needs and problems. A large number of
emotional responses as well as cognitive appraisals were assessed following each scenario. Blaming the "victims" for self-infliction of their fates
(BVSI) was one of the appraisals assessed. The zero-order correlation
between GBJW and BVSI was r = .50. (Further information is provided in
Montada, Schmitt, and Dalbert, 1986).

3.1.2. Study 2

A second study was conducted with similar objectives and essentially the same methodological approach as in Study 1. In this study, poor
people in the Third World, foreign guest workers, and unemployed people
in Germany were selected as "victim categories." Several subsamples were
drawn and combined to a heterogeneous sample of 865 participants (for
further information, see Montada & Schneider, 1989, 1991). A similar scale
as in Study 1 was used to assess the tendency to blame victims for

[1] Retest reliability was proven in a longitudinal study (referred to as Study 3 below) with a
large heterogenous sample.

[2] I take BVSI measures instead of derogating of victims as an indicator of blaming victims
because we have used that kind of measure in more studies. In those studies where both
BVSI and derogation measures were used, these variables proved to be correlated
(typically about r = .50).

self-infliction of their fate (BVSI). The zero-order correlation between GBJW and this scale was r = .39.

3.1.3. Study 3

This was a longitudinal follow-up of about half of the sample that participated in Study 2 using the same questionnaires. In this replication, the zero-order correlation between GBJW and BVSI scores was r = .44.

3.1.4. Study 4

This dealt with issues similar to those addressed in Studies 1, 2, and 3. The "victim categories" were people in the Third World and in Russia, and people who applied for asylum in Germany for economic reasons. The tendency to blame these needy people for self-infliction (BVSI) was assessed by a questionnaire of perceived responsibility for the existing needs: the needy people themselves, the state, other agents, or bad luck. The zero-order correlation between GBJW and BVSI was r = .29 (cf. Bartos, 1992).

3.1.5. Study 5

Responsibility attributions for rape were examined. BVSI scores were drawn from a scale of 22 items assessing the tendencies to blame rape victims for self-infliction, to excuse the perpetrators, and to deny the seriousness of the experience of rape. The zero-order correlation between GBJW and BVSI was r = .25 (cf. Knerr, 1986).

3.1.6. Study 6

The focus was on the tendency of 107 young adults to isolate AIDS virus carriers. The majority of the subjects were recruited at a technical college. An internally consistent scale to blame AIDS victims for self-infliction was constructed. It correlated significantly and substantially with GBJW (r = .50) for heterosexuals, but no correlation was found for homosexuals. (For further information see Montada & Figura, 1988).

3.1.7. Study 7

This was mainly a replication of Study 6 with a larger sample of young adults. Again, GBJW and the tendency to blame AIDS victims for self-infliction were substantially correlated: r = .58. (For further information see Montada, Hermes, & Schmal, 1990).

3.1.8. Study 8

This was designed to compare the relative impact of BJW and control motivation on the tendency to blame victims of traffic accidents. Two

TABLE 1. Correlations between BJW (GBJW) and the Tendency to Blame "Victims" for Self-Infliction of "Their Fate" (BVSI)

	Zero-order correlation"	Categories of "victims"/ Blaming the victim scores (BVSI)	Samples
Study 1	r = .50	1. Poor people in the Third World 2. Foreign workers 3. Physically handicapped BVSI: Scores aggregated across 9 items on self-infliction (3 for each category of victims)	n = 340, about half drawn as a random sample from an urban area, the other half from criterion groups expected to have either positive or negative attitudes toward one of the victim categories; mean age 36.1 years; 52% male, 48% female; higher levels of education a bit overrepresented
Study 2	r = .39	1. Poor people in the Third World 2. Foreign workers 3. Unemployed people BVSI: Scores aggregated across 9 items (3 for each category of victims).	n = 865 privileged with respect to education (university students), social security (civil servants with tenure), wealth (business owners, people living in wealthy neighborhoods); mean age 36 (18–86 years); 59% male, 41% female
Study 3	r = .44	Same as in Study 2	n = 434 randomly selected subjects from the sample in Study 2 for a longitudinal replication
Study 4	r = .29	1. Poor people in the Third World 2. Poor people in Russia 3. People seeking asylum for economic reasons BVSI: Drawn from a question-naire about responsibility for existing needs: the needy themselves, the state, other agents, bad luck.	n = 223 high school students; mean age 17.7 years; 44.8% female, 55.2% male
Study 5	r = .25	Rape victims BVSI: Drawn from a question-naire about responsibility attributions to victims, excuses of rapists, and denial of seriousness of rape consequences.	n = 334 university students (199 males, 135 females) and n = 25 members of womens' organizations; mean age, 24 years

Study 6	r = .50 (heterosexuals)	AIDS patients, HIV positives	n = 88 heterosexual members of a technical college and n = 19 homosexual or bisexual men/members of a technical college or a homosexual group; mean age, 26 years; 57% male, 41% female (2 participants with missing gender information)
	r = .01 n.s. (homosexual men)	BVSI: Questionnaire scale.	
Study 7	r = .58	AIDS patients, HIV positives	n = 231 mostly students at a university or technical college; mean age, 26 years; 58% female, 41% male (2 participants with missing gender information). Because the number of participants with a homosexual or bisexual orientation was too small (n = 9), no specific analyses were run.
		BVSI: Same as in Study 6.	
Study 8	r = .34	Traffic accident victims	n = 214 university students (Psychology, Law)
		BVSI: Questionnaire scale.	
Study 9	r = .36	Unemployed people	n = 405; random samples from two urban areas; mean age 45 years; 46% female, 54% male; 22% jobless
		BVSI: 5 items on self-responsibility of the unemployed	

[a]All coefficients without suffix are significant (p < .01).

measures of the tendency to blame victims for self-infliction (BVSI) were constructed (cf. Kordmann, 1991):

1. A questionnaire to assess the tendency to attribute self-responsibility or co-responsibility to accident victims without having detailed information about specific incidences. (Example item: Frequently, pedestrians who are involved in traffic accidents are responsible themselves.) The correlation between GBJW and this BVSI measure was r = .34.

2. A second measure of BVSI was designed which consisted of responsibility attributions on the basis of five vignettes containing detailed information about single cases relevant to the judicial appraisals of the cases. It might be that the information about responsibilities presented in the vignettes was too concrete and salient to allow the expression of a bias to blame victims. The correlation between BVSI scores and the five vignettes was also minimal so that no aggregated score could be formed. Consequently, the correlations with GBJW were spurious and inconsistent. They were significant for only one of the five vignettes. I will discuss this finding later.

3.1.9. Study 9

This was designed to assess and analyze responses to and appraisals of mass unemployment. Various attributions of responsibilities of the unemployed were used as measures of BVSI. The aggregated BVSI scores were correlated with GBJW (r = .36) (cf. Montada & Mohiyeddini, 1997).

Overall, the results of these studies consistently support the hypothesis that the BJW assessed with the GBJW scale is motivating a tendency to blame victims for having self-inflicted their hardships and losses. In order to be cautious with generalizations, I should point out some specific characteristics of these studies:

1. In all studies, most subjects were personally not affected by the victims' fate.
2. Subjects were not personally acquainted with the victims.
3. Subjects were not directly confronted with victims; instead, the victims as well as the kind of victimization was either described by vivid portrayals in scenarios or merely named in questionnaire items by abstract concepts. (By the way, across the nine studies, the level of correlations does not appear to depend on the vividness of the descriptions.) Whether the respondents identified themselves with the victims or whether they felt empathy with them and what impact identification or empathy with the victims

had on the correlation between GBJW and blaming the victims for self-infliction will be discussed later.

4. Moreover, with the exception of Study 8, no detailed information about causality of and responsibility for the victimization was given to the respondents which could have restricted biased attributions. In Study 8, this is true only for a first measure of BVSI which is listed in Table 1. For this measure, the typical correlation with GBJW was found. A second procedure to assess BVSI was employed which provided the respondents with more detailed information subjects about causality and responsibility of victims and perpetrators. This second procedure did not yield consistent attributions across the five scenarios and did not correlate consistently with GBJW. It might well be that the correlation between GBJW and the tendency to blame victims is higher when respondents are not required to consciously reflect and to weigh up the causal contributions and responsibilities of different agents or agencies when relevant information is provided. The nine studies that are presented here offer a hint of this possibility. In studies 4, 5, 8 and 9 the respondents rated responsibilities of various agents, possible including the victim. Causality and responsibility of agents, other than the victims had to be appraised as well. In these studies the mean correlation coefficient between GBJW and BVSI was r = .31, whereas in the other five studies, where only attributions of self-infliction were required, the mean correlation coefficient was r = .48.

With these reservations against an overgeneralization in mind, I do not hesitate to interpret the data as a convincing confirmation of the BJW hypothesis. The shared variance of GBJW and BVSI ranges from 6.3 to 33.6%. This is substantial, especially when considering that in all studies, both GBJW and BVSI scores were not normally distributed but displayed a tendency toward the negative pole of the scales (mean scores indicating a moderate rejection of GBJW and BVSI statements) and, consequently, variances were restricted.[3]

Nevertheless, the correlations are far from being perfect. (Of course, corrections for unreliability of both measures would still have raised the

---

[3] Looking at the mean scores one might prefer to interpret correlations between GBJW and BVSI in the following way: The less GBJW, the weaker subjects' tendency to blame victims for self-infliction. Of course, this is logically the same interpretation as the positively formulated one. Although the correlations are substantial, the larger part of the BVSI variance is not explained by GBJW so that the search for alternative and further predictors is reasonable.

correlations a bit.) This may have quite different explanations. I will only mention two hypotheses for which we can offer some data.

1. When answering the GBJW scale, an unknown number of respondents thought about other areas of the world than those where the victims focused on in a study were located and where their victimization occurred. If the scores on GBJW vary intraindividually depending on the area of the world focused on, then the scores of a number of subjects on GBJW may not be relevant to the attributions made on the BVSI measure. This mismatch of BJW and BVSI measures can be reduced by utilizing area-specific GBJW measures. This is demonstrated in Section 3.2.
2. The impact of BJW on BVSI might not be generally the same for all people but may be moderated by some other variable. By distinguishing facets of BJW (Section 2), I have referred to preferences for distribution principles. These may function as moderators of the correlation between GBJW and BVSI as will be discussed in Section 3.3. Another moderator may be are respondents perceived similarity to victims, sympathy for victims, and others. I will deal with these issues in Section 3.4.

3.2. Area-Specific Assessment of BJW: SPBJW and BVSI

As already stated, in the items of GBJW the belief in justice is assessed without any specification of areas of "the world of social life." Therefore, it is not known which parts or domains of the world are focused on by individual respondents when they generate their answers to the items of the scale. It is a reasonable assumption that various respondents think of different sections of the reality when they appraise justice. Consequently, many respondents may not think of those sections of the world that are focused on in the BVSI scales. Therefore, the question was, what would be the effect of assessing BJW with respect to those problem fields focused on in the BVSI measure to assess the tendency to blame victims. We know that a correspondence in content has an impact on the closeness of relationships between variables, cf. Schmitt, Dalbert, and Montada, 1985. Therefore, we developed area-specific measures of BJW for the Studies 1, 2, and 3 specifying the areas of Third World, Turkish guest workers, handicapped people, and the unemployed. In Table 2, (third column) the correlations between GBJW and SPBJW are listed. They are very similar in all three studies, ranging form $r = .61$ to $r = .65$. The correlation is substantial but not perfect. This means that it is reasonable to assume that different subjects either focus on different sections of "the world" when they answer the GBJW scale or that they attach varying weights to the specific areas focused on in SPBJW.

By comparing these area-specific measures (SPBJW) with the general measure (GBJW) we can test the hypothesis that the correspondence in context between predictor (BJW) and criterion (BVSI) raises the correlation coefficients (cf. Table 2). By using the same aggregation level as was used in the preceding description of Study 1 to Study 3 (cf. Table 1), it can clearly be demonstrated that SPBJW has a higher correlation with BVSI than GBJW. The results demonstrate that the correspondence in areas between BJW and BVSI measures increases the shared variance between 12.24 and 29.44%. In absolute terms, by using the area-specific measures (SPBJW), the shared variance with BVSI measures varies from 32.49 to 54.76% in the three studies.

3.3. BJW and Preferences for Principles of Distributive Justice

BJW was conceived as the belief that everybody gets what he or she deserves and that everybody deserves what he or she gets. That means, Lerner conceived the construct by primarily focusing on deservingness as a principle of justice. In Rubin and Peplau's scale (cf. Rubin & Peplau, 1973), explicit reference to deserving is made. However, it may also happen that some people think that the world or their world is a just one although they do not think of the deservingness principle as the standard, but instead, of another principle, e.g., the need principle or the equality principle.

In our scales (both the general and the area-specific ones) most items were neutral with respect to specific principles of justice. The attitudes to some of these principles—the need principle, the equality principle, and the equity principle meaning proportionality of input (achievement, investment etc.) and outcomes, the latter one representing the deservingness principle—were assessed separately in several studies.

These principles, too, were operationalized in either a general way (items were put together across various cases within various aspects of

TABLE 2. Comparison of the Correlations with Tendency to Blame Victims for Self-Infliction (BVSI) when BJW is Assessed Either with a General Scale (GBJW) or with Scales Specified to the Groups of Victims in Focus and to Areas of the World Relevant to Them (SPBJW)

	Correlation between BVSI[a] and BJW measures[b]		
	General measure GBJW	Specific measure SPBJW	Correlation between GBJW and SPBJW
Study 1[c]	r = .50	r = .57	r = .65
Study 2[c]	r = .39	r = .67	r = .61
Study 3[c]	r = .44	r = .74	r = .62

[a]Scores are aggregated across three categories of victims in each study.
[b]All coefficients are significant (p < .01).
[c]For a description of the study, see Table 1.

life) or area-specific (items were formulated specific to the focused problem areas). This design allowed us to look for relationships between the
BJW scales and the attitude toward specific principles of distributive
justice. It turned out that the preference for the equality principle was, in
general, uncorrelated with the BJW scales, but attitudes toward the need
and the equity principle covaried with BJW scales, though the correlation
with the attitude toward the need principle did not appear consistently
across various studies and was much lower than the attitude to the equity
principle.

Table 3 provides an overview of the results of several studies. The
data demonstrate that a substantial positive correlation exists between the
attitude toward the equity principle and the BJW scales[4] and—in the
median—a low negative correlation between the attitude toward the need
principle and the BJW scales. In two studies, the correlation between GBJW
and the need principle is positive. In sum, the correlation of BJW with
attitude toward the need principle is marginal and inconsistent, whereas
the correlation to the equity principle is positive. This makes sense. Given
the obvious extent of neediness in many areas of the world, it is easier to
preserve BJW when one prefers the equity and not the need principle.

The pattern of low correlations between BJW and preference for the
need principle means that they vary more or less independently from each
other. Consequently, some people with a strong BJW prefer the need principle. What does this psychic constellation mean? It is much easier to blame
victims by applying the equity principle than by applying the need principle. In fact, the correlation between BVSI and the equity principle is typically high and positive (e.g., $r = .71$ in Study 2) and negative between BVSI
and the attitude toward the need principle (e.g., $r = -.39$ in Study 2).
Especially in cases of missing or ambiguous information, it is all too easy
to blame victims for having made mistakes, for irresponsible or risky
behaviors, for not having prevented their losses and problems, and so forth.
The assignment of blame to victims supports the view that the victims'
hardships are deserved. However, when the need principle is applied, it is
not quite that easy to blame the victims for their existing needs.

Applying the need principle means that those who are in need may
justly claim help or support unless they themselves are objectively responsible for having caused their need. Therefore, when confronted with
hardships and problems of needy people, a preference for the need prin-

---

[4] Although BJW scores and preference for the equity principle substantially covary, they
assess different constructs. BJW measures and attitudes to equity contribute independently
to the prediction of emotional responses toward the victims, the prediction of cognitive
appraisals concerning the victims and their problems as well as to readiness to commit
oneself to the support of the victims (cf. Montada, Schmitt & Schneider, 1989, 1991).

TABLE 3. Correlations between BJW Measures
(GBJW, SPBJW) and Attitudes toward the
Equity Principle and the Need Principle

Study[a]		Correlations between variables[b]	
Study 2	GBJW	-Equity, general	$r = +.42$
		-Need, general	$r = -.15$
	SPBJW	-Equity, specific	$r = +.73$
		-Need, specific	$r = -.21$
Study 3	GBJW	-Equity, general	$r = +.39$
		-Need, general	$r = -.05$ n.s.
	SPBJW	-Equity, specific	$r = +.77$
		-Need, specific	$r = -.21$
Study 9	GBJW	-Equity, general	$r = +.30$
		-Need, general	$r = +.21$
Study 10[c]	GBJW	-Equity, general	$r = +.29$
		-Need, general	$r = +.10$ n.s.

[a]For a description of the studies, see Table 1.
[b]All coefficients without a suffix are significant ($p < .01$).
[c]This study was on the perception of "existential injustices" meaning disadvantages by bad luck (like being born with genetically caused handicaps); n = 128, mean age, 31.2 years, 30.5% male, 66.5% female, the rest missing data.

ciple should attenuate the usual impact of BJW and the tendency to blame victims whereas a preference for the equity principle should even strengthen the impact of BJW. Methodologically, these are moderator hypotheses. The expectation is that the regression of victim blame (BVSI) on BJW is moderated by the preference for a justice principle: It is strengthened by the preference for the equity principle and weakened by the preference for the need principle.

We have data sets which allow to test these moderator hypotheses. An example is given in Table 4 with data from Study 2. In 8 of 12 tests, a moderator effect was found, in seven out of eight cases, the effect is in the hypothesized direction. In five out of six tests, the preference for the need principle attenuates the effect of BJW on BVSI, whereas the amplifying effect of preference for the equity principle is significant in only two cases.

In one other data set (Study 9), these hypotheses were also tested but could not be confirmed. GBJW as well as attitudes toward the general need principle (NE) and the general equity principle (EY) contributed independently to the prediction of BVSI: NE negatively, EY positively. In this study, the moderating effects of EY and NE on the relationship between GBJW and emotional responses to mass unemployment were also tested. In some cases, the effects of EY, NE, and GBJW are additive, in others they are multiplicative in a meaningful way. For instance, resentment about (unjust) mass unemployment depends on NE (the more positive NE, the

TABLE 4. Four Regression Analyses of Blaming the Victims for
Self-Infliction (BVSI) to BJW, Attitudes toward the Justice Principles
Equity and Need, and the Interaction of BJW to Attitudes toward
Justice Principles[a]

	Categories of victims (BVSI)		
Predictors	Unemployed	Poor in the Third World	Turkish foreign workers
GBJW	—	.58	.24
Equity, general	.16	.98	.55
GBJW × Equity, general	.06	−.10	—
GBJW	.54	.59	.63
Need, general	—	—	—
GBJW × Need, general	−.04	−.05	−.06
SPBJW	.43	.22	—
Euity, specific	.24	.57	.23
SPBJW × Equity, specific	—	—	.07
SPBJW	.55	.68	.79
Need, specific	—	—	—
SPBJW × Need, specific	—	−.04	−.06

[a]Data are drawn from Study 2; numbers are significant b coefficients.

more resentment, beta = .51) and the interaction of GBJW and NE: GBJW
has less impact with increasingly positive NE. However, for subjects who
do not accept NE as an applicable justice principle, higher scores on GBJW
are associated with low scores on resentment. A second example: EY
amplifies the effects of GBJW on anger about jobless people (who are
choosy and do not accept every job).

3.4. Empathy, Identification, and Similarity of Fate

It was not a goal of the studies described above to investigate the
impact of empathy or identification with the victims on the correlation
between BJW and blaming victims for self-infliction. Nevertheless, some
data are informative with respect to this issue. The hypotheses are: (1)
Assuming a self-serving bias we could expect that respondents who
identified themselves with the victims, for instance, because they experienced similar victimization in the past or felt empathy with the victims
would be, on the average, less prone to state that the world is a just one.
(2) However, if they believed in a just world, we would expect that their
BJW would not lead to blaming of those victims for self-infliction with
whom they identified with or they felt sympathy for.

The first hypothesis can be tested in Studies 2 and 3 in which several
emotional responses to scenarios describing victims and their hardships

were assessed: Sympathy with the victims was one of them. Sympathy with the victims correlated negatively with GBJW, e.g., in Study 2 r = −.08, resp. r = −.35. The second hypothesis could also be tested in Study 2 by splitting the sample at the median of the sympathy scale. It turned out that the correlation between SPBJW and blaming victims for self-infliction was, in five of six comparisons, a bit higher for subjects with little sympathy for the victims than for subjects with more sympathy for the victims.[5]

The question of whether subjects identified themselves with victims or not cannot be tested directly in these studies since measures of identification were not assessed. In some studies, however, subsamples of respondents were available who were either sharing a similar fate as one of the victim categories (namely, unemployed people in Studies 2, 3, and 9) or who were bearing a risk for experiencing similar hardships and losses than the victims did (namely, people having an insecure job in Studies 2 and 3 as well as homosexual men who may bear a higher risk of AIDS infection than heterosexuals in Study 6).

It is open to question, however, exactly what effects BJW will have on BVSI in such cases. Theoretically, at least three hypotheses seem reasonable. (1) BJW motivates people to the blame victims for self-infliction regardless of whether that attribution of blame to other agents or factors (bad luck, for instance) would be self-serving. In that case, the effects of BJW would be consistent across various categories of victims including those who are perceived by the subjects as similar to themselves. In the case of a strong BJW deserved mishaps would be perceived and accepted as just. (2) Even blaming victims who are objectively similar to oneself may be self-serving because it is always possible to focus or to construe some crucial differences between oneself and others. Blaming similar others does not imply blaming oneself in order to defend ones' BJW. Instead, blaming similar others for having self-inflicted their mishaps (who, insofar, deserve them) may be associated with confidence that one's self has not deserved similar hardships which, therefore, in case of a strong BJW, are not expected to occur to oneself. In cases where they have already happened, they may be expected to be alleviated or compensated for in the future. (3) The victimization of similar others is perceived as unjust. A strong BJW would motivate claims for compensation, claims to blame those who are responsible, and/or efforts to support the victims.

As the psychology of BJW and the processing and coping with the bad fate of similar others offers various hypotheses, the empirical investigation is an exploratory one. In three studies, samples who had experi-

---

[5] In Study 9, the correlation between GBJW and BVSI was r = .33 for subjects above the median for sympathy versus r = .41 for subjects below the median.

TABLE 5. Belief in a Just World (GBJW, SPBJW) and Blaming the Victims for Self-Infliction (BVSI): Comparison of Subjects Who are Similar to Victims and Subjects Who are Dissimilar in Terms of Experienced Losses or Risks of Loss

		Correlations BJW–BVSI	
Study[a]	Categories of "victims"	Subjects similar to victims	Subjects dissimilar to victims
Study 2[b]	Jobless people	Jobless subjects (N = 24) GBJW r = −.15 n.s. SPBJW r = .08 n.s.[a]	Clergymen with tenure (N = 55) GBJW r = .33 SPBJW r = .54
Study 9	Jobless people	Jobless subjects (N = 55) GBJW r = .19 n.s.	Employed and other adults not seeking a job (N = 350) GBJW r = .54
Study 6	AIDS patients HIV positives	Homosexual and bisexual men (N = 19) GBJW r = .01 n.s.	Heterosexuals (N = 87) GBJW r = .50

[a]For further information about the studies, see Table 1 and text.
[b]For comparison: With jobless subjects, BJW is substantially correlated with BVSI to other categories of victims, like foreign workers: SPBJW–BVSI, r = .58.

enced similar losses as the victims (the unemployed in Studies 2 and 9) or who have a heightened risk for similar victimization (homosexuals with respect to AIDS infections in Study 6) were compared to samples of subjects dissimilar to the victims (Table 5).

In all three studies, the correlation between BJW and BVSI was not significant for subjects similar to the victims, whereas for dissimilar subjects, the correlations were significant and substantial. In Study 2, the available data suggests that the correlation between BJW and BVSI is only attenuated in case of similar victims (the unemployed) and it is not attenuated in cases of dissimilar victims (foreign workers living in poor conditions). In the sample of unemployed subjects, the correlation between GBJW and BVSI for foreign guest workers is r = .58.

The results suggest that BJW only disposes people to blame those victims who are dissimilar to themselves. What does this mean? The motivational function of BJW is moderated depending on the similarity of victim categories. According to a self-serving hypothesis, BJW does not dispose subjects to blame similar victims.

3.5. BJW and the Defense of Self-Interest

The covariations between BJW and BVSI measures are very consistent in our studies. (By the way, they remain substantial and significant when social desirability is controlled for. They also remain substantial and significant when control motivation is partialled out as was done in Studies 4 and

8.) The explanation imposing itself is that blaming the victims for self-infliction is serving subjects' justice motive as Lerner has suggested.

However, as already stated, from an objective standpoint self-infliction is frequently suspected without valid information and, insofar, attributions of responsibility and blame are biased and unfair. Therefore let us ask what may motivate the bias to blame victims. I will advance two hypotheses: (1) BJW is benign. It is a resource. Subjects tend to defend it against challenging observations, own experiences, and information. I will consider this hypothesis in Section 3.6. (2) BJW is a view of the world that justifies existing inequalities in the world that are favorable and advantageous for oneself; as a motivated view it justifies the maintenance of existing own advantages. I will consider this hypothesis first.

BVSI not only serves peoples justice motives but also their self-interests. Why? It is conventionally accepted that self-inflicted hardships and needs reduce the obligation of others to help, to support the needy, to share with them, or even to feel sympathy for them.

In our studies we found rich support for this hypothesis which is also well corroborated by research on helping (e.g., Bierhoff, 1980): BVSI measures are negatively correlated with the readiness to support the victims as well as with claiming support for them by powerful others: The correlation coefficient between BVSI measures and readiness to support measures range between r = −.25 and r = −.50 in Studies 2, 3, 4, and 9 for different categories of needy people.

The fact that BJW is correlated with BVSI measures raises the question of whether BJW has a facet of self-interest, too. How can this question be answered on an empirical basis? We have data indicating that BJW—at least Belief in Immanent Justice as assessed by GBJW and SPBJW—does not reflect an other centered (a victim centered) but an ego centered view of the world. More frequently, the associated motivational disposition is the defense of self-interest rather than consideration of needy others and their entitlements.

In Table 6 those covariates of BJW are listed that may be interpreted as indicators of a tendency to defend one's self-interest or to care for one's self-interest from our studies:

Justification of One's Own Advantages as Deserved relative to the "fate" of various categories of needy people was assessed in the three studies and proved to be substantially correlated with BJW.

Moral Outrage Because of Gross Social Inequalities in One's Own Favor. This is a response which does not justify own advantages but quite the contrary. The inequalities are emotionally criticized as unjust even though oneself is enjoying the good life. The correlations with BJW are negative.

Lack of Existential Guilt Feelings with respect to needy people means that subjects do not perceive the gross social inequalities in favor of

TABLE 6. Correlations of BJW Indicating the Defense of Self-Interests

Covariate	Study[c]	Measures of BJW	Correlation with BJW measure[a]
Justification of own advantages (Example item: I have deserved my better conditions in life.)	1	GBJW	r = .49
		SPBJW	r = .62
	2	GBJW	r = .42
		SPBJW	r = .67
	3	GBJW	r = .47
		SPBJW	r = .74
Lack of moral outrage about gross inequalities to one's own favor—lack is indicated by negative correlations (Example item: I feel outraged when I look at the huge differences between my own life and the misery of these needy people.)	2	GBJW	r = −.13
		SPBJW	r = −.36
	3	GBJW	r = −.16
		SPBJW	r = −.38
	9	GBJW	r = −.14
Lack of perception of own advantages as substantially interrelated to the disadvantages of others—lack is indicated by negative correlations (Example item: My better living conditions and the disadvantages of those people are interrelated to each other.)[b]	2	GBJW	r = −.22
		SPBJW	r = −.48
	3	GBJW	r = −.18
		SPBJW	r = −.41
Fear of losing own advantages (Example item: When I think about the misery of those people, I become anxious to lose my own current living conditions.)[b]	2	GBJW	r = −.06*
		SPBJW	r = −.06*
	9	GBJW	r = −.24
Contentment with own advantages (Example item: Considering this misery, I can be content with my living conditions.)[b]	2	GBJW	r = .27
		SPBJW	r = .26
	9	GBJW	r = .18
Anger at the victims (Example item: I feel angry at those people because they don't do anything to improve their situation.)	2	GBJW	r = .44
		SPBJW	r = .72
	9	GBJW	r = .29

Description		Measure	r
Lack of existential guilt—lack is indicated by negative correlations (Example item: When I see the needs of these people, I feel guilty because of my much better living conditions.)	1	GBJW	r = -.13
		SPBJW	r = -.34
	2	GBJW	r = -.06 n.s.
		SPBJW	r = -.27
	9	GBJW	r = .08
Lack of felt own responsibility to act in favor of the disadvantaged—lack is indicated by negative correlations (Example item: I feel responsible to do something to help these people.)	2	GBJW	r = .07*
		SPBJW	r = -.33
	11[d]	GBJW	r = -.20
Lack of readiness to prosocial commitments for less fortunate—lack is indicated by negative correlations (Example item: I am ready to involve myself actively in an organization supporting the needy people.) (Three categories of readiness to support in Study 9: (1) financial renunciations or donations, (2) political support, and (3) claims for support by law.)	2	GBJW	r = -.02 n.s.
		SPBJW	r = -.23
	4	GBJW	r = -.05 n.s.
	9	GBJW	(1) r = -.09 n.s.
			(2) r = -.47
			(3) r = -.10 n.s.
	11	GBJW	r = -.17 n.s.[e]
Tendency to isolate AIDS virus carriers	6	GBJW	r = .32[f]
	7	GBJW	r = .40

[a] All coefficients without suffix p < .01; *p < .05; n.s. not significant.

[b] Scores aggregated across 9 scenarios describing hardships of three categories of victims.

[c] For further information, see Table 1 or text.

[d] A study about justice and prosocial commitments, N = 323, 180 females, 143 males; age range 17–80; median 40; higher education somewhat overrepresented (Moschner, 1994).

[e] Coefficient for the control group of currently not prosocially committed subjects, N = 95.

[f] Heterosexual subjects.

themselves as difficult to justify. The correlations between SPBJW and Existential Guilt are negative as was expected, but only one of the few correlations between GBJW and Existential Guilt is significant.

Anger at the Disadvantaged because they do not care for themselves adequately can be understood as the opposite of sympathy with or pity for the needy. In a sense, this response is the emotional confirmation of blaming victims for self-infliction. Moreover, anger at the needy indicates a moral reproach meaning that they violate a social norm for self-responsibility. It is highly correlated with BJW.

Lack of Perceiving an Objective Interrelation between One's Own Advantages and the Disadvantages of the Needy was assessed in Studies 2 and 3. To give an example: mass unemployment may be considered to result from a distribution of work time and saleries advantaging one part of the population (the insiders) and disadvantaging another (the outsiders, the unemployed). BJW turned out to be negatively correlated with perceiving such relationships within societal or global distribution processes of wealth, employment, social security, etc. This may be interpreted as a tendency to defend one's own advantages by denying their interrelations with others' disadvantages.

Fear of Losing Own Advantages as a response to scenarios that describe hardships of needy others can be interpreted as an egocentric self-interested response. Contrary to this hypothesis, the correlations with BJW are either negative, though low, or not significant. It may be that this negative correlation reflects the fact that BJW offers feelings of security.

Contentment with One's Own Privileged Situation as a response to hardships of others was also taken as an indicator of egocentrism. It is moderately correlated with BJW.

Responsibility and Willingness to Support the Victims: "Felt Own Responsibility to Support the Needy" and "Readiness for Prosocial Commitment in Favor of the Needy." BJW seems to impede rather than motivate prosocial activities in favor of the needy, but most of the correlation coefficients are low.

Moral Exclusion of Victims: Quite the contrary is true for negative activities with respect to needy people. A positive correlation was found between BJW and the recommendation *to Isolate AIDS Patients.* (These studies were conducted in the late 1980s when the information was not yet sufficiently validated that casual contacts with AIDS patients and HIV positives are not very risky.) This can be interpreted as a tendency to exclude victims from one's own community of solidarity, a behavior that has also been called moral exclusion (Opotow, 1990).

Taken together, this pattern of correlations suggests that BJW is frequently associated with a tendency to defend one's own interests and not the interest of victims and needy others. Insofar as some of these indicators of self-interest imply some objective unfairness to the needy, we can say that BJW is not a pure manifestation of the justice motive.

However, the justice motive is frequently confounded with self-interest, for instance, in cases of relative deprivation where claims for justice aim at reducing relative disadvantages either for oneself or for one's group (the latter was called fraternal deprivation by Runciman, 1966). In a situation of relative deprivation, claims for justice serve self-interests, namely, the abolition of deprivation.

By examining cases where neither subjects themselves, their social group, or members of their social group are deprived, disadvantaged, or victimized should be an ideal way to study the justice motive that is not confounded with self-interest. All studies of observers' reactions to other peoples' harm, hardship, and losses seem adequate in this respect as long as the observers are not directly affected. Therefore, we looked at relatively privileged subjects and their reactions to others' relatively deprived living conditions (e.g. Studies 1, 2, 3, 4). And we could observe many obvious expressions that the privileged perceive gross inequalities to their own advantage as unjust. Many privileged people evaluate gross inequalities as unjust, they do not justify their own advantages, they feel existential guilt, they are morally outraged, and so forth (cf. Montada et al., 1986; Montada & Schneider, 1989, 1991). I am convinced that these are indicators of a justice motive that does not serve self-interests.

Our measures of BJW cannot be correlated with these indicators of a dynamic justice motive, if for no other reason than for reasons of face validity: The items used to assess BJW are statements that "the world—respectively some area of the world—is just." This implies a denial of existing injustices. (This denial is represented in high positive correlations between BJW measures and minimization of the seriousness of victims' described hardships.) The above mentioned fact that, on the average, the justice statements of the BJW measures are not accepted as true but are rather rated as more or less not true by the majority of the subjects in all of our studies may be taken as another indicator of an existing dynamic justice motive. However, this is not assessed by these measures of BJW in its pure form. My best understanding of these measures is that BJW is a hybrid of the justice motive and self-interest. And this corresponds to Melvin Lerner's concept the way I understood it.

Certainly, BJW does not purely represent self-interest. The concern for justice is evident. The highest mean correlation coefficients in Table 6 are with the variable "Justification of own advantages as deserved." Why should victims be blamed for self-infliction if not for the reason to fabricate subjective justice? Why do we have substantial correlations with the equity principle if this wasn't motivated by a concern for justice?

However, the blending of justice concerns and the concern for self-interest is not homogenous in BJW measures. I will demonstrate this by one replicated finding in our studies. As already listed in Table 6, SPBJW is correlated negatively with "Readiness to prosocial commitments." Mul-

TABLE 7. Changing Relationships between BJW and Readiness
for Prosocial Commitments for Victims When Preference for the
Equity Principle and BVSI are Partialled Out

Study	Zero-order correlation SPBJW-Prosocial commitment	b-weight of BJW when Equity and BVSI are entered in a regression equation
2	$r = -.23^a$	b = n.s.
3	$r = -.21^a$	$b = .21^a$
9	$r = -.09$ n.s. (financial support)	$b = .22^a$
	$r = -.47^a$ (political support)	b = n.s.

[a]Coefficients are significant ($p < .01$).

tiple regression analyses have repeatedly shown a suppressor effect meaning that the b-weight of SPBJW becomes positive when other predictors
are included into the regression equation, namely the preferences for the
equity principle and BVSI measures. By partialling out the preference for
the equity principle and the tendency to blame the victims makes another
facet of BJW visible: one of motivating prosocial activities (Table 7, cf. also
Montada & Schneider, 1989).

3.6. BJW as a Personal Resource in Case of Victimization

So far I have dealt with the impact of BJW on the processing of the
bad fate that other people are experiencing. Looking at various data sets
and theoretical analyses, BJW can be considered a spiritual resource
helping people to cope with observed hardships occurring to others. It
may be a benign thought to live within a just world, a thought providing
feelings of security for subjects who are not suffering hardships themselves and who do not feel guilty for norm violations for which they
deserve to be punished.[6] That BJW tends to be benign as well for observers
who are not themselves victims of losses and hardships may be deduced
from positive correlations between GBJW and SPBJW and life satisfaction
(Studies 2 and 3) or from correlations between SPBJW and the optimism
that one will not become a victim of cancer, unemployment, or an accident
(Maes & Montada, 1989).

[6] This is not contradicted by assuming that to believe the world is unjust can also serve for
coping with hardships, especially in cases of incontestable and uncorrectable injustice.
Accepting these as realities in an unjust world may counteract a justice motive and either
strengthen a self-interest motivation or the hope for an ultimate justice in heaven. Thus
avoiding illusions about the justice of the world may motivate hopes for a transcendental,
better world or it may give the freedom for an egoistic, selfish behavior.

Now changing the perspective, we can take a look at the victims. In the event that subjects are experiencing losses and hardships themselves, the effects of BJW may also be benign. The distinction between immanent and ultimate BJW made by Maes (1995, and in this volume) is helpful to generate hypotheses. (a) Immanent BJW may dispose the victims to look for their own failings which let the losses appear as deserved and a just balance. This view is not comfortable, but it may be preferred to the view that one was unjustly victimized, and it is more benign than to ruminate about the question "Why me?" (b) Ultimate BJW may dispose the subject to expect later compensation for current suffering. This is, of course, a comforting thought. If the suffering was inflicted by an agent who is responsible for preventing it, retaliation may be expected. This, probably, is a satisfying thought, too.

In case of losses perceived as undeserved, subjects' immanent BJW will be shaken. This should result in aversive emotional states like irritation (or bitterness) which can be avoided by reappraising the case. Playing down the seriousness of the losses or attributing some causal responsibility to oneself ("self-blame") or searching for some positive side-effects would be adequate coping strategies (cf. Montada, 1994).

Claudia Dalbert (1996, and in this volume) has dealt extensively with BJW as a resource in cases of victimization, disadvantage, or discrimination. She found a negative relationship between BJW and the appraisal of being undeservedly victimized (by unemployment, by having a handicapped child). By looking at indicators of resourcefulness in our studies, I can contribute a bit of information to this issue.

The following variables are suggested as *indicators of resourcefulness*: life satisfaction, self-esteem, lack of fear, and successful coping with victimization (in several specifications). In Table 8, the correlations of GBJW with these indicators assessed in three studies are listed. They are compatible with the hypothesis that BJW functions as a resource in cases of victimization. BJW helps to preserve life satisfaction and self-esteem; it helps the victims to cope successfully with their losses. Thus, we may state that BJW tends to be generally benign in cases of victimization.

4. SUMMARY AND OUTLOOK

The approach we chose was to operationalize BJW by assessment scales same as others did (cf. Rubin & Peplau, 1973; Furnham & Procter, 1992; Lipkus, 1991). Since the explanation of the phenomenon of blaming (innocent) victims was one of Lerner's intentions in developing his BJW theory, the relationships between measures of BJW and such phenomena constitute the primary validation criteria. The data presented in this chap-

TABLE 8. Belief in a Just World (BGJW) as a Resource in Cases of Victimization

Indicators of resource function	Study[a]	Kind of "victims"	Zero-order correlations between GBJW and indicator[b]
Life satisfaction	2	unemployed	r = .59
	3	unemployed	r = .10
	9	unemployed	r = .28
Fear for own future	9	unemployed	r = −.24
Lack of self-esteem (negatively formulated items, e.g., "Occasionally I feel useless.")	9	unemployed	r = −.43
Self-esteem (positively formulated items)	9	unemployed	r = .16 n.s.
Self-esteem, assertiveness	12[c]	paraplegics, quadriplegics	r = .25
Positive personality development	12[c]	paraplegics, quadriplegics	r = .26
Perceived social recognition	12[c]	paraplegics, quadriplegics	r = .12 n.s.
Positive emotions	12[c]	paraplegics, quadriplegics	r = .29

[a]For more information about the studies, see Table 1 and text.
[b]All coefficients without a suffix are significant (p < .01).
[c]Study on responsibility attributions and coping with lesions caused by accidents. N = 96 paraplegics and quadriplegics, cf. Montada, 1996.

ter demonstrate that the scales we have put together may be considered to be valid. The reader might be skeptical whether the—on the average—moderate levels of correlations really provide a convincing validation. I think they do unless one would insist on a completely a deterministic relationship. BJW theory of victim blame or victim derogation does not claim that everyone is blaming every victim for every case of victimization. I will only present some arguments from an interindividual differences perspective.

1. BJW may motivate active efforts to correct injustices instead of the subjective one of blaming the victim. The "choice" of the way to restore justice (objectively or subjectively) may depend on the perceived costs, the perceived responsibilities, the attitudes toward the victims, etc. Empirically, a hint for the hypothesis that some subjects may prefer objective corrections of injustices may be the finding that although the correlations between BJW and readiness to prosocial commitment are negative, they are not very high (cf. Table 6).

2. Even stating that a specific victimization means an injustice (implies a reproach) may subjectively be scored as a contribution to objective justice. In fact, the correlation between BJW and the evaluation of specific victimization as unjust is negative but also

not very high. For example, BJW and ratings of disadvantages as unjust are correlated $r = -.17$ for GBJW and $r = -.45$ for SPBJW in Study 2 meaning that some of the subjects who believe in a just world perceive the disadvantage of others as unjust.

3. BJW is not the single motive that may become operative in a situation: Empathy and altruism, anticipatory self-defense (in case of similarity to victims, cf. Section 3.4), the justice motive, and other motives may interfere and either muffle or trump BJW.

4. Assuming interindividual and intraindividual differences in the context of BJW we do not expect that everyone's BJW is challenged by the same cases (cf. Section 2 and 3.2).

5. BJW is not the only motivation causing people to blame and derogate victims for self-infliction and to derogate them. Others are, for example, the need for control, (some people would like to say that such mishaps would not occur to themselves), prejudices against victims, and pure self-interest (blaming victims in order to reject any responsibility for them). For this reason we should not expect that the entire variance of blaming the victim measures is explained by BJW.

For these reasons (cf. also Schmitt's chapter in this volume), I consider the data presented here to be an adequate validation. We should not expect that in every study with every sample and every case of victimization, a correlation of every BJW measure and every BVSI measure will be found. Of course, such a result would not be a falsification of BJW theory of victim blame phenomena when this theory is conceived of as a probabilistic one. In that case, validation research has three general aims: (1) to determine average probabilities (or closeness) of relationships for knowledge of the modal "impact" of the construct, (2) to discover and identify situational contexts, personality factors, and conditions which change the probabilities of relationships, and (3) to learn more about the psychological meaning of the variables under investigation, both the manifest (operationalized) and the latent ones. It is especially through pursuit of the second and third aim that scientific development of concepts and theories is driven. Empirical results which run counter to expectations are challenges for scientific development.

This is also true for research on BJW theory. When the correlation between a BJW measure and a BVSI measure was less than expected, researchers created hypotheses about why this might have happened. These hypotheses contribute to the development of a generative concept and theory when they are tested empirically. It doesn't matter whether they can be corroborated or not empirically, we still can say that we know then more than before.

In my group, as was done in others, we thought about various aspects of BJW partly outlined in Sections 2, 3.2, and 3.3 (cf. also the chapters by Maes and Mohiyeddini & Montada in this volume).

In Section 2 I distinguished several facets or specifications of BJW. We tried to represent these facets using specifying assessment scales, e.g., assessing BJW according to "areas of the world." This is also possible for other facets as the standards or principles of justice principles applied. Every useful specification of BJW should allow a better prediction of what events will be a challenge for this world view. Another line of development is the differentiation of variants as, for instance, Maes has done by distinguishing Immanent BJW from Ultimate BJW. This means a differentiation of the construct into two subconstructs with different motivational implications. The same is true for the variant Hope in a Just World (Mohiyeddini & Montada, this volume).

A third line of research was to test alternative hypotheses to explain blaming the victim comparatively with Lerner's BJW hypothesis, especially the control motivation hypothesis derived from Walster's and Shaver's work (cf. also Maes, 1994, 1996; Schmitt, in this volume) and the hypothesis of prejudice against victims (cf. Montada & Figura, 1988). By creating scales for assessing BJW as well as control motivation, and by searching for cases of victimization that provide a differential challenge to one of these motives (either to preserve subjective BJW or to preserve subjective internal control) helped to disentangle these frequently confounded motives and to identify their singularities. By doing this, the specific features of BJW will be more clearly delineated (cf. Schmitt in this volume).

BJW may have a second career in addition to the research on blaming the victim phenomena: It is the psychology of coping with self-experienced hardships, losses, and victimizations (cf. Dalbert, 1996). BJW was conceptualized by Lerner (cf. 1980) as a resource. Evidence is growing that it functions as a resource for victims in coping with injustices and adversities (cf. also Section 3.5).

Thinking about the future of BJW research, I first would like to state that the construct BJW has enriched the world of ideas in Psychology and the Social Sciences and that it has found a stable recognition which is proven by a continuous flow of publications focusing on or referring to BJW theory.

Presently, what are major tasks for future research on BJW? In my opinion, further exploration is necessary on the hypothesis that BJW is a blending of the justice motive with self-interest. By taking up Lerner's work on the justice motive as contrasting to self-interest, we have to take efforts to operationalize the justice motive (JM) in a pure form to investigate the relationships to BJW and their interplay in the prediction and explanation of phenomena. We are thinking of a construct that we have operationalized as Centrality of Justice (cf. also Schmitt in this volume). Currently, two scales are available which have already been tested in a series of studies. Overall, GBJW and Centrality of Justice (CJ) (example items are " I believe that I am more affected by an injustice that I have observed than most other people," and "I wouldn't have a close friendship with a person who doesn't have a strong sense of justice") are uncorrelated (e.g., r = .02 n.s. in Study 9). The pattern and direction of correlations of BJW and CJ tend, however, to be contrasting in justice-related criteria. Two examples are (data again from Study 9): Whereas GBJW is positively correlated with BVSI in case of unemployment (r = .36), CJ is negatively correlated (r = –.11, p < .05) and whereas GBJW is negatively correlated with outrage about mass unemployment (r = -.14), CJ correlates positively (r = .38).

The entire pattern of correlations suggest the following interpretation: CJ represents an openness or readiness to perceive existing injustices (according to own conceptions and standards), whereas GBJW represents readiness to deny existing injustices (again according to own conceptions and standards) at least in cases where the restoration of justice is costly or even outside the abilities and possibilities of an injustice. In terms of the psychology of coping: CJ seems to dispose subjects to appraise and envisage injustices, GBJW seems to dispose one to reappraisals aiming at preserving one's illusion of a just world. Therefore, in my opinion, CJ is a candidate for measuring the justice motive as Melvin Lerner has conceived it.

The relationship of both constructs to self-interest needs to be further clarified empirically. This affords the definition of self-interest in an operational manner and a validation process according to the standards of scale construction. This ultimate goal is a continuing contribution to the understanding of BJW with a growing network of related or contrasting variables as well as the further exploration of its dispositional power.

REFERENCES

Bartos, M. (1992). Gerechtigkeitsüberzeugungen, Kontrollüberzeugungen und handlungsleitende Kognitionen als Faktoren von Prosozialität. Unv. Dipl.arbeit, Univ. Trier.

Bierhoff, H.W. (1980). Hilfreiches Verhalten. Darmstadt: UBT.

Dalbert, C. (1996). Über den Umgang mit Ungerechtigkeit: Eine psychologische Analyse. Bern: Huber.

Dalbert, C., Montada, L., & Schmitt, M. (1987). Glaube an eine gerechte Welt als Motiv: Validierungskorrelate zweier Skalen. Psychologische Beiträge, 29, 596–615.

Furnham, A. & Procter, E. (1992). Sphere-specific just world beliefs and attitudes to Aids. Human Relations, 45, 265–280.

Knerr, I. (1986). Analyse von Einstellungen zu Vergewaltigungen. Unv. Dipl.arbeit, Univ. Trier.

Kordmann, P. (1991). Determinanten der Opferbeurteilung: Einflüsse von Gerechtigkeits- und Kontrollüberzeugungen auf den Attributionsprozeß. Unv. Dipl.arbeit, Univ. Trier.

Lipkus, I. (1991). The construction and preliminary validation of a global belief in a just world scale and the exploratory analysis of the multidimensional belief in a just world scale. Personality and Individual Differences, 12, 1171–1178.

Lerner, M.J. (1977). The justice motive. Some hypotheses as to its origins and forms. Journal of Personality, 45, 1–32.

Lerner, M.J. & Lerner, S.C. (eds.). 1981). The justice motive in social behavior. New York: Plenum Press.

Lerner, M.J. & Miller, D.T. (1978). Just world research and the attribution process: Looking back and looking ahead. Psychological Bulletin, 85, 1030–1051.

Maes, J. (1994). Blaming the victim—belief in control or belief in Justice? Social Justice Research, 7, 69–90.

Maes, J. (1996). Reaktionen auf die Viktimisierung anderer am Beispiel schwerer Krebserkrankungen: Der Einfluss von Gerechte-Welt- und Kontrollüberzeugungen. Unpublished doctoral thesis, Universitat Trier.

Maes, J. & Montada, L. (1989). Verantwortlichkeit für "Schicksalsschläge": Eine Pilotsstudie. Psychologische Beiträge, 31, 107–124.

Miller, D. T. (1977). Altruis and threat to a Belief in a Just World. Journal of Experimental Social Psychology, 13, 113–124.

Montada, L. (1992). Attribution of responsibility for losses and perceived injustice. In. L. Montada, S.-H. Filipp & M.J. Lerner (Eds.), Life crises and the experience of loss in adulthood (pp. 133–162). Hillsdale NJ: Lawrence Erlbaum.

Montada, L. (1994). Injustice in harm and loss. Social Justice Research, 7, 5–28.

Montada, L., Schmitt, M., & Dalbert, C. (1986). Thinking about justice and dealing with one's own privileges: A study of existential guilt. In H.W. Bierhoff, R. Cohen, & J. Greenberg (Eds.), Justice in social relations (pp. 125–143). New York: Plenum Press.

Montada, L. & Figura, E. (1988). Some psychological factors underlying the request for social isolation of Ais victims (Berichte aus der Arbeitsgruppe "Verantwortung, Gerechtigkeit, Moral" Nr. 50). Trier: Universität Trier, Fachbereich I - Psychologie.

Montada, L. & Schneider, A. (1989). Justice and emotional reactions to the disadvantaged. Social Justice Research, 3, 313–344.

Montada, L., Hermes, H., & Schmal, A. (1990). Ausgrenzung von AIDS-Opfern: Erkrankungsängste oder Vorurteile gegenüber Risikogruppen (Berichte aus der Arbeitsgruppe "Verantwortung, Gerechtigkeit, Moral" Nr. 55). Trier: Universität Trier, Fachbereich I - Psychologie.

Montada, L. & Schneider, A. (1991). Justice and prosocial commitments. In L. Montada & H.W. Bierhoff (Eds.) Altruism in social systems (pp. 58–81). Toronto: Hogrefe.

Montada, L. & Mohiyeddini, C. (1995). Arbeitslosigkeit und Gerechtigkeit (Berichte aus der Arbeitsgruppe "Verantwortung, Gerechtigkeit, Moral" Nr. 87). Trier: Universität Trier, Fachbereich I - Psychologie.

Opotow, S. (1990). Moral exclusion and injustice: An introduction. Journal of Social Issues, 46 (1), 1–20.

Rubin, Z. & Peplau, L.A. (1973). Belief in a just world and reactions to anothers lot: A study of participants in the national draft lottery. Journal of Social Issues, 29 (4), 73–93.

Runciman, W.G. (1966). Relative deprivation and social justice. London: Routledge & Kegan Paul.

Schmitt, M., Dalbert C., & Montada, L. (1985). Drei Wege zu mehr Konsistenz in der Selbstbeschreibung: Theoriepräzisierung, Korrespondenzbildung und Datenaggregierung. Zeitschrift für Differentielle und Diagnostische Psychologie, 6, 147–159.

Chapter 13

The Two Forms of Belief in a Just World

SOME THOUGHTS ON WHY AND HOW PEOPLE CARE ABOUT JUSTICE

MELVIN J. LERNER

The discussion that follows begins with the observation that the dominant view among contemporary investigators is that most adults have outgrown the childish belief they live in a just world (BJW). These BJW investigators have also assumed that one can assess the vestigial remnants of that belief as a stable meaningful individual difference variable. Beginning with the question of why this view of BJW has prevailed over the initial theory and research that portrayed BJW as a "fundamental delusion," I will raise and attempt to address several basic issues. Among these are whether, in fact, adults give up their BJW or merely employ various ways to maintain it in the face of contradicting evidence, and to what extent BJW actually influences people's lives. After reviewing relevant evidence and contemporary theories, I will offer evidence to the effect that people actually maintain and express the effects of two forms of BJW: One involves consciously held conventional rules of morality and rational social judgments, while the second is characterized by preconscious processes with primitive rules of blaming and automatic emotional

MELVIN J. LERNER • Department of Psychology, University of Waterloo, Waterloo, Ontario N2L 3G1, Canada.

Responses to Victimizations and Belief in a Just World, edited by Montada and Lerner. Plenum Press, New York, 1998.

consequences. Recognizing the two forms of BJW raises questions concerning what can and cannot be profitably studied with questionnaire research. Clearly, the highly creative and insightful contributions reported in the chapters in this volume are among the best examples of what can be learned. Finally, I will conclude with the scientific and personal implications of failing to recognize the differential properties and influences of these two forms of BJW.

1. BJW: CHILD'S FAIRY TALE OR "FUNDAMENTAL DELUSION"

1.1. Everyone Knows BJW Is a Childish Fantasy

It has been clear for several years that published research on the Belief in a Just World (BJW) has been predominantly influenced by Rubin and Peplau's (1973) portrayal of BJW as a child's fairy tale that people more or less outgrew leaving a relatively stable individual difference. That conception of BJW has prevailed over my initial characterization of BJW as a fundamental belief that people defended in various ways for the sake of their "security and sanity." I had initially proposed that, depending upon the circumstances, people would engage in more or less vigorous efforts to maintain their confidence that they lived in a world in which they could get what they deserved, eventually, if not immediately. I believed then, and still do, that the important dynamics appear in the various ways people protect that belief: Do they compensate the victim and punish the harmdoer, or derogate the victim, or try to persuade themselves they and the victim live in different worlds, or just simply deny the injustice by either not thinking about the event, or promising themselves that justice would eventually prevail in the next life, if not the present.? The available evidence clearly illustrates that each of those can occur, and provides some understanding of when people will manifest one or another of those coping reactions (Lerner, 1980; Lerner & Miller, 1978). If that is the case, however, why then is there the persistent interest in treating the BJW as a measurable dimension on which people reliably and steadfastly differ, that people defend in various ways.

The most plausible answer, however, is that the Rubin & Peplau assumptions seem to make sense. Most people can recall their own disenchantment from the child's world of fantasies and fairy tales. The reassuring myths that promised the "good" will be rewarded and the "wicked" punished eventually gave way to the overwhelming evidence that bad guys often win. Most people, if asked, would more readily agree that they live a "tough" world where what matters is power of one sort or another, rather than a "just " one where people get what they deserve. They might admit to being upset by injustices and wishing that justice would prevail, but now they realize that often does not happen. So people's own experiences seem to concur with Piaget's (1932) observation that children normally grow out of their belief in immanent justice. At the same time, most people would not claim that people never get what they deserve, and if pressed would be willing to place their beliefs somewhere on a dimension from rarely to very frequently. But, if you asked them point blank "do you believe you live in a just world where people always get what they deserve" they would probably tacitly, if not openly, question your sanity or intelligence for asking such a dumb question. But is it true that most sane, reasonably mature adults give up their belief, (or is it trust?), that they live in a world where people get what they deserve, not in every instance and not immediately, but certainly in matters that count, and eventually?

1.2."Normalizing" Injustices Means No Injustice Has Occurred

The available evidence from various sources suggests that, of course, people recognize the myriad instances in which innocent people suffer and bad guys win, but rather than giving up their belief in a just world they have developed various means of neutralizing the anger and anxiety generated by those occasions. The easiest way to do that is to remove the element of injustice from the loss or suffering by "normalizing " the event. The normalizing devices that people have available to them include cultural truisms such as the recently popular "Shit Happens!" Psychologically, what this means is that if something "bad" has happened to you through no fault of your own, you can take comfort in the recognition that such things eventually happen to everyone and thus you are not being unjustly singled out for victimization. You are only getting your fair share of what everyone experiences.

In writing this section I recalled a rather bizarre, but true, example of this normalizing process. Shortly after arriving in Canada and moving in to an upper middle class community very close to the University, my grade school age son was regularly hassled by a clump of older and bigger boys from the neighborhood. One day they taunted him by saying terrible things about his being an American by birth and, along with roughing him up a bit, to insure that he got the message they spit on him. When I approached the father of the main bully, a physician by trade, with this information, and strongly recommended several courses of action, his response was to reassure me that this was nothing at all to worry about since his own son, when he was my son's age, had gone through similar hazing from some of the very same older boys. The important point here, is that he was trying to establish that there was no "injustice" being done to my son, since being bullied and spat upon was simply part of the normal process of growing up in that rather posh neighborhood. And, since his son, an earlier "spittee" had been the main "spitter" in this case, my physician neighbor obviously had impeccable credentials as an expert on the local socialization process. Presumably, thus reassured, I could then look forward to my son, in the not too distant future, bullying and spitting on some other vulnerable smaller child. No injustices and victims here, just the normal process of growing up in that rather affluent community. And given his consensually supported perspective, that highly educated imbecile, thoughtless to the point of justifying and perpetuating cruelty, was probably right: If it is "normal," there is no injustice, no cruelty, no victims.

Similar dynamics may appear when people employ the well-documented coping mechanism of "downward comparison." Apparently victims can achieve comfort by comparing their fates with people who are worse off than they (Taylor, 1983). Again, the underlying mechanism appears to be based on the mental gymnastics that allow the person to undo the feeling they have been singled out for undeserved suffering. Instead, some other poor soul has.

1.3. Religious Beliefs Provide Ultimate Justice

Probably the most visible and openly recognized way that adults neutralize the personal impact of the injustices we all see and experience is the adoption of some form of religious beliefs. These may offer an explanation for why bad things often appear to happen to good people (Kushner, 1981) but more importantly they promise that the wicked will be punished and the virtuous rewarded, in heaven if not next week. The importance and prevalence of this belief in an omnipotent and omniscient justice restoring superhuman force watching over people's lives cannot be over-estimated. Highly sophisticated, mature, people find it acceptable, and at times, necessary to seek this form of comfort when confronted with undeserved suffering. I discovered a rather telling example of this in excerpts of an interview with Mario Cuomo, the intellectually gifted and effective political figure, that were published in the New York Times (Rosenbaum, 1995). When the interviewer asked if the death of his brother's child ,who had fallen through the ice of the canal behind the house, had led to questioning the existence of God, Cuomo responded: "What my brother, my sister-in-law, my whole family concluded then, is that either there is some explanation that eludes me at the moment, or there is none. If there is utterly no rationale then I'm not sure I can deal with the rest of my life. I'm not sure I can make myself sufficiently comfortable in this environment to go forward in it. Therefore I must accept the thesis that there is some justification. That in the long run it does work out, even if I don't understand at the moment" (p. 58).

One could not ask for a more explicit statement of why many people, intelligent mature adults, must believe in a just world. Cuomo describes the essential function that the belief in a just world provides in their coming to terms with tragic injustices in the real world.

At the same time, I would wager that if one asked him directly whether or not he believes he lives in a just world, he would probably answer, "Of course not. Only very young children believe in Santa Claus."

1.4. Adult's Irrational Self-Blame

Now, if one still has doubts that most people, adults, are strongly motivated to believe that people get what they deserve then consider the evidence that Rubin & Peplau reported in their initial BJW article (Rubin & Peplau, 1973). They recruited young men of draft eligible ages to participate in a study during the actual occasion of the draft lottery. These vulnerable young men were seated in small groups around tables with their birth dates visibly displayed on cards in front of them. They all understood that if their dates of birth were among the first third drawn they would almost certainly be drafted with the clear expectation they would then go to Vietnam. If their birth dates were within the middle third there was a possibility of being drafted, but if in the bottom third they would almost certainly not be called. Both before and immediately after learning of their fates they each completed a series of questionnaires and scales, including a measure of self-esteem. Rubin and Peplau found remarkable, but quite understandable, post lottery changes in their subjects' self-esteem. Those who had "won" the lottery tended to show increases in self-esteem, and, even more remarkable, they found that the majority (71%) of those who learned that they were virtually certain to be drafted lowered their self-regard. What could have possibly led to this self-derogation? Certainly, by conventional rules of reasoning and morality there is no way these "victims" of the lottery could have found fault with themselves for having their birth date appear early in the drawing. Their self derogation appears to be an example of the automatic preconscious influence of the attributionally primitive script: "bad things happen to bad people."

Of course, other possible explanations may come to mind, especially those focusing on mood elicited cognitions (Forgas, 1995). However, additional data reported by Rubin & Peplau, reveal that the lottery victims, while derogating themselves, did not consistently exhibit pessimistic or negative mood congruent reactions. Not everything or everyone was viewed negatively. For example, the victims tended to view the beneficiaries of the lottery more positively than those who were expected to be drafted.

Other experiments have revealed similar irrational self blaming reactions. Probably the most familiar of these are associated with the "transgression compliance" effects (see, e.g. Freedman, Wallington, & Bless, 1967). Apparently, having subjects believe they have accidentally harmed someone will measurably increase their willingness to comply with subsequent requests to help a third party. For example, in several experiments, the subjects' harmdoing followed from the innocent act of pulling out a chair in response to the experimenters instructions to take a seat while awaiting their further participation. Unknown to the subject, it had been arranged for the innocent act of moving the chair to cause unseen stacks of data cards to spill on to the floor. The experimenter then commented that the accidental spilling of the cards would cause the cards owner, a graduate student, considerable time and effort to reassemble and thus delay his thesis research. Meindl & Lerner (1984) confirmed that such an accident makes subjects feel rather sad and guilty.

But, why would these inadvertent causal agents experience self blame and guilt ? It was clearly an unforeseeable accident, and they did not intend to do harm, they were just trying to sit in the only available chair, as instructed by the experimenter. McGraw (1987) reported considerable evidence confirming that such accidental harm doing often leads to as much, if not more, guilt than foreseeable or intentionally caused harm.

2. HOW EXPLAIN "IRRATIONAL SELF-BLAME?"

2.1. Anomalous Overriding of Rational Self-Interest

How can one explain such findings? This is particularly problematic because the conventional rules of morality absolve anyone of culpability when the consequences of their acts were unforeseeable by any reasonable person, and there was no evidence of recklessness or lack of consideration, and certainly no dishonorable intentions (Shaver, 1985). If societal rules of morality judge the inadvertent agent of accidental harm to be entirely innocent, what could possibly elicit the guilt and lowered self-esteem? Obviously, if those painful reactions do not originate from any external source, they must be self-inflicted. But that would seem to contradict the assumption, held by most psychologists, that people are pre-eminently motivated to avoid pain and gain pleasure. In support of that assumption, there is considerable evidence that whenever possible people attempt to portray themselves and their efforts in the best possible light. e.g, the ubiquitous self-serving bias in attributions (Miller & Ross, 1975).

2.2. Control Motive

If people are motivated to avoid pain, then why is it so common for people to blame and condemn themselves when societal rules clearly say they have done no wrong? One attempt to find pain avoidance, or self interest, in these self blaming reactions refers to a control based motive (Bulman & Wortman, 1977). Presumably, to avoid the loss of control, which they associate with long term benefits, people are willing to accept the short term pain of unwarranted self blame. There is no consistent body of empirical support for this conjecture, and the example of the self-derogation exhibited by the victims of an explicitly random draft lottery studied by Rubin & Peplau (1973) seems to clearly contradict any underlying motivation to preserve a sense of control: Control over what, the outcome of future lotteries?

2.3. Correspondence Bias

The explanation offered here is that the perception of bad outcomes automatically elicits preconsciously held scripts. In peoples minds, bad outcomes automatically imply someone has done something bad. This is similar in some respects to the "Correspondence error" that appears to be common to social cognitions, generally. Apparently, because of the cognitive set with which they enter most situations, people automatically assume that the outcomes associated with a person's acts reveal his/her motivation. And, it is only if and when observers engage in subsequent efforts to further analyze the possible influences of external circumstances that they may arrive at more sophisticated causal attributions (Gilbert & Malone, 1995). In other words, in the absence of special efforts people will automatically blame someone for bad outcomes. What is not sufficiently understood is whom they will blame. It is as if people walk around with preconscious cognitively primitive scripts that have two readings, or there are two very similar scripts: "bad outcomes happen to bad people," and "bad outcomes are caused by bad people." Of course, those are not mutually exclusive cognitions and conceivably the predominant effect in any given encounter might depend upon contextual factors, such as the focus of attention, and salience.

2.4. Persistence of Developmentally Earlier Blaming Process

It is important to note, however, that although derogating one's self or blaming others may elicit radically different emotional experiences, e.g., guilt versus anger, the attributional process in both cases is remarkably similar in form. Both involve directly generalizing from the evaluation of

the outcome, "bad," to the evaluative judgment of the actor's—perpetrator's or victim's—personal characteristics, "bad." What is obviously missing in these evaluative judgments are the mediating, and thus moderating,
influences of sophisticated causal analysis and conventional criteria for
assigning blameworthiness. In the cognitively primitive blaming process
the questions of whether the consequences of the person's actions were
foreseeable or controllable, and whether the actor had honorable or dishonorable intentions are simply irrelevant. It is as if, as Piaget (1932) and
others demonstrated, in the normal developmental process children learn
the more sophisticated conventionally appropriate rules for arriving at
moral judgments. But, contrary to Piaget's observations, in the course of
becoming adults, children do not give up or lose their earlier more primitive outcome based blaming process. Instead, the evidence clearly indicates that those early counter-normative scripts become part of the
preconscious processes that continue to influence their social judgments
and emotional reactions. This occurs even as they consciously know better
than to react so irrationally.

3. TWO FORMS OF THE JUSTICE MOTIVE AND BELIEF IN A JUST WORLD

3.1. Rational, Normatively Conventional

In brief, it seems that what might be referred to as the "belief in a just
world" appears in peoples lives in at least two rather different ways. In
terms of conscious thought processes and public utterances most adults do
not believe that everyone gets what he or she deserves. When further
probed they would probably state that they would prefer if that were more
typical of their society, and that they are easily upset when they become
aware of gross violations of rules of fairness and decency. They would
maintain, however, that their emotional reactions follow from their rational
analysis of the causes and responsibilities for someone's apparent suffering.
If their analysis of the evidence indicates that the victim is primarily
responsible and blameworthy for his or her own suffering than obviously
no injustice has occurred. If a perpetrator or external circumstances are
primarily responsible then they will feel sympathy for the innocent victim.
Weiner and his students have generated numerous experimental demon-
strations of people thoughtfully employing this normative rational process
in arriving at the attribution of responsibility which then elicits their emotional reaction of sympathy or anger toward a victim (see, e.g. Weiner, 1993).
So people, in general, may consciously admit to serious doubts about the
extent to which justice prevails in their society, but they have no reluctance

to admit that they care about justice and they follow sensible, rational, rules of deserving in assessing when an injustice has or has not occurred.

3.2. Experiential Counternormative Scripts

However, when actually confronted with clear, and especially, dramatically vivid instances of victim's suffering, people often exhibit one or a combination of an array of reactions that appear to have in common that they do not at all follow the rules of rational assignment of blame, and they eliminate, or at least reduce, the element of injustice-undeserved suffering. This might include blaming an objectively innocent victim, even themselves, or persuading themselves that the victim will be compensated and the perpetrator punished at a later time, or simply refusing to recognize or think about the event. In addition people will not be aware of what is driving their reactions. They will not be able to consciously describe the irrational counter-normative processes, reasons, underlying their reactions (Nisbett & Wilson, 1977).

Although the actual reasons are not that well understood, they appear to have two sources. One is the automatic application of very simple causal schemas, or scripts that initially appeared very early in their lives and persist throughout adulthood—bad outcomes are caused by bad people. The other is emotion driven, possibly a combination of anxiety and anger. People attempt to reduce their injustice induced anxiety by re-establishing justice, often in irrational ways such as blaming an innocent victim, or embracing a justice promising ideology. When these reactions appear, they are naturally framed in ways that do not directly violate conventional rules of logic or morality, e.g. the person who derogates a victim will generate a culturally plausible basis for that condemnation; however, when examined under controlled circumstances it is possible to demonstrate that the condemnation, or avoidance of a victim was driven by the injustice based threat, and the normatively plausible reasons were generated after the fact (Lerner, 1980; Lerner & Miller, 1978) as justifications. In some circumstances, no rational explanation can be offered and the person refers to inherently despicable characteristics, or simply faith in an omnipotent force that promises to restore justice. For the most part, then, the underlying dynamics that insure that people get what they deserve reflect irrational, counter-normative processes that take place, preconsciously, out of the person's awareness.

3.3. Experimental Example of Two Forms of Reactions to Victims

An early experiment by Simons and Piliavin (1972) illustrates the operation of both the conscious, conventionally rational processes and the influence of the preconscious "irrational" processes on observer's reaction to the suffering of an objectively innocent victim. Replicating the experimental context of prior experiments that found victim derogation (see, e.g. Lerner, 1980), these investigators had undergraduate students watch an 8 minute video tape of another student who received painful electric shocks when she made unavoidable errors in a paired-associate learning task. In one set of experimental conditions, the observers were led to believe they were watching an actual ongoing event over closed circuit television and their purpose for watching was to look for cues of emotional arousal as part of their participation in an experiment. After watching the tape these observers were led to believe there would be a second session of the victim being shocked, and in the interim they were to complete some ratings, among which were a series of bipolar adjectives that described the kind of impression the victim gave of herself (e.g. kind–cruel, intelligent–unintelligent, likable–dislikable, etc.). Other observers were told that they were watching a video tape of one session of a learning task that had occurred the previous day. As expected the observers who were in the midst of observing an innocent student suffer two sessions of electric shocks ascribed reliably more negative characteristics to the victimized young woman than did those who believed there had been only one session of suffering and it was over. As in the earlier research, the more undeserved suffering the more negative the evaluations of her character.

Although essentially replications of previous findings, these ratings of the victim's characteristics take on much more significance when compared with those given by similar observers in the other experimental conditions. In one set of additional conditions the observers were reminded of the societal norms concerning how people are supposed to react to victims. They were told twice before making their ratings of the victim that: "This experiment studies the way people react to other people who, through no fault of their own, fall victim to some uncontrollable outside force or action. Victims of a hurricane or earthquake are examples, another would be a person attacked by a stranger on a city street" (Simons, 1968). After being instructed to remember how people are supposed to respond to truly innocent victims, the observers showed no evidence of derogating the victim. Also, in additional conditions, when the observers were instructed that the victim was merely an actor portraying a suffering victim, they did not derogate the portrayed victim and more importantly they predicted that observers who thought her suffering was real would not disparage or condemn her (see also, Lerner, 1987).

These findings illustrate, rather clearly, that observing the suffering of an innocent victim can elicit derogating reactions. However, disparaging innocent victims does not fit the normative expectations concerning how people are supposed to react. Also, people are not at all aware that they and others would be so irrational as to react negatively to an innocent victim. Their consciously held beliefs and expectations are that people will react with compassion to innocent victims, and only reject those who may have brought about their own misery.

Thus, there appears to be two levels at which people react to such events, with two different processes and consequences. The conscious level of discourse that reflects societal rules concerning rational processing of information and conventional morality, and a pre-conscious level where relatively simple scripts and emotion driven associations prevail. Issues of justice and morality appear at both levels however the specific rules and application differ radically. When given the time, and opportunity, under relatively dispassionate circumstances, people will exhibit relatively rational assessments of the causal contingencies and arrive at normatively appropriate moral judgments (Nisbett & Wilson, 1977). However, when fully engaged, and especially when motivationally or affectively aroused, people's reactions will reflect more automatic and intuitive judgments of culpability and blameworthiness, often by mere association: "Bad outcomes are caused by bad people, and bad things happen to bad people." Whatever the contributing psychological processes—cognitive balance, affective generalization of some form, hard wired emotion specific attributions—they resemble and have the effect of maintaining the belief in a just world, where people get what they deserve, or rather, deserve what they get.

The kind of quandary Mario Cuomo and many others have faced, described earlier, begins with their conscious resistance to accepting the most available justifications for why the child should have died and the family suffer from his death. They refuse to believe, and with good reasons, what their initial intuitive feelings tell them: that some member of their family or the child had done something terribly wrong. Instead, if they cannot find someone to blame people often actively seek comfort by going beyond the immediate context. Religious faith promises that ultimately no injustice has occurred. Shweder & Miller (1985) discovered that in the Brahmin village they studied people naturally maintain the moral order in their lives by assuming that such tragic events were caused by earlier transgressions, possibly in a previous life. In this manner, according to Shweder & Mille, the villagers never have any doubt that they live in a just world where people get what they deserve.

3.4. Contemporary Theoretical Models of Two Underlying Processes

Contemporary psychologists from various sub-disciplines, social, cognitive, clinical, personality theory, developmental, have generated considerable data and attempted to formalize the distinction between two modes or channels of processing information (see e.g. Chaiken & Trope, Forthcoming), very similar to what we discovered in our efforts to understand how the belief in a just world appears in people's lives. For example, Shweder & Haidt (1993) point out that theories of "cognitive intuitionism" distinguish between two kinds of moral judgments: those based upon moral intuitions and those arrived at by moral reasoning. The intuitive responses are automatically elicited by rapid appraisals based upon pattern matching of available cues. Although the person often experiences the consequences of that appraisal process as emotions of anger, shame, or guilt, and judgments of what is right or good, the process itself occurs preconsciously and is "introspectively opaque." That is, people are not aware of and cannot consciously retrieve the psychological bases for those reactions: they are intuitively valid. By contrast, Shweder & Haidt propose that moral reasoning involves relatively slow ex post facto manipulation of conscious thoughts according to rules of propositional and abstract reasoning.

Epstein and his colleagues (see e.g. Epstein, Lipson, Holstein, & Hub, 1992) make a very similar distinction between two conceptual systems, "experiential" and "rational," that people employ in processing all the information they receive. According to Epstein the experiential system preconsciously encodes information in concrete images and metaphors, and makes associationistic connections, while the conscious "rational system" is more process oriented and encodes reality in abstract symbols while making cause and effect connections. Moreover events are experienced passively in the experiential system and although people may be seized by their subsequent emotions, what they experience is accepted as self-evidently valid. As with the moral intuitions described by Shweder & Haidt all of this occurs preconsciously. Whereas, in the "rational system," as described by Epstein, events are experienced consciously with people in control of their thoughts and reactions require justification via logic and evidence. This is clearly directly comparable to Shweder & Haidt's description of "moral reasoning."

Clearly, we have good reason to believe there are at least two radically different ways people respond to important events happening to themselves or others. One is the preconscious, intuitive, often based upon emotion driven associations. The other involves conscious, thoughtful rational processing of the available information. The theories and related data suggest that people's subsequent reactions will very greatly depending upon which of these systems predominately influence the person's subsequent reaction. The extant theories also suggest some theoretical guidelines concerning when, under what circumstances either of these or some blending of the two are most likely to occur. For example, if people are emotionally removed from the event, and are given time and the incentive to engage in thoughtful reasoning, it is most likely that they will consciously reproduce the normatively appropriate responses. On the other hand, in the absence of the time and incentive, and especially if they are emotionally aroused, and feel compelled to respond immediately one is more likely to find signs of the counter normative experiential system influencing their reactions.

4. METHODOLOGICAL AND THEORETICAL IMPLICATIONS

4.1. Another Experimental Example: People Care Much More about Justice Than They Think

It is extremely important, crucial, for investigators to recognize that people are not aware of how the preconscious system influences their own or other peoples behavior. As a consequence peoples' expectations and social predictions will typically mimic the conscious normative system; although their reactions, in ongoing encounters, with little opportunity to pause and reflect upon their course of action. will often be radically different. For example, Dale Miller (1995, 1997) found that young men when given the opportunity were much more motivated by the prospect of earning a fair wage and 33% additional pay be used to reduce the suffering of a poverty stricken family, than the chance to keep the additional pay for themselves. At the same time similar young men, when asked how they and their friends would react to various pay incentives predicted directly self-interested preferences. They predicted that if any of their pay were given to the family that would function as a deterrent and reduce the attractiveness of the job (Miller, 1975, 1977). In this case, the normatively appropriate response in the context of working for wages was to act in a rationally self-interested manner, not volunteer 33% of one's pay to strangers, no matter how bad off they were. In fact, though, the opportunity to get a decent wage and help those miserable victims proved to be intuitively compelling. It just felt right, so they did it. The important point is that if Miller had only provided his subjects with vignettes or a survey questionnaire their reactions would have led him to conclude that people, at least when it comes to earning wages, are primarily self-interested, with virtually no concern for the welfare of victims. Studying their behavior in vivo led to a radically different conclusion: people care much more about justice for themselves and victims than maximizing their own pay.

4.2. Justice as Rational Self-Interest

Before getting any further into the question of how particular research methods influence the kinds of data that are generated, let us take a stab at locating the belief in a just world in a more fully elaborated theoretical context. To begin with, it appears that people are motivated, want, to see justice prevail. But, why is that? The most commonly accepted answers, refer to a form of enlightened, or, rational self-interest. People have reasoned that it is to their own best interests, in the long run, to live in a predictable, and controllable, just world. And, they have learned to anticipate painful consequences if they are caught violating rules of fairness, including punishing themselves for failing to live up to an internalized ideal. In this manner, social psychologists portray justice as having a more or less consciously manipulated instrumental role in interpersonal relations. Supposedly, people follow rules of justice if and when that promises them less pain and more pleasure than ignoring those rules (Walster, Walster, & Berscheid, 1978). Similarly, it has been proposed that in all situations people select those rules of fairness that promise to optimize their outcomes as defined by other values and goals (see Messick & Cook, 1983; Walster et al., 1978). It is just that simple: justice appears in peoples' lives as the rational use of social rules to optimize one's desired outcomes. The eminent philosopher–political theorist Russell Hardin (1996) does not hesitate to assert that in all encounters in the real world mutual self-interest, or benefit, "trumps" justice. Every time!

That approach raises as many questions as it answers. If Hardin and the others cited above are correct, then why do people keep messing around with notions of justice? Why is justice such an omnipresent and sanctified part of peoples lives at all levels of personal and social organization? In terms of cultural values, it is the primary, virtually sacred value, as evidenced by the fact that justice can and often does legitimize the intentional sacrifice of all other desired resources including life, liberty, and the pursuit of happiness. Also, justice, in the form of specific rules of entitlement (obligations and privileges), defines the role relationships in all social institutions. In addition, people remain exquisitely sensitive and continually responsive to issues of deserving and justice as they go about acquiring and distributing desired resources. Finally, it is all too common for individuals to sacrifice themselves in the name of justice. Is all of this an accident of our Hellenic, Judeo-Christian, cultural history? The cross-cultural evidence strongly indicates that is not the case (see, e.g. Shweder & Miller, 1985).

4.3. Justice as the Inevitable Consequence of the Human Endowment and a Stable Environment

That only leaves a few alternatives. One is that "justice" must be one hell of a good idea for it to capture and dominate so much of people's lives. But if that is the case why do very smart rational people like Hardin (1996) find it so inadequate on logical grounds and so easily "trumped" by more mundane considerations?

The other obvious candidate is that people can't help themselves. People develop a commitment to justice quite naturally, inevitably, out of the interaction between their genetically based human potential and a relatively stable physical and social environment (Lerner, 1987). One possible element in this process is the natural tendency for the developing human organism to create a stable conception of their environment. Their cognitive-perceptual system populates their world with "objects" and ways of moving about i.e. rules for how to get from here to there. Along with naturally creating a stable environment, people are also appetitive: Things taste, feel, look, good, bad, better or worse. As a consequence, through their memory and cognitive constructions they imbue the stable objects in their environment with evaluative properties, desirable-undesirable, better or worse.

In the course of acting on the environment, people elect one or another path-how to get from here to there- to acquire a particular desired object-outcome. If that path has been imbued with stable qualities, ie. the person is subjectively certain of how to move in the desired direction, and if those actions do not succeed in producing the outcome, the person will experience an "injustice." Having done all that is necessary to acquire x, the person feels entitled to x. "It should have happened." The subsequent failure should not have occurred. The essential element is the subjective certainty that the person has met all the requirements, correctly followed the appropriate path. If the subjective probability is less than certain, then the subsequent failure may be frustrating or disappointing, but will not be experienced as an injustice.

It is inevitable that people have desires and that they learn ways to fulfill those desires. The sense of being entitled to them, is a product of subjective certainty that a particular path will be successful: "It should have happened, I did everything necessary to get it." That sense of a violated entitlement will be experienced as an "injustice" if another person or agency is blamed for not receiving what one deserves. But, what leads to such subjective certainty? I am not certain, but probably generalizing from past successful experiences, absolute and convincing assurances from reputable sources, etc. Could it be that simple? I think so. Both simple and inevitable.

And, of course, it is also much more complicated, because people imbue objects in their world with value—relatively good and bad people, groups, ways of behaving, personal attributes. And in their preconscious they are linked by association—good people, good acts, desirable attributes, with good outcomes. Although these associative links have been described by Heider (1958) and gestalt theorists (see, e.g. Asch 1952), the emotional and motivational aspects are still relatively unknown. For example, if one begins with Heider (1958) how does one get from the cognitive tendency or aesthetic and attitudinal preference to associate good outcomes with good people and good acts i.e. cognitive balance, to the finding that the experience of an injustice is the most reliable determinant of the emotion of anger. In other words, how would Heider explain the experience of imbalance leading to anger? One group of theorists find the conceptual link in some form of inherited evolutionary functional process: The emotion of anger is functional in promoting the re-establishing of justice because it impels the person to act on the environment and in particular against humans (Smith & Ellsworth, 1985).

But how does one derive the emotional and motivational experience of an injustice—which can also produce sadness as well as anger (Keltner, Ellsworth, & Edwards, 1993) from the preference for "balanced cognitions"? The answer may be found in people's need for, or is it investment in, the fundamental structure of their world. It is the threat to that structure, the way people organize all their experiences, that generates the person's emotions. When very bad things happen to good people, or follow from good, appropriate acts, it is not simply perceived as a bit of inconsistency with ones expectations, or imbalance with one's preferred ordering of events. If the person's cognitions definitely implied that bad outcomes "should not" have occurred, then the person's "world" will be shaken, threatened to a greater or lesser extent. The injustice based emotions will then follow.

4.4. How Does This Theory of Justice Differ from Rational Self-Interest?

Do these theoretical conjectures locate justice within the domain of self-interested motivations? Possibly "yes," depending upon what is meant by the term self-interest in this context. For example, the answer is, "not at all," if by self-interest one means the search for economic, material, and symbolic resources. Does it mean that the justice related reactions including the emotions have affective consequences so that the person is emotionally upset when confronted with an injustice and "feels better" in some way if justice is restored. In that case, the answer is, "yes." But at the same time it is crucial to recognize that what elicits the "upset" or what makes the person feel better are the perceptions of justice and injustice. Those perceptions are not driven or responsive to other motivational agenda—the desire for more pleasurable outcomes, material or symbolic. To be sure, how the person subsequently reacts to the experience of the injustice may well be influenced by various agenda, including individual profit, or mutual benefit and wanting to do that which is normatively acceptable. It is a safer bet, however, that the subsequent response will be tailored not to directly violate the rules of entitlement and thus elicit the experience of another injustice.

4.5. Where Do Stable Individual Differences Fit in This Theory?

What about stable individual differences in the way people react to injustices, in particular, their belief in a just world? It would be no surprise to find that individuals, no less than cultures, generate belief systems that neutralize the threats associated with perceiving undeserved suffering, and once having adopted those beliefs they try to defend them. Since Rubin and Peplau's (1973) initial work, there has been good reason to believe that people who agree with BJW type statements, indicating that people generally get what they deserve, are somewhat more likely to reject victims—not all victims, not all the time—but somewhat more often than those who are in less public agreement with the BJW items. And people who agree with those items are somewhat more optimistic about their ability to cope with threatening events: bad things will not happen to them. And there are many other findings that make sense theoretically (see other chapters in this volume). But it must be remembered that the BJW statements are essentially counter-normative in the sense that strong agreement would indicate an unrealistic, naïve, child like faith that people always deserve what they get. So one can expect to find a relatively low general level of public agreement with these items, and the empirical associations will by and large be based upon relative degrees of disagreement and marginal acceptance (Miller & Ratner, 1996).

The belief in ultimate justice, as one finds in religious systems, will probably turn out to be another stable and quite meaningful variable (aee e.g., Maes, this volume). As discussed in Lerner (1980), there is good reason to believe that faith in a benevolent justice maintaining force can offer considerable comfort to people, and preclude their engaging in other forms of justice maintaining reactions. For example, there is evidence that religious faith can eliminate the need for people to blame victims for their suffering (Sorrentino & Hardy, 1974) and can enable victims to tolerate their own terrible fates (Lerner, 1980).

But it is important to recognize that what is being assessed by these reactions to questionnaire items, may have no simple direct relation to the preconscious processes that generate the justice judgments and their associated emotions—what might be termed the "justice motive." In essence, the responses to questionnaire items reveal the beliefs people have adopted for various reasons including the need to cope with injustice experiences. However, those beliefs tell us little, if anything, about the processes involved in generating those experiences. It is obvious that people simply cannot consciously retrieve, nor talk about those processes.

But careful systematic observations can enable us to test theoretically important hypotheses about the structure and dynamics of the justice motive. Early experiments, for example, revealed quite clearly that it was information about the extent of the victim's undeserved suffering that was driving the observer's evaluation of the victim, rather than some personal failing that the victim was exhibiting (see e.g. Lerner, 1980; Lincoln & Levinger, 1972; Simons & Piliavin, 1972). On the other hand, if one had asked the observers to give the reasons for their reactions, or make predictions as to whether they would derogate an innocent victim, we would have found exactly what Weiner (1993), and his students have repeatedly found: no decent, sane, person would reject an innocent victim. To admit to doing so would be completely contrary to our societal norms. Every good citizen would insist that they would only react negatively toward those victims who bought about their own suffering through their misdeeds. That is part of our conventional morality. Unfortunately, in reality people do often blame and condemn innocent victims for many reasons, including the threats to their beliefs in a just word posed by the suffering of those innocent victims.

4.6. What about the Use of Questionnaire Research Methods in Studying the Two Forms of BJW?

Can questionnaire studies ever reveal the operation of the "experiential" preconscious processes? Of course, they can. And many of the chapters in this volume reveal highly creative, and worthwhile examples. But the simple rule is that such studies will not succeed as long as the nature of the questions, or the experimental context lead the respondent to generate a normatively appropriate response. Such norm eliciting contextual factors can be as subtle as requiring the respondent to engage in a thoughtful choice between alternatives with differing pay-offs, or the anticipation of having to explain the bases of one's choices to an important audience. In both cases people feel compelled to generate a normatively defensible "rational choice," rather than express their automatic, rather thoughtless, though meaningful preferences.

This is illustrated nicely by Bazerman, White and Lowenstein (1995), who described the findings of a series of experiments which assessed people's preferences for fair outcomes in comparison with unfair but greater outcomes. One such example involved the preferences for a situation in which they and another person would each receive 400 dollars, versus one where they would receive 500 while the other would have 700 dollars. In a variety of such studies involving differing contexts, the respondents preferred the fair but lesser outcomes (400/400) to the larger unfair ones (500/700), but only if they made separate desirability ratings. However, when simultaneously presented with both sets of distributions and asked to choose between the two they overwhelmingly chose the one that optimized their outcomes, e.g. receiving 500 while the other received 700 dollars. Bazerman et al., reasoned that by requiring the subjects to make the explicitly comparative choice between the two distributions they had made salient the two issues of fairness and maximizing profit. As a consequence the respondents felt constrained to make the self-optimizing choice because It was the normatively appropriate, rational thing to do. But, without that imposed demand to be rationally self-interested they actually preferred having the lesser but fair outcomes.

Another example of the normative demands overriding the experiential reaction was described in a recent article by Jennifer Lerner, Goldberg & Tetlock (forthcoming). They found that subjects, after being angered by witnessing a terrible injustice, were inclined to blame and punish someone in the next situation who had negligently caused harm to others. The greater their anger at the initial injustice the more punitive their subsequent response. That clearly "irrational" reaction was eliminated however, if subjects were informed, in advance, that a post-doctoral student would subsequently interview them concerning their reactions. In that case the subjects' blaming reactions were closely linked to their ratings of the harmdoers responsibility and negligence, rather than their own anger. Apparently, the anticipated interview led the observers to find rational reasons for their judgments rather than allowing their lingering anger to directly express itself in "irrationally" blaming and punishing the next harmdoer they happened to confront.

The general rule is quite clear: Once aware of the normatively appropriate responses, people will tend to modify or override whatever other impulses or preferences they experience to respond in ways that meet the normative rules. One can probably imagine some exceptions, especially when the non-rational response is very familiar and not flagrantly bizarre or contemptible according to conventional standards. Noteworthy examples of this would be the "regret" and "counterfactual" findings (see Kahneman and Miller, 1986) as well as Rozin's demonstration of the intrusions feelings of disgust (Rozin, Markwith, & McCauley, 1994). In the main, though, when investigators give their emotionally unaroused respondents the time and incentive to generate a thoughtful response, the chances increase that those respondents will express their understandings of the conventionally appropriate ways to think, feel, and act (Nisbett & Wilson, 1977).

4.7. Once Again: How Important Is BJW the Justice Motive in Peoples' Lives?

But if the preconscious experiential processes are so easily overridden by more sensible considerations how important are they in people's lives? How much influence does the preconscious, intuitive, "justice motive" have on what people do? Without even attempting complete answers to those questions, it might be useful to consider two important examples in contemporary society. In these cases, the emotional consequences of the preconscious processes are too compelling and persistent to be easily "normalized" by conscious rational processes.

Professional consultants (Levenson, 1994; Smith, 1994), have identified an unexpected undesirable byproduct of the corporate reorganizations that are a common part of contemporary corporate policies. Corporate management in response to competitive market forces often dismiss a significant part of their labor force and institute more efficient procedures. Typically, the decisions of whether and how to go about the reorganization process are arrived at after careful, thoughtful deliberations, and the dismissal of any employees is understood to be necessary for the welfare of the corporate stake holders, including the remaining employees. This entire process is not only considered normatively legitimate it is viewed as morally justified in a rational utilitarian sense. What has been discovered, however, is that subsequent to the dismissal of the otherwise adequate employees, a significant portion of the management develops serious feelings of guilt and remorse. It is important for our purposes to note that the guilt reactions were not anticipated during the decision process. That is quite understandable since according to societal norms management would be doing no wrong. If that is the case, then why the subsequent guilt? The answer, of course, is that it was only after the reorganization that they began to learn of the dismissed, and now unemployed, workers deprivation and suffering. The awareness of that suffering automatically elicited the perception of themselves as the harmdoers. Whatever justification they could consciously marshall, in their preconscious, they were the "cause" and were to blame for that undeserved suffering. As an anthropologist friend observed: "In the preconscious the lesser of two evils is still evil."

This same pattern of rational decision making eventuating in unanticipated guilt feelings has been observed among daughters who have placed their parents in nursing homes (Brody, 1985; Mullen, 1992).

Although the daughters typically have provided the necessary care and met their parents needs for several years, they still feel as if they have failed their parents. The unanticipated guilt appears even though everyone, including the professional advisors, had concurred that the placement would be best for all concerned, including the deteriorating parents. In these cases, the rational, normatively desirable considerations are not sufficient to override the irrational, but persistent, guilt feelings that are elicited by the awareness that the parents are "abandoned" to the care of strangers in a nursing home, and they are miserable.

5. SUMMARY

In essence, I began this chapter by highlighting the Rubin & Peplau (1973) assumption that in the normal course of development most people outgrow the belief they live in a world where people get what they deserve. What remains in adulthood is a relatively stable individual difference reflecting the extent to which they maintain any such trust in the justness of their world. I contrasted their view with my notion that the belief in a just world was a "fundamental delusion"—fundamental in the sense that it is essential for most people's sense of security and sanity, and "delusional" to the extent that it was a set of factually false beliefs that were motivationally defended. The early research my colleagues, students, and I conducted was designed to reveal how witnessing undeserved suffering would motivate observers to find or invent evidence that would eliminate the injustice of what they had seen. Additional studies revealed the conditions under which people would employ alternative ways of defending their belief in a just world. And yet other research revealed how the processes underlying that essential belief may lead to personally painful self-condemning reactions.

All the evidence seemed to indicate that children do not normally outgrow the justice motive or belief in a just world, but rather they learn the conventionally accepted rules for deciding what is just and how to rationally arrive at sensible judgments of deserving. As a result most adults live with two systems of morality. One is the underlying, vestigial, pre-conscious "justice motive" that operates according to relatively simple, cognitively primitive, rules of association and organization. These preconscious processes are "introspectively opaque," and often associated with emotional reactions of anger, shame, guilt, etc. The second moral system, superimposed on the earlier one, consists of the consciously available conventional, rational rules of moral judgments and reasoning. Both systems can and do involve issues of deserving and justice; however the intuitive preconscious processes follow radically different, counter normative rules. Fortunately we have some notions about the conditions under which one or the other of these is most likely to influence the person's reactions on a particular occasion. But much remains to be known, especially with regard to how these two systems interact over time.

One thing we know for certain. It is crucial that investigators recognize the differences between these two systems, the preconscious "experiential" and conscious "rational" and how they differentially influence people's reactions. The failure to do that in past research, has led to seriously mistaken conclusions about how much and in what ways people care about justice. And those errors not only perpetuate inadequate theories of human motivation, they also invite personal and collective decisions with tragic consequences.

REFERENCES

Asch, S.E. (1952). Social psychology. New York: Prentice Hall.

Bazerman, M.H., White, S.B., & Lowenstein, G.F. (1995). Perceptions of fairness in interpersonal and individual choice situations. Current Directions in Psychological Science, 4, 39–42.

Brody, E. (1985). Parent care as normative family stress. The Gerontologist, 25, 19–29

Bulman, R.J., & Wortman, C.B. (1977). Attributions of blame and coping in the real world: Severe accident victim's reactions to their lots. Journal of Personality and Social Psychology, 35, 351–363.

Chaiken, S. & Trope, Y. (Eds) (forthcoming). Dual process theories in social psychology. New York: Guillford

Epstein, S., Lipson, A., Hostein, C., & Hub, E.(1992). Irrational reactions to negative outcomes: Evidence for two conceptual systems. Journal of Personality and Social Psychology, 62, 328–339.

Forgas, J.P. (1995). Mood and judgment: The affect intrusion model (AIM). Psychological Bulletin, 117, 39–66.

Freedman, J.L., Wallington, S.A., & Bless, E. (1967). Compliance without pressure: The effects of guilt. Journal of Personality and Social Psychology, 7, 117–124.

Gilbert, D.T. & Malone, S.P. (1995). The correspondence bias. Psychological Bulletin, 117, 21–38.

Hardin, R., (1996) Distributive justice in the real world. in L. Montada & M.J. Lerner (Eds.) Current societal concerns about justice (pp. 9–24). New York: Plenum Press

Heider, F. (1958). The psychology of interpersonal relations New York: John Wiley & Sons.

Kahneman, D., & Miller, D.T. (1986). Norm theory: Comparing reality to its alternatives. Psychological Review, 93, 136–153.

Keltner, D., Ellsworth, P.C., & Edwards, K.(1993). Beyond simple pessimism: Effects of sadness and anger on social perception. Journal of Personality and Social Psychology, 64, 740–752.

Kushner, H.S.(1981). When bad things happen to good people New York: Schocken.

Lerner, J., Goldberg, J. & Tetlock, P. (forthcoming). Sober second thought: The effects of accountability, anger, and authoritarianism on attributions of responsibility. Personality and Social Psychology Bulletin.

Lerner, M.J. (1980). The belief in a just world: A fundamental delusion New York: Plenum Press.

Lerner, M.J. (1987). Integrating societal and psychological rules of entitlement: The basic task of each social actor and fundamental problem for the social sciences. Social Justice Research, 1, 107–125.

Lerner, M.J., & Miller, D.T. (1978). Just world research and the attribution process: Looking back and ahead. Psychological Bulletin, 85, 1030–1051.

Lincoln, H. & Levinger, G. (1972). Observers' evaluations of the victim and the attacker in an aggressive incident. Journal of Personality and Social Psychology, 22, 202–210.

Levenson, H. (1994). Why the behemoths fell: Psychological roots of corporate failure. American Psychologist, 49, 428–436.

McGraw, K.M. (1987). Guilt following transgression: An attribution of responsibility approach.Journal of Personality and Social Psychology, 53, 247–256.

Meindl, J. & Lerner, M.J. (1984). Exacerbation of extreme responses to an outgroup. Journal of Personality and Social Psychology, 47, 71–84.

Messick, D. M. & Cook, K.S. Eds. (1983). Equity theory: Psychological and sociological perspectives New York: Praeger.

Miller, D.T. (1975). Personal deserving vs. justice for others: An exploration of the justice motive, Doctoral dissertation. University of Waterloo.

Miller,D.T. (1977). Personal deserving and justice for others: An exploration of the justice motive. Journal of Experimental Social Psychology, 13, 1–13.

Miller, D.T. & Ratner, R.K.(1996). The power of the myth of self-interest. In L. Montada & M.J. Lerner (Eds) Current societal concerns about justice (p. 25–48). New York: Plenum Press.

Miller, D.T. & Ross, M. (1975). Self-serving biases in the attribution of causality: Fact or fiction? Psychological Bulletin, 82, 213–225.

Mullen, J.T. (1992). The bereaved caregiver: A prospective study of changes in well-being. The Gerontologist. 32, 673–683.

Nisbett, R.E. & Wilson, T.D. (1977). Telling more than w can know: Verbal reports on mental processes. Psychological Review, 84, 231–257.

Piaget, J. (1932). The moral judgment of the child. New York: Harcourt, Brace.

Rosenbaum, R. (1995). Staring into the heart of darkness. New York Times Magazine, June 4, 36–46.

Rozin,P., Markwith, M., & McCauley, C.(1994). Sensitivity to indirect contacts with other persons: AIDS aversion as a composite of aversion to strangers, infection, moral taint, and misfortune. Journal of Abnormal Psychology, 103, 495–504.

Rubin, Z., & Peplau, L.A. (1973). Belief in a just world and reactions to another's lot: A study of participants in the national draft lottery. Journal of Social Issues, 29, 73–93.

Shaver, K.G. (1985). The attribution of blame: Causality, responsibility, and blameworthiness. New York: Springer-Verlag.

Shweder, R.A. & Haidt, J. (1993). The future of moral psychology: Truth, intuition, and the pluralist way. Psychological Science, 4, 360–365.

Shweder, R.A., & Miller, J.G. (1985). The social construction of the person: How is it possible?. Chapter 3 in K.J. Gergen & K.E. Davis. (Eds.) The social construction of the person. New York: Springer-Verlag.

Simons, C. (1968). The effects of deception manipulations within an experiment on reactions to victims of misfortune. M.A. thesis. University of Pennsylvania.

Simons.C., & Piliavin, J. (1972). The effect of deception on reactions to a victim. Journal of Personality and Social Psychology, 21, 56–60.

Smith C.A., & Ellsworth, P.C. (1985). Patterns of cognitive appraisal in emotion. Journal of Personality and Social Psychology, 48, 813–838.

Smith, L. (1994). Burned-out bosses. Fortune, 130, No.2 (July 25), 44–52.

Sorrentino, R.M. & Hardy, E.(1974). Religiousness and derogation of an innocent victim. Journal of Personality, 42, 372–382.

Taylor, S.E. (1983). Adjustment to threatening events: A theory of cognitive adaptation. American Psychologist, 11, 1161–1173.

Walster, E., Walster, G.W., & Berscheid, E. (1978). Equity: Theory and reseach. Boston: Allyn and Bacon.

Weiner, B. (1993) On sin versus sickness: A theory of perceived responsibility and social motivation. American Psychologist, 48, 957–965.

Index

Printed in the United Kingdom by
Lightning Source UK Ltd., Milton Keynes
137323UK00009B/150/P

UNIVERSITIES AT MEDWAY LIBRARY